In Vitro Fertilization

Elizabeth S. Ginsburg • Catherine Racowsky
Editors

In Vitro Fertilization

A Comprehensive Guide

Springer

Editors
Elizabeth S. Ginsburg, MD
Division of Reproductive Endocrinology and Infertility
Department of Obstetrics and Gynecology
Brigham and Women's Hospital
Boston, MA
USA

Catherine Racowsky, PhD
Division of Reproductive Endocrinology and Infertility
Department of Obstetrics and Gynecology
Brigham and Women's Hospital
Boston, MA
USA

ISBN 978-1-4419-9847-7 ISBN 978-1-4419-9848-4 (eBook)
DOI 10.1007/978-1-4419-9848-4
Springer New York Heidelberg Dordrecht London

Library of Congress Control Number: 2012952100

Printed on acid-free paper

Springer is part of Springer Science+Business Media (www.springer.com)

To our husbands and children for their constant support and love and to our patients, who inspire us continually to move our field forward.

Elizabeth S. Ginsburg, MD
Catherine Racowsky, PhD

Preface

In vitro fertilization (IVF) gained recognition as a realistic treatment for infertility with the birth of Louise Brown in 1978. Since then, the evaluation of male and female infertility has been refined and the field has made tremendous strides. Commercial development of human menopausal gonadotropins greatly improved the efficiency of ovarian stimulation, and purification of FSH products and continued advancements, including the use of GnRH analogs, has led to the development of a variety of ovarian stimulation regimens. Improvements in ultrasound technology allowed ultrasound-guided oocyte retrievals to replace the laparoscopic approach, decreasing the invasiveness of the technology. Improvements in embryo transfer catheters and techniques led to improved overall treatment efficacy. Intracytoplasmic sperm injection was developed and then rapidly adopted, effectively bypassing even the most severe male factor infertility. Advances in the IVF laboratory led to increasingly efficient culture of embryos to day 2, 3, and finally day 5/6, with culture to the blastocyst stage of development. Micromanipulation technology led to the ability to perform embryo biopsy, with preimplantation genetic diagnostic methods assessing the normality of an entire embryo through analysis of even a single cell; these technologies are currently in rapid phases of development. Throughout, adjunctive treatments, such as acupuncture, to enhance IVF outcomes have continually been studied.

The future of IVF is exciting. Embryo cryopreservation has slowly moved from slow freezing as established in the early 1990s to vitrification, with increasingly successful survival and pregnancy rates. This has led to the ability to successfully cryopreserve oocytes, allowing fertility preservation to move closer to standard of care treatment for women facing loss of ovarian function due to surgery and cancer treatment. Increasing maternal age has led to increased utilization of donor oocytes, and combined with improvements of cryobiology, the field may be moving slowly towards the establishment of oocyte banks. In addition, the increasing acceptance of third-party reproduction has led to increasing utilization of gestational carriers for women with abnormal or absent uteri, or those at high risk of carrying a pregnancy.

The economics of assisted reproductive technology (ART), restrictive ART regulation in some countries, globalization of the world economy, and widespread availability of information through the Internet has led to increasing cross-border reproduction, with individuals or couples obtaining care in countries other than their own. While ART procedures too often result in multiple gestations and high levels of stress in some patients, great efforts are being made to move more aggressively towards elective single embryo transfer and to provide emotional support for patients.

It is truly incredible how rapidly the field of assisted reproductive technologies has developed and grown over the last 20 years; many of the authors of the chapters of this book have been part of this evolution. The goal of this book is to provide a practical resource for clinical and laboratory staff of in vitro fertilization programs, and to provide a thorough understanding of ART for those beginning to familiarize themselves with these procedures. We look forward with anticipation to the future.

Boston, MA, USA Elizabeth S. Ginsburg
Boston, MA, USA Catherine Racowsky

Contents

Contributors

G. David Adamson, MD Fertility Physicians of Northern California, San Jose, CA, USA

Michael M. Alper, MD Department of Obstetrics & Gynecology, Harvard Medical School, Waltham, MA, USA

Manish Banker, MD Department of Infertility, Nova IVI Fertility and Pulse Women's Hospital, Ahmedabad, Gujarat, India

Sara E. Barton, MD Division of Reproductive Endocrinology and Infertility, Department of Obstetrics and Gynecology, Brigham and Women's Hospital Boston, MA, USA

Charles L. Bormann, PhD Department of Obstetrics, Gynecology, and Reproductive Biology, Brigham and Women's Hospital, Harvard Medical School, Boston, MA, USA

Paul R. Brezina, MD, MBA Division of Reproductive Endocrinology and Infertility, Department of Gynecology and Obstetrics, Johns Hopkins Medical Institutions, Baltimore, MD, USA

Ying C. Cheong, MD Department of Obstetrics and Gynaecology, Princess Anne Hospital, University of Southampton, Southampton, UK

Marie-Madeleine Dolmans, MD, PhD Department of Gynecology, Cliniques Universitaires Saint-Luc, Université Catholique de Louvain, Brussels, Belgium

Alice Domar, PhD The Domar Center, Boston IVF, Waltham, MA, USA

Jacques Donnez, MD, PhD Department of Gynecology, Cliniques Universitaires Saint-Luc, Catholic University of Louvain, Brussels, Belgium

Rony T. Elias, MD Center for Reproductive Medicine, Weill Cornell Medical College, New York, NY, USA

Elizabeth S. Ginsburg, MD Division of Reproductive Endocrinology and Infertility, Department of Obstetrics and Gynecology, Brigham and Women's Hospital Boston, MA, USA

Jill Gross, MS Boston IVF, Waltham, MA, USA

Brooke Harnisch, MD Department of Urology, Boston Medical Center, Boston, MA, USA

Pascale Jadoul, MD Department of Gynecology, Cliniques Universitaires Saint-Luc, Université Catholique de Louvain, Brussels, Belgium

William G. Kearns, PhD Department of Gynecology and Obstetrics, Johns Hopkins Medical Institutions, Baltimore, MD, USA

The Center for Preimplantation Genetics, LabCorp., Rockville, MD, USA

Joshua U. Klein, MD Division of Reproductive Endocrinology and Infertility, Department of Obstetrics and Gynecology, New York Presbyterian Hospital, Columbia University Medical Center, New York, NY, USA

Juergen Liebermann, PhD Fertility Centers of Illinois, Chicago, IL, USA

Nick S. Macklon, MD Division of Human Development and Health, Princess Anne Hospital, University of Southampton, Southampton, UK

Roberta Maggiulli, BSc., PhD GENERA Centre for Reproductive Medicine, Clinica Valle Giulia, Rome, Italy

Devin Monahan, BSc Ronald O. Perelman and Claudia Cohen Center for Reproductive Medicine, Weill Cornell Medical College, New York, NY, USA

Queenie V. Neri, MSc, BSc Ronald O. Perelman and Claudia Cohen Center for Reproductive Medicine, Weill Cornell Medical College, New York, NY, USA

Khanh-Ha Nguyen, MD Department of Obstetrics & Gynecology, Beth Israel Deaconess Medical Center, Boston, MA, USA

Robert D. Oates, MD Department of Urology, Boston University School of Medicine, Boston, MA, USA

Gianpiero D. Palermo, MD, PhD Ronald O. Perelman and Claudia Cohen Center for Reproductive Medicine, New York, NY, USA

Pravin Patel, MD Department of Endoscopy, Nova IVI Fertility and Pulse Women's Hospital, Ahmedabad, Gujarat, India

Catherine Racowsky, MD Division of Reproductive Endocrinology and Infertility, Department of Obstetrics and Gynecology, Brigham and Women's Hospital, Boston, MA, USA

Kevin S. Richter, PhD Shady Grove Fertility Reproductive Science Center, Rockville, MD, USA

Laura F. Rienzi, BSc., MSc GENERA Centre for Reproductive Medicine, Clinica Valle Giulia, Rome, Italy

Zev Rosenwaks, MD Ronald O. Perelman and Claudia Cohen Center for Reproductive Medicine, Weill Cornell Medical College, New York, NY, USA

Mark V. Sauer, MD Center for Women's Reproductive Care, Columbia University Medical Center, New York, NY, USA

Glenn Schattman, MD Department of OB/GYN, The Center for Reproductive and Infertility, Cornell Weill Medical Center, New York Presbyterian Hospital, Weill Medical College, Cornell University, New York, NY, USA

Robert J. Stillman, MD Shady Grove Fertility Reproductive Science Center, Rockville, MD, USA

Eric Surrey, MD Colorado Center for Reproductive Medicine, Lone Tree, CO, USA

Michael Tucker, PhD IVF Laboratory, Shady Grove Fertility RSC, Rockville, MD, USA

Filippo Ubaldi, MD., MSc GENERA Centre for Reproductive Medicine, Clinica Valle Giulia, Rome, Italy

Matthew D. VerMilyea, PhD Penn Fertility Care, University of Pennsylvania, Philadelphia, PA, USA

Eric A. Widra, MD Shady Grove Fertility Reproductive Science Center, Washington, DC, USA

Pre IVF Evaluation of the Infertile Woman

1

Khanh-Ha Nguyen and Michael M. Alper

Introduction

A thorough but focused history, physical exam, and evaluation of the infertile female patient is paramount before proper counseling regarding treatment options can be offered. The initial consultation aims to collect the information needed to guide appropriate testing but is also an important step in establishing a relationship with the patient which, in turn, supports the demanding nature of infertility care. This is crucial as the patient proceeds through stressful and potentially time-consuming treatment, disappointment from unmet expectations, and often financially burdensome choices. The decision to proceed to in vitro fertilization (IVF) may result after the complete evaluation or when simpler and less expensive fertility treatment has failed. In both situations the patient may not be psychologically, emotionally, or financial prepared for IVF and this dilemma underscores the importance of establishing a positive rapport as a component of the pre-IVF evaluation of the infertile woman or couple.

KHD. Nguyen, M.D.
Department of Obstetrics & Gynecology,
Beth Israel Deaconess Medical Center,
Boston, MA 02215, USA
e-mail: kdnguyen@bidmc.harvard.edu

M.M. Alper, M.D. (✉)
Department of Obstetrics & Gynecology,
Harvard Medical School,
130 Second Avenue, Waltham, MA 02451, USA
e-mail: michael.alper@bostonIVF.com

Clinical Approach to the Infertile Woman

History taking is directed at identifying contraindications to pregnancy, risk factors for infertility guiding laboratory and imaging assessment, and the need for referral to other services such as social work or anesthesia consultation. After a complete evaluation, the cause of infertility for most patients will fall into one of several diagnostic categories which have remained stable over the past decade (see Fig. 1.1) [1]. The infertility specialist is in the ideal position to optimize the health of the patient prior to pregnancy and to offer preconception screening for potentially devastating diseases that can occur in the offspring such as cystic fibrosis, spinal muscular atrophy, and other genetic conditions. While there are standard guidelines for minimum preconception counseling and testing, recommendations regarding management options for specific reproductive conditions including recurrent pregnancy loss or endometriosis are less clear. When possible, both partners of a couple should be present for the initial consultation, especially when treatment decisions may be made.

Risk Factors for Infertility

Obtaining medical history directed at causes for infertility is imperative as it can easily identify risk factors for infertility and lead to an efficient

E.S. Ginsburg and C. Racowsky (eds.), *In Vitro Fertilization: A Comprehensive Guide*,
DOI 10.1007/978-1-4419-9848-4_1, © Springer Science+Business Media New York 2012

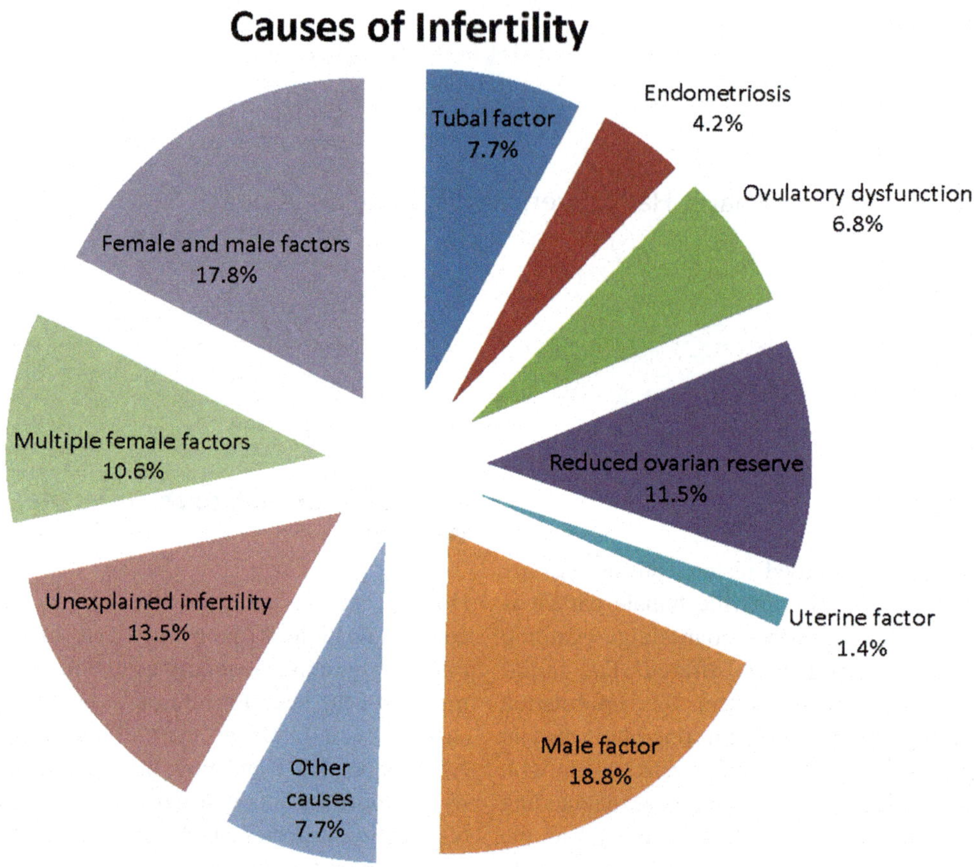

Fig. 1.1 Causes of infertility among couples who had assisted reproductive technology cycles using fresh autologous eggs or embryos in 2009. *Source*: Adapted from the Centers for Disease Control and Prevention [1]

evaluation. Age alone is one of the major risk factors for infertility. Ovulatory dysfunction can be suspected from a history of irregular menstrual cycles. When accompanied by symptoms of hyperandrogenism, polycystic ovarian syndrome (PCOS) may be suspected. Signs of hyperprolactinemia such as nipple discharge, headache, and visual changes should be considered in the review of symptoms. Uterine, cervical, or tubal risk factors may be assessed with a history of pelvic infection or recurrent miscarriages, prior surgical intervention such as curettage and cervical cryotherapy or conization, intrauterine device use for contraception, or ectopic pregnancy. Exposures to tobacco smoking, excessive alcohol use, stress, poor diet, intensive exercise, and extremes of weight are all risk factors that should be screened for in the initial consultation.

Women presenting with signs and symptoms consistent with endometriosis, or endometrial implants outside the uterus, may have more difficulty achieving pregnancy. While staging endometriosis standardizes the description and severity of disease, it does not predict fecundity and does little to guide management in the setting of the infertile patient [2]. IVF is considered the most effective fertility treatment in patients with endometriosis [3]. The role of laparoscopic ablation or resection of implants and cystectomy of endometriomas is often reserved for cases of repeated IVF failures and could improve IVF outcomes.

Celiac disease is an enteropathic immune disorder of gluten intolerance. Approximately 1 in 133 persons have this condition and are unable to digest foods containing or coated with gluten such as wheat, rye, barley, medicines, and lip balms [4]. When ingested, an immune-mediated destruction of the intestinal villi prevents proper absorption of nutrients into the bloodstream causing typical nonspecific symptoms of constipation, diarrhea, abdominal pain, vomiting, and weight loss. As a multifactorial genetic condition, manifestations of this disease are highly variable between persons and throughout a lifetime even among families. It is associated with HLA-DQ2 and HLA-DQ8 and coexisting autoimmune disease is common. It is often chronically present but can be activated by stressful events such as surgery, pregnancy, or infections. Celiac disease may present in conjunction with unexplained infertility or recurrent miscarriage. The National Institutes of Health has recommended testing patients presenting with these reproductive problems for anti-tissue transglutaminase (tTGA) or anti-endomysium (EMA) IgA antibodies [4]. Presence of these antibodies should be followed by referral to a gastroenterologist, with endoscopic confirmation of villous atrophy and treatment with nutrition counseling and diet modification.

Contraindications to Pregnancy

Contraindications to pregnancy may be ascertained in the review of the medical, surgical, and social history. Conditions which may place the patient at unacceptably high risk for pregnancy-related complications, such as morbid obesity, history of cardiac malformation, and recent exposures to infectious diseases, should be screened for in the history. Undiagnosed or undertreated diseases such as hypertension, diabetes, autoimmune disorders, abnormal uterine bleeding, and malignancy should also be considered in the patients' answers to review of systems. A careful review of current medications may uncover those drugs known to cause human fetal toxicity or adverse effects in animal studies. The decision to continue any medication should consider the benefits and risks of continuing treatment in a woman planning conception.

In many circumstances, these contraindications may be overcome with timely diagnosis and appropriate treatment or monitoring to allow subsequent fertility treatment. This may require a multidisciplinary approach with maternal fetal medicine, oncology, and other medicine or surgical specialists.

Preconception Counseling

The American College of Obstetricians and Gynecologists (ACOG) has published complete guidelines for preconception counseling and antepartum care for all women [5]. The annual routine female health assessments such as medical history, screening for adult disease, Pap smear, breast exam with or without mammogram (recommended in women aged 40 and higher or earlier with a positive family history), and physical exam including vital signs should be up-to-date. In addition, several areas of assessment deserve special attention in the setting of IVF.

Women with body mass index (BMI) of 30 kg/m^2 or more are at increased risk of having medical and obstetrical complications such as increased risk of gestational diabetes, preeclampsia, large or small for gestational age fetuses, surgical delivery, and children with neural tube defects. For these reasons, morbidly obese women must undergo maternal fetal medicine consultation during preconception planning and prior to IVF treatment. Supplementation with 1.0 mg folic acid daily (routine dose is 0.4 mg daily) may be considered although the benefit of this dose in non-diabetic obese patients is not established [6]. Multiple studies have shown that addressing nutritional issues and improving obesity result in better pregnancy outcomes and live birth rates in IVF [7]. In a retrospective review of 4,609 women undergoing their first IVF cycle, those with a BMI greater than 30 kg/m^2 had significantly lower odds of clinical pregnancy and live birth [8]. Obesity appears to be related to higher gonadotropin requirements during stimulation, poor oocyte quality and lower fertilization rates [9, 10]. Weight reduction supervised by a nutritionist as well as more aggressive approaches such as bariatric surgery may be indicated before starting IVF treatment. The delay in conception attempts that will occur when awaiting potentially beneficial weight loss must be weighed against the lower pregnancy rates expected as women age. A delay of at least 12 months after bariatric surgery is recommended prior to pregnancy.

Screening for genetic and familial conditions is part of a routine history review but, for several reasons, is especially important in patients undergoing IVF. A family history of premature ovarian insufficiency or mental retardation can prompt Fragile X carrier screening by FMR1 gene premutation analysis and consideration of expediting IVF treatment, or counseling on donor oocyte for IVF. Offering carrier screening for cystic fibrosis and spinal muscular atrophy is recommended by ACOG and the American College of Medical Genetics (ACMG) for all women considering conception [5]. Patients of Ashkenazi Jewish ethnicity may also choose screening for common genetic diseases in this population such as Gaucher disease and Tay-Sachs disease [11]. If the patient or her partner is found to be a carrier for a genetic condition, there is opportunity to offer preimplantation genetic diagnosis (PGD).

The presence of multiple family members having blood clots at young ages without surgery or unrelated to trauma can reveal those patients who should be screened for thrombophilia diseases and who are at high risk of thrombosis during ovarian stimulation and pregnancy as well as being at risk for recurrent pregnancy loss (RPL).

Prenatal Panel

The following tests are considered routine prenatal testing for all women planning pregnancy or already pregnant: hemoglobin levels, blood group and Rhesus type, antibody screen, urinalysis with microscopic examination (in pregnancy), immunity to rubella, rapid plasma reagin (RPR) for syphilis, hepatitis B virus surface antigen, and hepatitis C antibody. When indicated due to ethnicity or risk factors, hemoglobin electrophoresis (for sickle cell anemia and thalassemias), testing for immunity to varicella, chlamydia, and gonorrhea screening, antibody screen for toxoplasmosis due to cat feces exposures, and Mantoux test for tuberculosis should also be performed. Physicians should be educated on the local regulations regarding testing and reporting human immunodeficiency virus (HIV). Preconception immunization is preferred when a patient is found to be susceptible to rubella. However, the inactivated influenza, tetanus, hepatitis B, and pneumococcus vaccines are considered safe in pregnancy and should be administered to patients at risk.

All patients should be offered carrier screening for gene mutations in CFTR (cystic fibrosis) and gene dosage of SMN1 and 2 (spinal muscular atrophy, or SMA). Because detection levels vary among different ethnicities and depend on the type of molecular genetic test performed, residual risk should be discussed in counseling and interpretation of results. For example, ACOG recommends a 23-mutation panel for the CFTR gene based on prevalence of those mutations in the Caucasian population. However, the same panel has a sensitivity of only about 50% when used in the Asian patient population. Results obtained from standard SMA screening report only whether a patient has two genes for SMN detected for example and a reduced risk. There is still a 2% chance that those two genes are present in *cis*, or on the same chromosome. In these situations, the patient would be a carrier for SMA and there is a possibility of transmitting the other chromosome which has no SMN1 genes.

Other ethnicity-based genetic testing includes Tay-Sachs disease, Canavan disease, and familial dysautonomia in Ashkenazi Jews. Additional carrier testing for other genetic diseases common in this ethnic group is available; however, pretest genetic counseling is imperative prior to extended panel screening to determine residual risk, manage patient expectations, and to discuss implications of a positive carrier status [11]. French Canadians, Old Order Amish and Cajuns in whom specific mutations exist with high carrier frequency should also be offered screening for Tay-Sachs disease.

Indications for Additional Referrals

Patients with chronic illnesses should undergo maternal fetal medicine consultation prior to undergoing fertility treatment. Such consultations will prepare them for any particular risks of pregnancy related to their condition, as well as the risks their condition may confer on the pregnancy and fetus (e.g., hypertension, diabetes). The consultation is also helpful to alert the IVF physician as to whether a flare in the condition may be expected, and when during pregnancy monitoring for the condition should begin.

Any patient with obesity, history of narcotic use, malignant hyperthermia, or history of anesthesia complications should be referred to an anesthesiologist prior to the day of the oocyte retrieval. Oocyte retrievals are typically done under intravenous general or monitored anesthesia care and are generally safe procedures unless there is a question of airway difficulty or ability to provide adequate anesthesia; in situations where there is concern about a difficult airway, use of spinal anesthesia may be considered.

As of 2008, the Centers for Disease Control (CDC) estimates that approximately 25% of Americans have some form of acute situational or chronic psychiatric illness [12]. In particular, antidepressants are most frequently used by those in reproductive age (18–44 years old) and women are more likely than men to be taking antidepressants. Women taking medications for psychiatric disorders require specific preconception consultation with a psychiatrist regarding management during pregnancy and risks of those medications on the developing fetus. Although untreated maternal psychiatric illness is not advocated, known risks of drugs like lithium (congenital heart malformations), valproic acid (neural tube defects), and benzodiazepine (floppy infant syndrome) should be discussed as well as the unknown risk of other birth defects and long-term neurocognitive deficits in less-studied drugs.

Referral to a mind body center or support group can accomplish both the goals of stress management and well-balanced lifestyle. Nutrition and appropriate levels of exercise can be addressed and is important for all women planning conception, and are especially important in the setting of obesity and metabolic conditions such as PCOS.

Laboratory and Imaging Assessment

While the approach is slightly different when the infertile female patient presents as a single woman, as a partner in a same sex couple, or as a partner in a heterosexual relationship, three basic components of the female patient workup are essential: ovarian reserve testing, uterine and tubal evaluation, and appropriate preconception screening. As the evaluation has evolved over time, some tests such as the post-coital test to assess cervical mucus and endometrial biopsy for histological dating have proven to be unreliable measures of fertility [13, 14]. Likewise, laparoscopy is no longer routine since it rarely provides additional information that would change treatment. Figure 1.2 represents the clinical algorithm we recommend for evaluation of the infertile woman.

Ovarian Reserve Testing

Once oogonia are established in the ovaries, they undergo the dramatic process of atresia throughout the woman's lifetime from a maximum number of six to seven million at 20 weeks gestational age to less than a million at the time of puberty [16]. After reproductive maturity, recruitment of cohorts of follicles containing developing oocytes occurs continuously with only one dominant follicle containing a mature oocyte released for fertilization each month, with the remaining follicles in each cohort undergoing atresia. Ultimately the number of follicles available, or the "ovarian reserve," becomes limited over time as the woman approaches transition into menopause when there is an end of follicular recruitment and development.

Tests of ovarian reserve are used to determine the quantity of oocytes that may be present in ovaries. Although some have suggested that they predict oocyte quality, this has not been found to

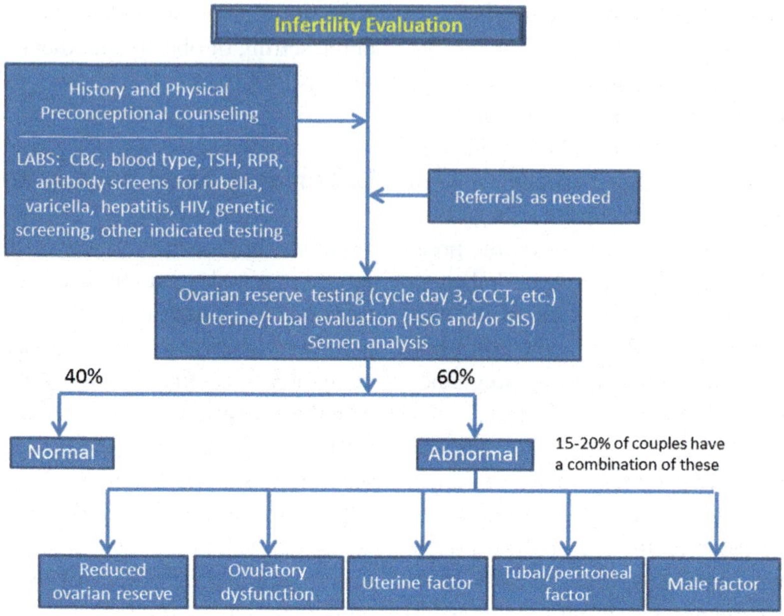

Fig. 1.2 Clinical algorithm for evaluation of the infertile woman. *Source*: Adapted from [15]

be true. It is now clear that these tests are rather poor predictors of pregnancy outcomes and are simply better indicators of how well the ovaries may respond to gonadotropin stimulation in IVF. They provide the physician with prognostic information to counsel patients on reasonable expectations from IVF treatment including number or quality of oocytes and embryos, resulting pregnancy rates, and possibly cancelation of ovarian stimulation or when IVF with autologous oocytes would be futile in the case of premature ovarian insufficiency [17].

Obtaining follicle stimulating hormone (FSH) and estradiol (E2) levels on menstrual day 2–4 is a relatively simple blood test of ovarian reserve, and such testing is available in virtually all commercial laboratories. Clinical interpretation of the values depends on reference ranges established for each assay given inherent intra- and inter-assay variability [18]. An FSH level of 10 mIU/mL or less with an E2 level less than 70 pg/mL is generally considered normal and reflective of ovaries that should respond well to ovulation induction. When E2 is greater than 70 pg/mL, the negative feedback effect on the hypothalamus and pituitary gland can spuriously lower the FSH level which can be misinterpreted as low or normal. Thus, measuring both hormones on the same blood sample is important.

As with other tests of ovarian reserve, basal FSH levels are associated with ovarian response to stimulation, especially when stratifying by age which, in turn, correlates much better with oocyte quality [19]. Thus when the patient is young (less than 35 years old) with a high basal FSH level, fewer oocytes may be expected at retrieval and higher cancelation rates are expected. However, because those oocytes are likely to be chromosomally normal, or "good quality," implantation and ongoing pregnancy rates are generally better than for a patient older than 35 who also has normal FSH levels [20]. Furthermore, regardless of the variability in FSH levels in different menstrual cycles in a single patient, a single elevated FSH is a poor prognostic indicator, and when found in an infertile patient, aggressive ovarian stimulation should be planned.

The clomiphene citrate challenge test (CCCT) is a provocative test to assess ovarian reserve. Cycle day 3 serum levels of FSH and estradiol are determined. Clomiphene citrate 100 mg per day is then taken orally by the patient from cycle days 5–9. A repeat FSH level is determined on cycle day 10. It is believed that as a weak estrogen agonist and antagonist, clomiphene citrate blocks estrogen receptors in the hypothalamus inducing increased release of GnRH and subsequently of FSH and luteinizing hormone (LH) from the pituitary gland. In women with normal reserve and the ability to produce robust levels of E2 and inhibin B from the follicular cohort, clomiphene citrate is competitively blocked from the estrogen receptors allowing the FSH levels to remain at a low level on day 10. In contrast, when the ovarian reserve is low with inadequate E2 and inhibin B production, FSH levels remain elevated on day 10. The CCCT is considered abnormal with FSH levels >10 mIU/mL on either day, or an E2 level of >70 pg/mL on day 2–4. Further, in women under age 40 undergoing IVF, the presence of only one elevated FSH level in the CCCT predicts that the live birth rates will be only half of those of women with normal CCCT [21]. In the setting of advanced age, or a family history of premature ovarian insufficiency, prior ovarian surgery, or short cycle lengths, the CCCT may reveal reduced ovarian reserve in 75% of these women who otherwise had normal basal FSH levels.

Follicular levels of inhibin B alone have been shown to be lower in poor responders compared to normal responders during the CCCT [22]. However, this test has limited routine clinical value because it does not appear to correlate with pregnancy outcomes in IVF and there is marked assay variability [23, 24].

Other provocative tests of ovarian reserve include exogenous FSH ovarian reserve test (EFORT, described by Fanchin et al. [25]), EFORT with inhibin B, and gonadotropin releasing hormone (GnRH) agonist stimulation test. Similar to the CCCT, they all measure the ability of the ovarian follicular cohort to respond to stimulation with an appropriate rise in E2 and inhibin B with normally suppressed FSH release.

Ultrasound for antral follicle count (AFC) may provide information regarding the number of possible follicles in a cohort that may be recruited during exogenous gonadotropin stimulation for IVF. This requires a transvaginal ultrasound examination performed between cycle days 2–4, or randomly in an amenorrheic patient. Follicles 2–3 by 10 mm in diameter are measured and included in the count. A young patient with PCOS or hypothalamic amenorrhea would be expected to have a very high AFC and robust response to ovarian stimulation. There is no universally recognized threshold for an abnormal AFC (less than 6 is typically considered poor), but it does allow planning of gonadotropin dosing and choosing protocols that have better success in poor responders and result in a lower likelihood of cycle cancelation [26, 27]. Total AFC appears to directly correlate with number of oocytes retrieved, pregnancy rate, and live birth rate [28]. Meta-analysis of multivariate model studies on ovarian reserve testing show AFC alone is equivalent to or better than other tests for this purpose [17].

Measuring serum anti-Mullerian hormone (AMH) has become more popular recently due to the ease of determining levels regardless of menstrual cycle day, concurrent use of oral contraceptives, existing pregnancy, and reasonable inter-assay correlation. Because it is secreted by the granulosa cells of the preantral follicles (an AMH level greater than 1 ng/mL is considered normal), it is a reliable surrogate for the number of follicles available for stimulation [29, 30]. Patients with PCOS and abundant preantral follicles have higher AMH levels (>3 ng/mL). As expected, AMH levels decrease with age and antral follicle count [31].

No one test of ovarian reserve is clearly superior, as shown in an extensive review of all studies on ovarian reserve testing by Broekmans et al. [32]. Abnormal laboratory testing, low antral follicle count, or documented poor response to aggressive ovulation induction, regardless of ovarian reserve testing results, are all considered consistent with the diagnosis of reduced ovarian reserve. When the diagnosis includes diminished or poor ovarian reserve, several adjunctive treatments in ART may be considered in preparation of an IVF cycle. These options are covered in Chap. 5.

Uterine Cavity and Tubal Evaluation

Assessment of intrauterine cavity and tubal patency is fundamental to the pre-IVF evaluation. A

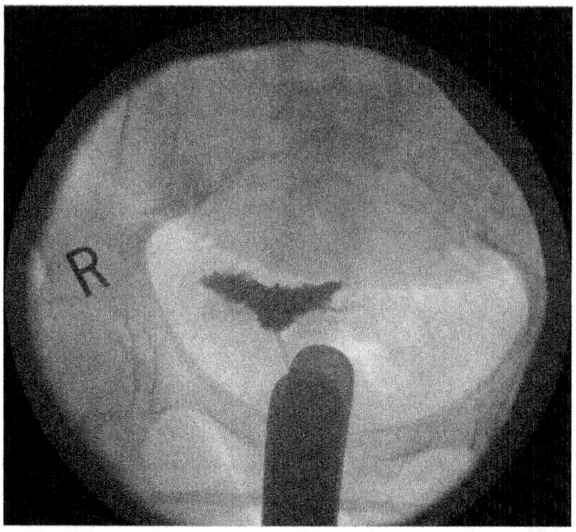

Fig. 1.3 Abnormal HSG: Irregular endometrial cavity and bilateral blocked fallopian tubes. A smooth endometrial contour is expected in a normal uterus in the early or mid-follicular phase but may be subject to lining irregularities when the HSG is performed in the late-follicular or luteal phase. No radiocontrast media infiltrated into the fallopian tubes may represent either tubal occlusion from adhesion, mucous plugs, prior pelvic infectious disease or tubal spasm

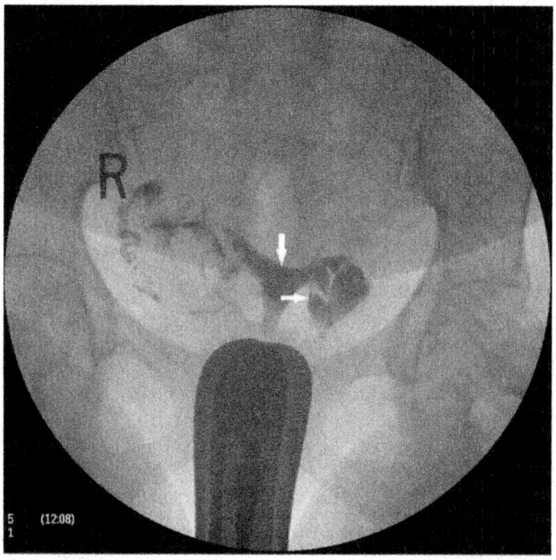

Fig. 1.4 Abnormal HSG: Arcuate uterine fundus and left hydrosalpinx

hysterosalpingogram (HSG) is routinely accomplished during the follicular phase by X-ray imaging after intrauterine instillation of a water-based radiocontrast media. Occlusion of both fallopian tubes on HSG with or without distal dilation representing a hydrosalpinx account for roughly 20% of infertile women and is a major age-independent reason for treatment with IVF. The rate of infection after an HSG procedure is low (1–3%) but can be as high as 11% with a documented hydrosalpinx which warrants post-procedure prophylactic antibiotic treatment [33]. Further, the American Society of Reproductive Medicine (ASRM) recommends removal of hydrosalpinges by salpingectomy when diagnosed prior to IVF to improve implantation and live birth rates [34]. Improvement in IVF pregnancy rates are more likely after salpingectomy when hydrosalpinges were evident as fluid-filled structures on ultrasound, rather than mildly dilated tubes seen only during dye instillation during the HSG.

HSG can be used to diagnose intrauterine pathology that may contribute to infertility and which should be treated prior to IVF. Endometrial polyps, fibroids with cavitary involvement, adhesions, Asherman's syndrome, and anatomical Mullerian variants such as uterine septa, fusion anomalies (unicornuate and bicornuate), and T-shaped cavity, caused by in-utero exposure to diethylstilbestrol (DES) in the past, are easily seen. These abnormalities can be further defined by saline infusion sonogram (SIS), 3D ultrasound, or magnetic resonance imaging (MRI) which allow improved multidimensional appraisal of the intrauterine cavity before proceeding to surgical intervention if indicated. Figures 1.3, 1.4, 1.5, 1.6, 1.7, and 1.8 provide examples of uterine and tubal pathologies diagnosed with these imaging modalities. Finally, the process of instilling radiocontrast media during the HSG may have some therapeutic effect in the setting of a normal uterine cavity and fallopian tubes. About one-third of patients with normal HSG findings will become pregnant over the subsequent 6 months, suggesting that small but significant adhesions or mucus plugs may have been freed during HSG allowing proper fertilization and implantation [35].

Endometrial biopsy is no longer a part of the routine evaluation of the infertile female patient unless it is indicated for other clinical reasons such as dysfunctional uterine bleeding or concern for endometrial carcinoma in a persistently anovulatory patient with PCOS. Initially, the histological dating of the endometrium with biopsy was deemed physiologically appropriate since progesterone-

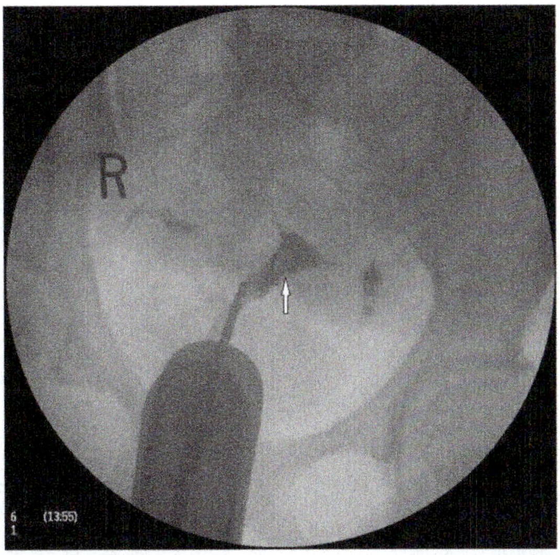

Fig. 1.5 Abnormal HSG: Persistent filling defect in the center of the endometrial cavity with normal patent fallopian tubes

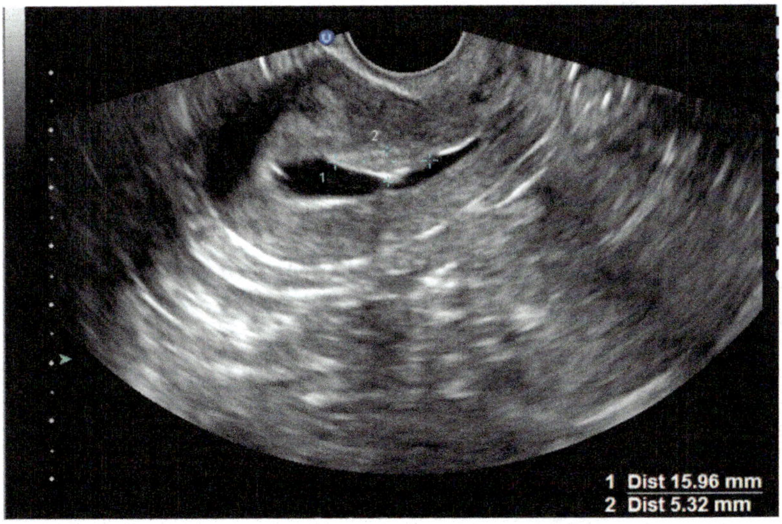

Fig. 1.6 Abnormal SIS: Follow-up of the persistent filling defect noted in Fig. 1.5 by SIS reveals an anterior endometrial polyp

induced maturation of the endometrial lining is important to document the adequacy of luteal phase changes necessary for implantation. An endometrial biopsy was considered abnormal and "out of phase" when there was greater than 2 days' discrepancy in the histologic and chronologic dating. Unfortunately, chronological dating was often inaccurate especially in irregular cycles and those with variability in luteal phase length. There was significant incongruous histology interpretation even among well-experienced pathologists. Most importantly, the results did not correlate with ability to achieve pregnancy and, interestingly, was abnormal more frequently in fertile women [13].

Operative hysteroscopy is not typically a part of the initial infertility evaluation and is reserved for treatment of uterine or tubal pathology. For example, some centers have started to use hysteroscopic placement of Essure® for tubal occlusion and treatment of hydrosalpinges prior to IVF, though care must be taken to ensure that the coils do not protrude into the endometrial cavity

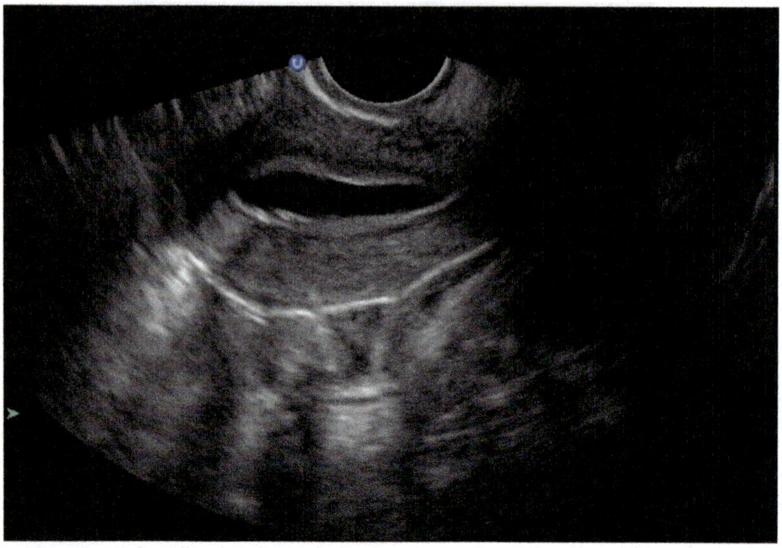

Fig. 1.7 Normal SIS

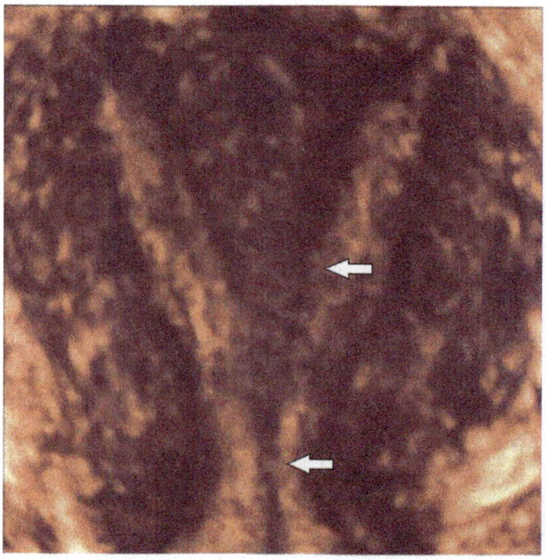

Fig. 1.8 Abnormal 3D ultrasound: 3D ultrasound clearly delineated a broad-based uterine septum extending from the fundus to the vagina with two cervices. This imaging modality was useful in differentiating a uterine didelphys versus uterine septum which could not be defined by other methods such as HSG or SIS. The implications of the correct diagnosis in this case could lead to different treatment recommendations and management. Appropriate tools should be considered when evaluating uterine pathology

[36]. In patients planning IVF, office hysteroscopy may be used for cavity assessment; however, it is appropriate to ensure that there is no ultrasound evidence of cystic adnexal masses consistent with possible hydrosalpinges prior to starting ovulation induction. In patients with recurrent pregnancy loss or recurrent implantation failure after IVF, hysteroscopic evaluation may be considered to evaluate occult pathology that is not otherwise visible on conventional imaging

Other Laboratory Testing and Evaluations

When ovulatory dysfunction is suspected, further evaluation is warranted to determine the underlying etiology. For example, the infertile woman presenting with irregular menstrual cycles may or may not have symptoms of hyperandrogenism. However, underlying PCOS may be diagnosed by laboratory assessment of total and free testosterone, androstenedione, and dehydroepiandrosterone sulfate (DHEAS) combined with ultrasound evaluation of the ovaries based on the revised Rotterdam criteria established in 2003 [37]. Patients with PCOS are at risk of metabolic syndrome, with attendant long-term health sequelae, emphasizing the need to optimize their health prior to IVF and pregnancy. Further testing for glucose intolerance, fasting lipid panel, blood pressure, and occult endometrial carcinoma should be performed.

It is important to evaluate the patient specifically for other conditions that can present with ovulatory dysfunction such as thyroid disorders, Cushing's disease, adrenal or ovarian tumor, nonclassical adrenal enzyme deficiency, insulin resistance, or a prolactin-secreting tumor. Testing should include thyroid stimulating hormone (TSH), possibly anti-peroxidase antibodies (as positive antibodies predict future hypothyroidism in a patient currently euthyroid), morning 17-hydroxyprogesterone level, and prolactin. Prolactin may be elevated in a patient with a history of head and neck trauma, hypothyroidism, breast stimulation, or in those taking medications known to increase prolactin secretion. Head imaging is important to rule out a pituitary tumor or compression tumor that may cause elevated prolactin levels. When to treat subclinical hypothyroidism in pregnancy and whether a target TSH level should be maintained to titrate medical therapy is controversial among guiding national societies with most groups leaning towards early treatment given the relative low risk and possible benefit to fertility and fetal neurocognitive development [38]. Recent data suggest that levels should be less than 3.0 μU/mL.

When the evaluation of ovulatory dysfunction leads to the diagnosis of eugonadotropic ovarian dysfunction, relatively simple and noninvasive approaches to fertility treatment can be explored such as weight reduction (when obesity is present), insulin-sensitizing agents (metformin), and/or ovulation induction with clomiphene citrate or letrozole prior to proceeding to IVF. The diagnosis of hypogonadotropic ovulatory dysfunction is supported when there is low or normal cycle day 3 FSH (suggestive of hypothalamic dysfunction) or low body weight. Although normal BMI can be as low as 18.5 kg/m^2, many patients diagnosed with hypothalamic hypogonadotropic ovulatory dysfunction have a BMI $<$ 20 kg/m^2. MRI assessment of the head is warranted in this clinical situation to rule out hypothalamic or pituitary tumors.

A history of recurrent pregnancy loss may prompt karyotype analysis of both partners to determine the presence of balanced translocations and inversions known to increase risk of this complication. As mentioned earlier, all patients with recurrent pregnancy loss and unexplained infertility should be tested for celiac disease by the presence of positive serum anti-TTG and anti-EMA antibodies. Because the association between inherited thrombophilias and adverse pregnancy outcomes such as recurrent early pregnancy loss, fetal loss, preeclampsia, fetal growth restriction, and placental abruption is unclear, there are no guidelines currently for screening. Likewise, large randomized clinical trials examining benefits of treatment in the setting of the infertile patient undergoing IVF are lacking. Consideration of treatment with aspirin or low molecular weight heparin should be individualized to each patient.

When IVF Is the Next Step in Treatment

Preparing the infertile woman for IVF involves a detailed discussion and consent process which must be documented and should include:

1. Steps of an IVF cycle including how the ovaries will be stimulated, side effects of medications, control of follicular maturation, monitoring, and expected length of gonadotropin stimulation
2. Alternatives to IVF
3. Oocyte retrieval process and risks of surgery and anesthesia
4. Risk of ovarian hyperstimulation syndrome and ovarian torsion
5. Current data on risk of cancer from treatment, if any
6. Risk of genetic disease and congenital anomalies or other disorders in the baby potentially related to IVF
7. Expected pregnancy rates and failure rates based on age-related decreased fecundity and increased aneuploidy
8. Pregnancy complications seen after IVF including ectopic pregnancy, premature delivery, lower birth weight, and placentation abnormalities
9. Regular insemination or intracytoplasmic sperm injection (ICSI)
10. Length of culture and number of embryos to transfer
11. When other treatment should be considered such as assisted hatching and preimplantation screening
12. Risk of multiple pregnancy
13. No guarantee of success
14. If IVF is futile or when donor oocyte for IVF is indicated

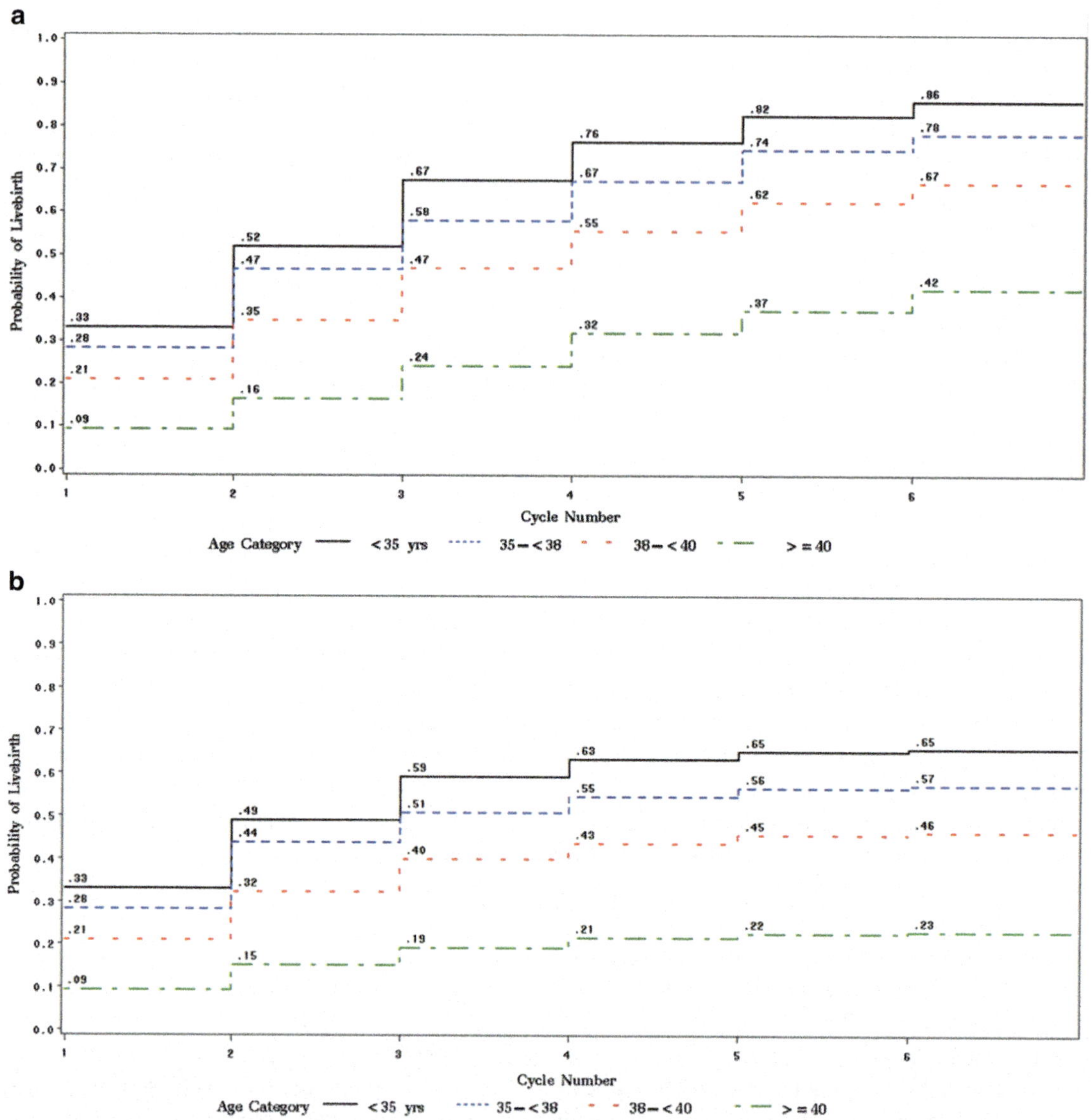

Fig. 1.9 Cumulative live births over six IVF cycles using optimistic and conservative models in 6,164 patients undergoing 14,248 cycles stratified by ages <35 years, 35 to <38 years, 38 to <40 years, and ≥40 years. Panel A represents optimistic Kaplan-Meier curves assuming women who did not return for subsequent IVF cycles have the same chance of live birth as those who did return for IVF treatment. Panel B represents the same patients assuming women who did not return for subsequent IVF had no chance of live birth. Log rank test comparing these two curves showed statistically significant difference for every age strata ($p<0.001$) [40]. Reprinted, with permission, from Elsevier. Malizia BA, Hacker MR, Penzias AS. Cumulative live birth rates after in vitro fertilization. *N Engl J Med* 2009; 360(3): 236–43, Fig. 2

15. Disposition of the unused embryos including freezing, donation, discarding, or use for research
16. Supplementation with progesterone when prescribed

Setting Expectations

Age is overall the most significant prognostic factor in a woman's ability to become pregnant. It is also important in predicting response to ovarian

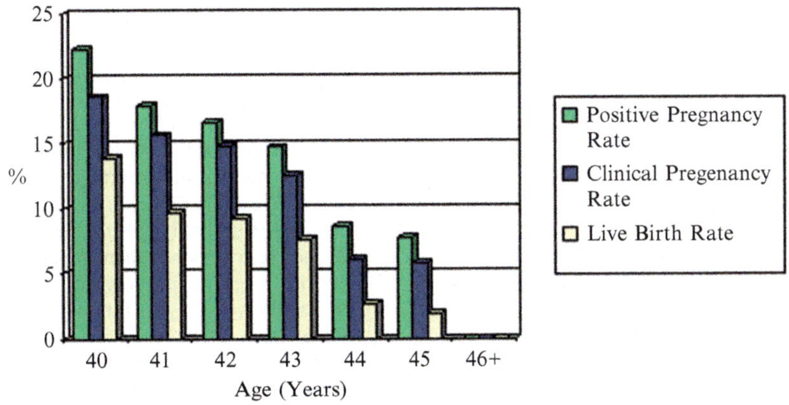

Fig. 1.10 Pregnancy outcomes after the first IVF cycle in 1,263 women over age 40 at a large university-affiliated infertility center [39]. Reprinted with permission. Klipstein S, Regan M, Ryley DA, Goldman MB, Alper MM, Reindollar RH. One last chance for pregnancy: a review of 2,705 in vitro fertilization cycles initiated in women age 40 years and above. *Fertil Steril* 2005;84(2):435–45, Fig. 2

stimulation and outcomes after IVF, affecting the rate of positive pregnancy test, clinical pregnancy, and live birth. IVF has been shown to overcome age-related effects of infertility especially in the less than 39 year-old age strata but is less likely to be effective in those older than age 40 (Fig. 1.9). Beyond age 43, the live birth rate falls dramatically to approximately 5% compared to 20% per cycle start in a 40 year-old woman (Fig. 1.10). It is important to give patients reasonable expectations with each IVF cycle based on their age, reason for infertility, ovarian reserve test results, and quality and number of embryos being transferred. The ASRM has established clear guidelines on the number of embryos to transfer based on age and the presence of excess embryos to cryopreserve in order to balance reasonable chances of pregnancy against risks of high-order multiple pregnancy [41]. Physicians have an ethical obligation to counsel those patients with futile chances of pregnancy using their own oocytes and to potentially offer a closure cycle after risks, benefits, and alternatives have been thoroughly discussed [39]

Summary

With a comprehensive and directed evaluation prior to infertility treatment, which includes proper preconception counseling, and a discussion of risk factors related to infertility and prenatal health, the infertile woman can be guided to optimize her chance of conceiving. In many circumstances, these steps alone can improve inherent fertility. IVF offers additional advantages for patients with specific reproductive issues such as tubal factor, diminished ovarian reserve, and known carrier status of a genetic disease. IVF can also help overcome nonspecific reasons for infertility when all evaluative testing is normal in the woman or when the male partner has poor semen parameters. Finally, additional information can be gained from each stimulated cycle for IVF such as oocyte yield, fertilization efficiency, and embryo development which should be considered in the pre-IVF evaluation for the subsequent cycle.

References

1. Centers for Disease Control and Prevention, American Society for Reproductive Medicine, Society for Assisted Reproductive Technology. 2009 Assisted reproductive technology success rates: national summary and fertility clinic reports. Atlanta, GA: US Department of Health and Human Services; 2011. http://www.cdc.gov/art/ART2009/PDF/ART_2009_Full.pdf. Accessed 2 Jan 2012.
2. Olive DL, Lindheim SR, Pritts EA. Endometriosis and infertility: what do we do for each stage? Curr Womens Health Rep. 2003;3(5):389–94.

3. Senapati S, Barnhart K. Managing endometriosis-associated infertility. Clin Obstet Gynecol. 2011;54(4):720–6.
4. NIH Consensus Statement on Celiac Disease. NIH Consens State Sci Statements. 2004; 21(1):1–22. http://consensus.nih.gov/2004/2004CeliacDisease118html.htm. Accessed 16 Mar 2012.
5. American Academy of Pediatrics Committee on Fetus and Newborn and the American College of Obstetricians and Gynecologists Committee on Obstetric Practice. Antepartum care. Guidelines for perinatal care. 6th ed. Elk Grove Village, IL: American Academy of Pediatrics; 2007.
6. American College of Obstetricians and Gynecologists. Obesity in pregnancy. ACOG Committee opinion no. 315. Obstet Gynecol. 2005;106:671–5 (reaffirmed 2008).
7. Rittenberg V, Seshadri S, Sunkara SK, Sobaleva S, Oteng-Ntim E, El-Toukhy T. Effect of body mass index on IVF treatment outcome: an updated systematic review and meta-analysis. Reprod Biomed Online. 2011;23(4):421–39. http://web.ebscohost.com.ezp-prod1.hul.harvard.edu/ehost/pdfviewer/pdfviewer?sid=fa6e24c2-0db0-4fcc-9049-cec786f4bbc6%40sessionmgr4&vid=2&hid=13. Accessed 2 Jan 2012.
8. Moragianni VA, Jones SML, Ryley DA. The effect of BMI on outcomes of first assisted reproductive technology cycles. Fertil Steril. 2012;98:102–8.
9. Shah DK, Missmer SA, Berry KF, Racowsky C, Ginsburg ES. Effect of obesity on oocyte and embryo quality in women undergoing in vitro fertilization. Obstet Gynecol. 2011;118(1):63–70.
10. Depalo R, Garruti G, Totaro I, et al. Oocyte morphological abnormalities in overweight women undergoing in vitro fertilization cycles. Gynecol Endocrinol. 2011;27(11):880–4.
11. American College of Obstetricians and Gynecologists. Preconception and prenatal carrier screening for genetic diseases in individuals of eastern European Jewish descent. ACOG Committee opinion no. 442. Obstet Gynecol. 2009;114(4):950–3.
12. Pratt LA, Brody DJ, Gu Q. Antidepressant use in persons aged 12 and over: United States, 2005–2008. NCHS data brief, no 76. Hyattsville, MD: National Center for Health Statistics. 2011. http://www.cdc.gov/nchs/data/databriefs/db76.htm. Accessed 1 Feb 2012.
13. Coutifaris C, Mayers ER, Guzick DS, et al. Histological dating of timed endometrial biopsy tissue is not related to fertility status. Fertil Steril. 2004;82:1264–72.
14. Grimes DA. Validity of the postcoital test. Am J Obstet Gynecol. 1995;172:1327.
15. Bayer SR, Alper MM, Penzias AS, editors. Boston IVF handbook of infertility. 3rd ed. New York: Informa Healthcare; 2011.
16. Fritz MA, Speroff L, editors. Clinical gynecologic endocrinology and infertility. 8th ed. Philadelphia, PA: Lippincott Williams and Wilkins; 2011.
17. Verhagen TE, Hendriks DJ, Bancsi LF, Mol BW, Broekmans FJ. The accuracy of multivariate models predicting ovarian reserve and pregnancy after in vitro fertilization: a meta-analysis. Hum Reprod Update. 2008;14(2):95–100.
18. van Rooij IA, Bancsi LF, Broekmans FJ, Looman CW, Habbema JD, te Velde ER. Women older than 40 years of age and those with elevated follicle-stimulating hormone levels differ in poor response rate and embryo quality in in vitro fertilization. Fertil Steril. 2003;79(3):482–8.
19. Abdalla H, Thum MY. An elevated basal FSH reflects a quantitative rather than qualitative decline of the ovarian reserve. Hum Reprod. 2004;19(4):893–8.
20. Toner JP. Age = egg quality, FSH level = egg quantity. Fertil Steril. 2003;79(3):491.
21. Yanushpolsky EH, Hurwitz S, Tikh E, Racowsky C. Predictive usefulness of cycle day 10 follicle-stimulating hormone level in a clomiphene citrate challenge test for in vitro fertilization outcome in women younger than 40 years of age. Fertil Steril. 2003;80(1):111–5.
22. Hofmann GE, Danforth DR, Seifer DB. Inhibin-B: the physiologic basis of the clomiphene citrate challenge test for ovarian reserve screening. Fertil Steril. 1998;69(3):474–7.
23. Urbancsek J, Hauzman E, Klinga K, Rabe T, Papp Z, Strowitzki T. Use of serum inhibin B levels at the start of ovarian stimulation and at oocyte pickup in the prediction of assisted reproduction treatment outcome. Fertil Steril. 2005;83(2):341–8.
24. Hall JE, Welt CK, Cramer DW. Inhibin A and inhibin B reflect ovarian function in assisted reproduction but are less useful at predicting outcome. Hum Reprod. 1999;14(2):409–15.
25. Fanchin R, de Ziegler D, Olivennes F, et al. Exogeneous follicle stimulating hormone ovarian reserve test (EFORT): a simple and reliable screening test for detecting "poor responder" in in-vitro fertilization. Hum Reprod. 1994;9:1607–11.
26. Frattarelli JL, Levi AJ, Miller BT, Segars JH. A prospective assessment of the predictive value of basal antral follicles in in vitro fertilization cycles. Fertil Steril. 2003;80(2):350–5.
27. Chang MY, Chiang CH, Hsieh TT, Soong YK, Hsu KH. Use of the antral follicle count to predict the outcome of assisted reproductive technologies. Fertil Steril. 1998;69(3):505–10.
28. Erdem M, Erdem A, Guler I, Atmaca S. Role of antral follicle count in controlled ovarian hyperstimulation and intrauterine insemination cycles in patients with unexplained subfertility. Fertil Steril. 2008;90(2):360–6.
29. Visser JA, de Jong FH, Laven JS, Themmen AP. Anti-Müllerian hormone: a new marker for ovarian function. Reproduction. 2006;131(1):1–9.
30. van Rooij IA, Broekmans FJ, te Velde ER, et al. Serum anti-Müllerian hormone levels: a novel measure of ovarian reserve. Hum Reprod. 2002;17(12):3065–71.
31. Seifer DB, Baker VL, Leader B. Age-specific serum anti-Mullerian hormone values for 17,120 women presenting to fertility centers within the United States. Fertil Steril. 2011;95:747–50.
32. Broekmans FJ, Kwee J, Hendriks DJ, Mol BW, Lambalk CB. A systematic review of tests predicting

ovarian reserve and IVF outcome. Hum Reprod Update. 2006;12(6):685–718.
33. Pittaway DE, Winfield AC, Maxson W, et al. Prevention of acute pelvic inflammatory disease after hysterosalpingography: efficacy of doxycycline prophylaxis. Am J Obstet Gynecol. 1983;147:623–6.
34. Practice Committee of the American Society for Reproductive Medicine in collaboration with The Society of Reproductive Surgeons. Salpingectomy for hydrosalpinges before in vitro fertilization increases the success rate. Fertil Steril. 2008;90:S66–8.
35. Alper MM, Garner PR, Spence JE, et al. Pregnancy rates after hysterosalpingography with oil- and water-soluble contrast media. Obstet Gynecol. 1986; 68:6–9.
36. Galen DI, Khan N, Richter KS. Essure multicenter off-label treatment for hydrosalpinx before in vitro fertilization. J Minim Invasive Gynecol. 2011;18(3):338–42.
37. Rotterdam ESHRE/ASRM-Sponsored PCOS Consensus Workshop Group. Revised 2003 consensus on diagnostic criteria and long-term health risks related to polycystic ovary syndrome. Fertil Steril. 2004;81(1):19–25.
38. Gharib H, Tuttle RM, Baskin HJ, Fish LH, Singer PA, McDermott MT. Subclinical thyroid dysfunction: a joint statement on management from the American Association of Clinical Endocrinologists, the American Thyroid Association, and the Endocrine Society. J Clin Endocrinol Metab. 2005;90(1):581–7.
39. Klipstein S, Regan M, Ryley DA, Goldman MB, Alper MM, Reindollar RH. One last chance for pregnancy: a review of 2,705 in vitro fertilization cycles initiated in women age 40 years and above. Fertil Steril. 2005;84(2):435–45.
40. Malizia BA, Hacker MR, Penzias AS. Cumulative live-birth rates after in vitro fertilization. N Engl J Med. 2009;360(3):236–43.
41. The Practice Committee of the Society for Assisted Reproductive Technology and the Practice Committee of the American Society for Reproductive Medicine. Guidelines on the number of embryos transferred. Fertil Steril. 2008;90:S163–4.

2 Pre-IVF Evaluation of the Infertile Man

Brooke Harnisch and Robert D. Oates

Introduction

Azoospermia and severe oligospermia are found in approximately 1% of all men and 15% of infertile men [1]. Men with azoospermia should undergo a comprehensive medical history, physical examination, and one or more semen analyses [2]. Depending on the presumptive diagnosis, further evaluation including genetic testing, hormonal assays, and/or imaging tests may be warranted. If at all possible, approaches to initiate, restore, or preserve natural fertility are attempted. When these methods fail, assisted reproductive technologies (ART) including in vitro fertilization and intracytoplasmic sperm injection (IVF-ICSI) may then be employed as primary or adjunctive therapies. The latter technology can effectively bypass the natural process of fertilization allowing for a single viable sperm to fertilize a single oocyte outside of the reproductive tract [3]. Previously considered sterile men can now father healthy children. As a result, it is important to have a firm understanding of which etiologies of azoospermia and severe oligospermia would benefit from these technologies and the work-up and surgical techniques involved before proceeding. One of the most important reasons for examination of the infertile male prior to any in vitro interventions being initiated is to identify any underlying medical conditions, diseases or syndromes that had not heretofore been recognized and/or treated. This information will not only best position couples in trying to achieve a successful pregnancy but also focus on the health of the male patient and future offspring.

B. Harnisch, M.D
Department of Urology, Boston Medical Center, Boston, MA 02118, USA
e-mail: brooke.harnisch@bmc.org

R.D. Oates, M.D. (✉)
Department of Urology, Boston University School of Medicine, 725 Albany Street, Suite 3B, Boston, MA 02118, USA
e-mail: robert.oates@bmc.org

Medical and Surgical History: What Can Be Learned?

Medical history begins with questioning regarding the duration of infertility, frequency, and timing of sexual intercourse, prior conceptions by either partner, and whether the couple has had prior fertility evaluation. Additionally, for the male specifically, erectile function/dysfunction and ejaculatory ability should be ascertained as prior illnesses such as transverse myelitis may lead to failure of the emission phase of the ejaculatory reflex without having other recognizable neurological consequences. Longstanding insulin-dependent diabetes can adversely affect vasal peristalsis, seminal vesicle contraction, and bladder neck closure eventuating in low-volume oligoasthenic semen specimens, retrograde ejaculation, or complete failure of the ejaculatory process [4]. Past medical and surgical history including onset of puberty, childhood conditions like viral orchitis

E.S. Ginsburg and C. Racowsky (eds.), *In Vitro Fertilization: A Comprehensive Guide*,
DOI 10.1007/978-1-4419-9848-4_2, © Springer Science+Business Media New York 2012

and cryptorchidism, genetic conditions, past genital and perineal trauma, and past retroperitoneal or inguinal surgery should be fully elucidated. Patients may have a genetic condition, e.g., adult polycystic kidney disease, von Hippel Lindau disease, and cystic fibrosis, that may not only impact the couple's fertility potential but have implications on the health of the offspring. In these instances, the couple may benefit from genetic counseling in combination with preimplantation genetic diagnosis [5]. A history of chronic respiratory illness or sinusitis may suggest a diagnosis of primary ciliary dyskinesia or cystic fibrosis [6].

Cryptorchidism is present in 1–3% of newborns. Although future fertility in cases of unilateral cryptorchidism is the norm, consequent infertility in adulthood is not unusual, even when orchiopexy is performed within the first few years of life—a helpful but not completely protective strategy [7–10]. At the extreme, azoospermia may be found in 10% of patients with a history of unilateral cryptorchidism and 32% of men born with bilateral undescended testes [11]. Of these men with resultant severe oligospermia, it is unlikely that semen parameter improvement can be obtained with any specific or empirical maneuver as this is generally a reflection of baseline poor spermatogenic capability [12]. If the patient is azoospermic, TESE oftentimes leads to sperm retrieval (see below). Patients with cyrptorchidism have an increased risk of testicular cancer above the normal population, so history and physical examination in these patients is paramount [13].

A history of unilateral testicular torsion can be found in 0.025% of males. Although semen parameters when compared to controls are normal, correctable contralateral testis pathology (perhaps an obstructive process) may be present and may lead to severe oligospermia or azoospermia [14–16].

Although vasectomy is the most common reason for obstruction of the ductal system, congenital and/or iatrogenic causes may be present. Up to 40% of men with obstructive azoospermia may have a reversible pathology [17–19]. Prior epididymitis, hernia repair (especially with mesh), and hydrocele repair are all historical clues that may suggest vasal or epididymal obstruction. As microsurgical reconstruction is often successful in restoring sperm to the ejaculate with resultant natural conception when performed by a fully trained urologist with an interest and expertise in male reproductive medicine and surgery, the proper diagnosis should always be made prior to simply resorting to sperm aspiration coupled with ART [20, 21]. The same holds true for couples in whom the male partner has had a vasectomy in the past, when reconstruction is successful and sperm are present in the ejaculate, then each and every month the couple has a chance for pregnancy achievement [22–24]. Thus vasectomy reversal should be the first option for these couples as it maximizes the opportunity for attainment of pregnancy.

Anabolic steroid use, whether illicit or prescribed (topical gels), is on the rise in men of all ages [25]. The spermatogenic process requires that testosterone is produced by Leydig cells that are located in the interstitium, immediately adjacent to the seminiferous tubules. When circulating exogenous androgen is present, it suppresses pituitary elaboration of LH thereby stifling testicular generation of testosterone. In consequence, spermatogenesis is reduced or abolished [26, 27]. Historical clues to current or past use include a history of body building and/or weight lifting (see below for typical endocrine pattern). Men should be encouraged to discontinue usage because a rebound of spermatogenesis will occur, spermatozoa will return to the ejaculate, and natural conception is likely. Most often, assisted reproduction will not be required. Every male should be asked specifically whether he is taking illegal anabolic steroids or legally prescribed testosterone. It is interesting that physicians that prescribe testosterone replacement or supplementation are not always aware of the deleterious effects on the creation of spermatozoa. In a recent study by Ko et al. which surveyed 387 urologists regarding their practice patterns in evaluating and treating the infertile male, 25% of those responding would continue patients on testosterone therapy even if they were actively pursuing pregnancy [28].

In patients with a prior malignancy, the type of cancer as well as the surgical, chemotherapeutic or radiation treatment protocols employed are all important determinants of future and/or present spermatogenic potential. If the patient is severely oligospermic several years later, as a corollary to his primary end point of cure, it is unlikely that any treatment, medical or surgical, will be effective in enhancing spermatogenesis. If the patient is persistently azoospermic years after chemo or radiotherapy for either benign or malignant disease, individual spermatozoa may be found at the time of TESE in up to 70% and serve as the source of sperm in combination with ICSI (see below) [29].

Patients should be questioned regarding their habit history as smoking has been shown to cause abnormal semen parameters, lower fertilization rates and increased embryo and pregnancy loss [30–32]. Additionally, studies have shown that offspring from men who smoke have an increased chance of developing certain childhood malignancies such as brain tumors and acute lymphoblastic leukemia. [33–35] As Santos et al. stated, "It is concluded that physicians should strongly advise their patients to quit smoking before undergoing medical treatment or assisted reproduction techniques to achieve pregnancy" [36].

Other lifestyle factors like food intake, obesity, medications and alcohol use should always be explored in the infertile male. Even though there are conflicting reports about these issues, it is always best to optimize general health, diet, exercise, and sleep [37–39]. Even though there is no consensus on the impact of obesity on semen parameters, the rapid weight loss and metabolic derangements that occur after bariatric surgery may significantly impair sperm production capacity [40].

The Physical Examination: What Can the Eyes and Fingers Tell Us?

On initial inspection of the patient, the general appearance should be noted, including height, weight, dysmorphic features, and level of virilization [2]. Is the patient undervirilized with lack of beard growth, decreased muscle mass, and eunichoid body proportions which may indicate a hypothalamic or pituitary endocrinopathy? Is the patient overvirilized with an excessive muscular bulk, possibly a clue to anabolic steroid use? Are there surgical scars that hint at hernia repair, hydrocele repair, or orchidopexy for cryptorchidism? On genital examination, is the penis of normal length, without curvature, and are there meatal anomalies such as hypospadias or epispadias? Is the testis size >20 cm^3 with a firm but not hard consistency [41]? Since the seminiferous epithelium makes up the bulk of the testis volume, when spermatogenic failure is present, the overall testis size will be reduced. Are there testicular masses, areas of induration, or tenderness?

Attention is then turned to the reproductive ductal structures, including the vasa deferentia and epididymides. If there is dilation or fullness felt on careful palpation, an obstructive process may be present as seen post vasectomy, after bilateral inguinal hernia repairs or possibly after an inflammatory process of the genitourinary tract. This is an incredibly important finding as microsurgical reconstruction can restore sperm to the ejaculate and allow the couple to achieve a natural conception [42]. Congenital bilateral absence of the vas deferens (CBAVD) is identified when the vasa are unable to be palpated. In CBAVD, there is always at least the caput of the epididymis but occasionally the corpus and tail can be present as well. The spermatic cord is inspected for varicoceles, hydroceles, spermatoceles, or lipomas. Varicoceles are found in 14% of healthy men but in 40% of infertile males [43].

The Semen Analysis, Azoospermia, and Severe Oligospermia

At least two semen analyses should be done, according to the World Health Organization Laboratory Manual for Examination and Processing of Human Semen [44]. No single parameter should be used in isolation to determine fertility or infertility. Slightly substandard semen parameters do not suggest a particular or specific diagnosis such as varicocele or certain medication usage. However, in severe oligospermia or azoospermia, an algorithmic approach can be used to define the etiology in many cases.

Azoospermia can be classified as Nonobstructive Azoospermia (NOA) due to failure of spermatogenesis or Obstructive Azoospermia (OA) due to blockage/occlusion of the reproductive ductal system (epididymides, vasa deferentia, seminal vesicles, and ejaculatory ducts). The etiology of NOA can either be "primary" at the level of seminiferous tubules or "secondary" at the level of the hypothalamus and pituitary. In the former, FSH is elevated as a compensatory response due to reduced spermatogenesis and in the latter, FSH output is markedly reduced or absent and a potentially normal spermatogenic compartment is not stimulated. This distinction usually can be made either anatomically and physiologically, or via clinical parameters (history, testis size and consistency, semen volume/pH) and serum follicle-stimulating hormone (FSH) levels [45].

A novel way to begin to think about and determine the etiology of azoospermia in an infertile male is based on semen volume and semen pH [45]. There are three main contributors to the ejaculate: alkaline seminal vesicle fluid which comprises 70%; acidic prostatic fluid which constitutes 20%; the remaining 10% is sperm-rich fluid from the vas and epididymis. The seminal vesicle and vas discharge their contents via the ejaculatory duct—one trio on each side. Typically, the alkaline seminal vesicle fluid overwhelms the prostatic contribution such that the end result of a normal semen specimen is a pH >7.2 and volume >1.5 ml [46]. Azoospermic semen specimens can, therefore, be defined as low volume, low pH (approximately 0.6 cm^3 and a pH of 6.5; consisting of only prostatic fluid) or normal volume, normal pH (approximately 1.5 cm^3 and a pH >7.2; consisting of testicular fluid via the vas, seminal vesicle secretions, and prostatic fluid) (Figs. 2.1 and 2.2). In the low volume, low pH azoospermic male, there are two diagnostic possibilities: the seminal vesicles are absent, aplastic or dysfunctional (e.g., CBAVD) or unable to empty (e.g., complete bilateral ejaculatory duct obstruction; EDO). In the normal volume, normal pH azoospermic male, the seminal vesicles are anatomically and functionally adequate and empty through patent ejaculatory ducts. In these situations, either the testes do not produce spermatozoa due to spermatogenic failure or sperm production is adequate but there exists a blockage to sperm flow at the level of the scrotal or inguinal vas ("proximal" to the ejaculatory ducts such that the seminal vesicles are able to discharge their fluid through the ejaculatory ducts but there is no sperm arriving into the vasal ampulla). History and physical examination are often all that are needed to elucidate the exact diagnosis. In CBAVD, the semen volume and pH are low and the vasa are not palpable [47]. In complete EDO, the semen volume and pH are low and careful scrotal examination reveals that both the vas and epididymis are full and firm, indicative of an obstructive process downstream to the site of palpation [48]. In spermatogenic failure, the semen volume and pH will be normal and the testes may be small and soft while the ductal structures are palpably without abnormality. In an epididymal blockage secondary to prior inflammation, the semen volume and pH will be normal and the testes will be natural in terms of size and consistency while the proximal epididymis will be full and firm (indicating downstream obstruction) and the vas distal to the blockage will be palpably delicate and normal. Just the combination of mind and fingers can make the vast majority of diagnoses in azoospermic males. Scrotal ultrasound is neither necessary nor helpful—all that needs to be known is easily able to be palpated.

Hormonal Assays: When, in Whom, and How Do They Help

The initial endocrine evaluation begins with serum follicle-stimulating hormone (FSH), luteinizing hormone (LH) and total testosterone. Indications to obtain these studies include: sperm concentration <10 million/ml, impaired sexual function, and/or clinical concern for an endocrinopathy [1]. But not all patients require hormonal studies. For example, the male with CBAVD and normal testis size, as determined by physical examination, will not benefit from

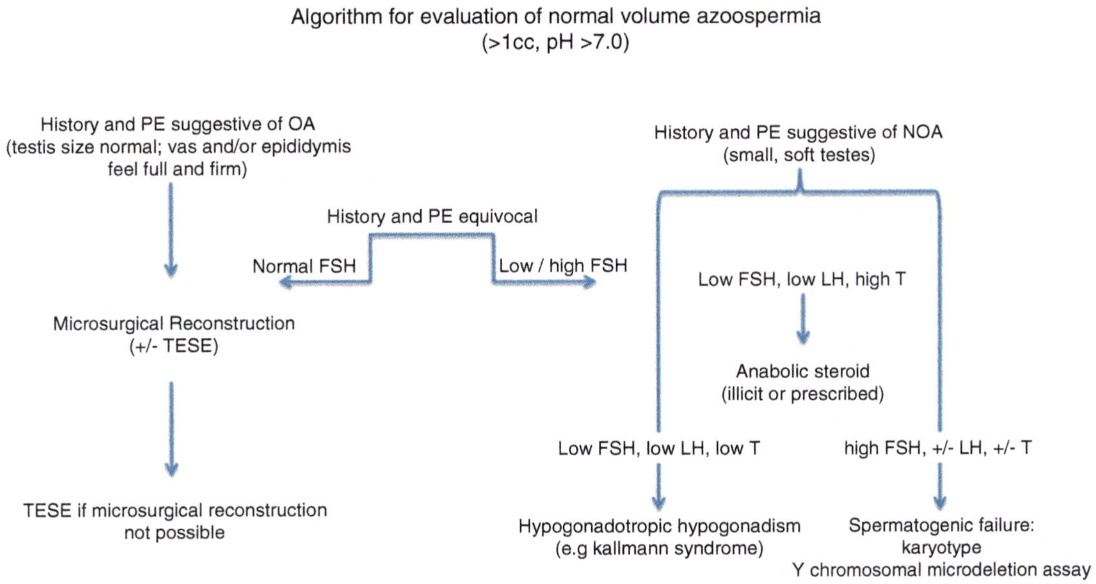

Fig. 2.1 Algorithm for the evaluation of the male with a normal volume, normal pH azoospermic semen analysis. Coupled with the history and physical examination, the etiology can often be determined as either obstructive or nonobstructive. When history and physical examination alone are not definitive, hormonal assays and, on occasion, genetic assays can be used as supplemental diagnostic tools. *FSH* follicle-stimulating hormone, *LH* luteinizing hormone, *NOA* nonobstructive azoospermia, *OA* obstructive azoospermia, *TESE* testicular sperm extraction

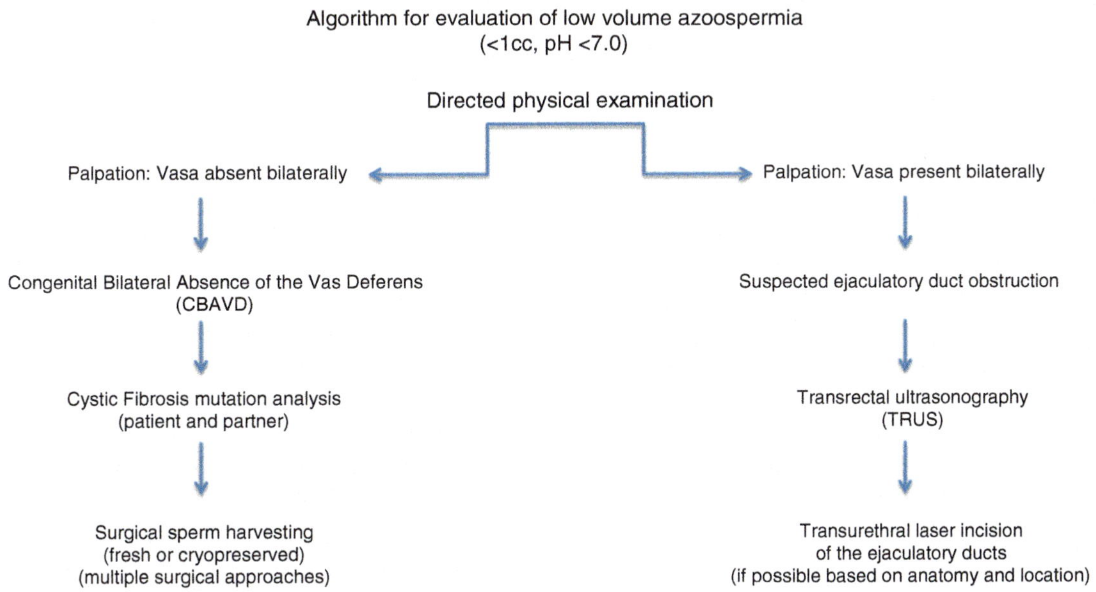

Fig. 2.2 Algorithm for the evaluation of the male with a low volume, low pH azoospermic semen analysis. The physical examination is the key to diagnosis. When the vasa are not palpable bilaterally, by definition the diagnosis is Congenital Bilateral Absence of the Vas Deferens (CBAVD). Both partners require CF mutation analysis and ultimately surgical sperm harvesting coupled with ICSI will be the treatment plan. If the vasa are palpable, they may also feel full and firm and Bilateral Ejaculatory Duct Obstruction would be suspected which can be confirmed with transrectal ultrasonography. Transurethral laser ablation may be accomplished as definitive treatment if a dilated ejaculatory duct or midline cyst is available for surgical entry

Table 2.1 Hormonal parameters expected based on clinical condition/disorder

Hypogonadotropic circumstances	*FSH*	*LH*	*Testosterone*
1. Congenital (e.g., Kallmann syndrome)	Reduced	Reduced	Reduced
2. Anabolic steroid (illicit or prescribed)	Reduced	Reduced	Elevated
3. Opiate (oral or injectable; illicit or prescribed)	Reduced	Reduced	Reduced
Hypergonadotropic conditions	*FSH*	*LH*	*Testosterone*
1. 47, XXY Klinefelter syndrome	Elevated	Elevated	Reduced/Normal
2. Bilateral cryptorchidism	Elevated	Elevated/Normal	Reduced/Normal
3. Prior ablative chemotherapy	Elevated	Normal	Normal
4. Spermatogenic failure: Y microdeletion	Elevated	Normal	Normal
5. Spermatogenic failure: unknown	Elevated	Normal	Normal

endocrinological evaluation. To review briefly, under stimulation by hypothalamic GnRH, the anterior pituitary releases FSH and LH. In the adult, FSH is regulated via negative feedback by inhibin B (the alpha subunit produced by Sertoli cells and the beta subunit secreted by the germinal epithelium) [49]. As spermatogenesis decreases, inhibin B decreases and FSH increases in compensatory fashion. In a male with optimal spermatogenesis, the amount of FSH normally produced by the pituitary is most often in the lowest aspects of the assay's "reference range." When FSH levels began to rise out of these lower reaches up to the mid or high levels of the "reference range," or even beyond, this is a clear indication of reduced spermatogenic potential, decreased testicular inhibin secretion and consequent compensatory pituitary elaboration of FSH. The "reference range" upper limit value is of no biological significance. In other words, to make the diagnosis of spermatogenic compromise or failure, the absolute value of measured FSH does not need to "exceed the upper levels of normal" [50, 51].

In hypogonadotropic hypogonadism, e.g., Kallmann syndrome, FSH, LH and testosterone are extremely low, if not undetectable. This diagnosis is usually confirmed in the teenage male who is not virilizing [50]. At that time, these young boys often receive testosterone supplementation simply to stimulate tanner stage progression. In adulthood, when fertility is desired, they must be taken off of exogenous androgen and intratesticular testosterone secretion and spermatogenesis induced via a sequenced combination of hCG and FSH injection therapy [52]. In the adult male with 47, XXY Klinefelter syndrome, LH and FSH are both elevated while testosterone is in the low/normal range reflecting abnormalities in both the spermatogenic and androgenic compartments of the testes. In anabolic steroid users, or those men on testosterone supplementation, pituitary LH and FSH output is suppressed resulting in poor or absent intratesticular testosterone manufacture. As described above, this leads to consequent diminished or absent spermatogenesis. Opiate usage may also suppress hypothalamic GnRH secretion resulting in blunted pituitary LH and FSH output and, therefore, poor testicular testosterone and sperm production. Coupled with history and physical examination, in the appropriate circumstances, a directed endocrinological panel can be of great help (Table 2.1).

Genetic Assays: When, in Whom, and How Do They Help

It is recommended that patients with NOA or severe oligospermia ($<5\times10^6/cm^3$ of spermatozoa) undergo genetic testing with Y chromosome microdeletion and karyotype [45, 53]. All patients with CBAVD should undergo cystic fibrosis mutation analysis [54].

Anomalies of chromosome number and/or structure are found in 10–15% of men with non-obstructive azoospermia and 5% of oligospermic men [45, 55, 56]. These include numerical abnormalities such as 47, XXY Klinefelter syndrome or 46, XX male syndrome. Structural abnormalities including Robertsonian translocations, reciprocal translocations, and pericentric inversions may be found in a small percentage of these men.

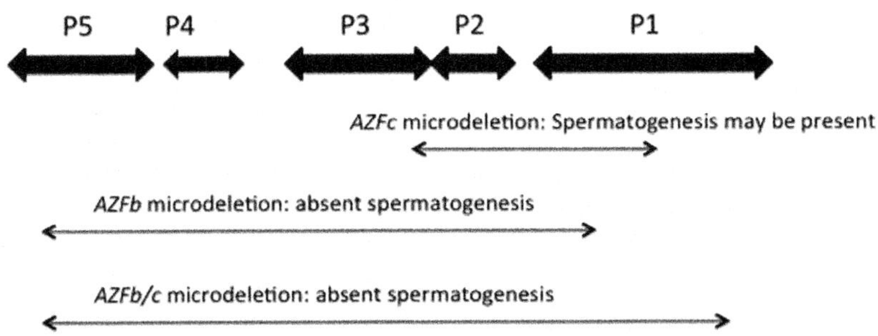

Fig. 2.3 The most common clinically relevant microdeletions that occur within the expanse bordered by the P5 and P1 palindromes. The *AZFa* microdeletion is located upstream on Yq closer to the centromere

Table 2.2 Potential for spermatogenesis depending on karyotypic/genetic etiology

Assay	Result	Spermatogenic potential
Karyotype	Translocation: Balanced Reciprocal	Presence of spermatogenesis depends upon chromosomes involved
	46 XX male syndrome	Absent spermatogenesis: no benefit from micro-TESE
	47, XXY Klinefelter syndrome	50% chance of finding spermatozoa on micro-TESE
Y Chromosomal Microdeletion	*AZFa* microdeletion	Absent spermatogenesis: no benefit from micro-TESE
	AZFb microdeletion	Absent spermatogenesis: no benefit from micro-TESE
	AZFb/c microdeletion	Absent spermatogenesis: no benefit from micro-TESE
	AZFc microdeletion	Severe oligospermia; 70% chance of retrievable sperm on micro-TESE
Cystic Fibrosis Mutation Analysis	CBAVD	Normal spermatogenesis

Depending on the chromosomal abnormality, some patients may produce ejaculate sperm or only small amounts of testicular sperm that can be surgically harvested to use in IVF-ICSI. For example, when testis tissue is extracted from males with 47, XXY Klinefelter syndrome, spermatozoa can be found in 50–60% of cases [57]. Over 100 chromosomally healthy babies have been conceived in this manner [58]. In 46, XX male syndrome, no sperm are present within the testes of these patients and so surgical exploration in an attempt to harvest spermatozoa is not warranted. However, in patients with chromosomal translocations, preimplantation diagnosis can be used to achieve a healthy pregnancy [59].

Within the Y chromosome, there are eight palindromic stretches on the long arm (P8–P1) [60–62]. Each palindrome is itself comprised of repetitive and duplicate subregions termed amplicons. This molecular geography predisposes to non-allelic homologous recombination (NAHR: intrachromosomal recombination between homologous repetitive sequences) [63]. NAHR may result in deletion of the intervening, variably sized pieces of the long arm of the Y chromosome (Fig. 2.3). These regions on the Y chromosome are the home for genes involved in spermatogenesis (DAZ, BPY, CDY1, etc.) [62]. As such, a PCR-based Y chromosomal microdeletion assay is used to search for microdeletion possibilities including (as they are known clinically): *AZFa*, *AZFb*, *AZFb/c*, and *AZFc*. For patients with an *AZFa*, *AZFb*, or *AZFb/c* microdeletion, there will be no sperm found in the ejaculate or in the testis tissue due to a complete absence of spermatogenesis [64–68] (Table 2.2). Since the Y chromosomal microdeletion assay, in these particular circumstances, is prognostic, the patient will not benefit from microsurgical TESE and should not be subjected to an invasive operative procedure nor should his partner undergo a planned simultaneous stimulation cycle in anticipation of IVF-ICSI (as some programs routinely do).

Conversely, in the setting of an *AZFc* microdeletion, if small numbers of sperm are not seen in the ejaculate, 70% of men undergoing TESE will have retrievable spermatozoa capable of generating pregnancy [69–71]. However, all sons conceived by either ejaculate or testicular spermatozoa will inherit that same *AZFc* microdeleted Y chromosome and their future spectrum of spermatogenic deficiency when they reach reproductive adulthood will be either severe oligospermia or azoospermia [72]. Couples need to be informed of this prior to undergoing ART so that, with this knowledge in hand, they can decide whether to use preimplantation genetic screening for the identification and transfer of only female embryos. Such an approach will prevent this anomaly from continuing on in that couple's family tree and burdening their sons with reproductive deficiency or sterility.

Cystic fibrosis (CF) mutation analysis is required in all patients with CBAVD, a disorder which is found in 2–3% of infertile Caucasian men [47, 73]. The genetic basis of CBAVD is the same as that which underlies CF: mutations in the genes encoding for the cystic fibrosis transmembrane conductance regulator (CFTR) on chromosome 7q31.2. CFTR is responsible for proper epithelial transmembrane sodium/chloride balance and is regulated by cAMP [74]. In CF, defective CFTR eventuates in viscous respiratory and pancreatic secretions leading to the known clinical manifestations and sequelae of the disease. The ultimate clinical expression of CFTR dysfunction is dependent on the combination of paternally and maternally inherited CFTR mutations. The two most common CFTR mutations found in men with CBAVD are delta F508 and 5T [54, 75]. If both mutations are deemed "severe," the patient will be on the more affected end of the phenotypic spectrum (profound pulmonary and pancreatic disease as well as bilateral vasal absence) while those whose mutations, in combination, affect the total CFTR pool to a much lesser degree will be located on the less severely affected end of that spectrum, perhaps with CBAVD as the only recognizable clinical consequence. If the combination of mutations impairs CFTR function somewhere in between those two endpoints, the clinical presentation may be intermediate as well (e.g., CBAVD and some mild, life-long sinus issues) [76]. Since the seminal vesicles are generally atrophic, aplastic or small and nonfunctional, the semen volume is low and the pH is acidic—the ejaculate comprised of just prostatic fluid. This is why men with CBAVD will have a low volume, low pH azoospermic semen specimen, an instant clue to the diagnosis.

Partners of patients with CBAVD should undergo cystic fibrosis mutation analysis and the couple should be referred to a genetic counselor [1]. If she is a carrier, then PGD should be used in combination with IVF/ICSI to prevent offspring from inheriting any form of CF mutation disease, the most concerning being clinical cystic fibrosis with its devastating pulmonary and pancreatic manifestations (Fig. 2.4).

A small percentage of men with CBAVD will not have a CFTR mutational basis. However, these patients often have unilateral renal agenesis thought to be due to a genetic anomaly affecting mesonephric duct development (responsible for both the reproductive ductal and ureteral derivatives). Couples should be aware that it is possible that their offspring could inherit a more severe bilateral renal agenesis phenotype [77]. The exact genetic anomaly is unknown.

Surgical Therapy: What Procedures Are Helpful in the Oligospermic or Azoospermic Male

Severe oligospermia or azoospermia with a varicocele: In the setting of reduced semen parameters and a large, clinically palpable varicocele, microsurgical varicocelectomy should be offered as the first option [78]. Many men will experience an improvement in sperm density and function (70%) and approximately 60% of couples will go on to conceive on their own without additional intervention [43]. Small varicoceles or ones detected only by scrotal ultrasonography and not by palpation should not be surgically

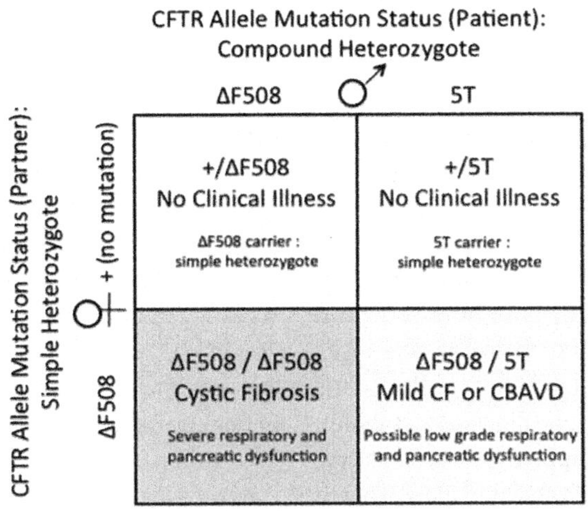

Fig. 2.4 Punnett square demonstrating the possible outcomes if the male with CBAVD has two recognizable Cystic Fibrosis mutations (e.g., delta F508 and 5T) and the female partner is a carrier (simple heterozygote; e.g., delta F508). In this circumstance, preimplantation diagnosis can be used to transfer only embryos that are simple heterozygotes and to prevent the transfer of embryos that will be delta F508 homozygous

corrected as the benefits are minimal, if at all. In men with an obvious varicocele and nonobstructive azoospermia (without a genetic anomaly that precludes sperm production such as an *AZFb/c* microdeletion), varicocelectomy should be performed 3–4 months prior to any anticipated adjunctive procedures. Approximately 30% of men will have an improvement in their overall level of spermatogenesis such that sperm return in small quantities to the ejaculate [79, 80]. It is not truly the anticipation (although possible) that the degree of spermatogenic recovery will be so dramatic that natural pregnancy will be likely; rather, varicocelectomy provides a way to maximize whatever reproductive potential exists. If spermatozoa are subsequently seen in the ejaculate, they can be used as the source of sperm for an ICSI cycle. If, 4 months later, the male is still azoospermic and requires microsurgical TESE, then whatever potential he has within his seminiferous tubules will have been maximized and, thereby, the possibility of finding sperm on TESE will have been optimized. If no sperm are eventually found on well-performed TESE, at least the couple will know and understand that every possible way to augment spermatogenesis was carried out prior to the definitive and final operative intervention of TESE.

Azoospermia in the setting of vasal or epididymal occlusion: If the azoospermic male has normal spermatogenesis but has a blockage of the ductal system from prior epididymitis or, more commonly vasectomy, microsurgical reconstruction should be carried out. This procedure should be performed by urologic surgeons practiced in that surgical discipline as rates of success are indeed linked to expertise and ability of the surgeon [23]. The intent is to return sperm to the ejaculate and allow the couple the opportunity to achieve conception naturally each and every month [18, 20, 42]. The patency rates following vasectomy reversal are approximately 95% and the naturally conceived pregnancy rates are approximately 50%, although multiple factors influencing these figures may result in even better results in subgroups of couples [81–83]. If the couple chooses to utilize ICSI if the reconstruction is technically not possible (as determined at the time of surgery), or is unsuccessful in returning sperm to the ejaculate, testis tissue can be harvested and cryopreserved at the time of surgery as a future source of sperm if the need arises.

Azoospermia in the setting of Congenital Bilateral Absence of the Vas Deferens: After appropriate genetic evaluation of both partners with CF mutation analysis, microsurgical epididymal sperm aspiration can be accomplished [84–87]. The caput of the epididymis is always present in cases of CBAVD and the efferent ducts can be microsurgically opened as they travel immediately underneath a thin layer of tunical tissue that bridges the testis and caput epididymis. Fluid obtained can be completely free of red blood cells and frequently provides the "newest" sperm that have been produced as the fluid that exists comes from the rete testis (intratesticular ductal system that collects the effluent from each seminiferous tubule). Cryopreservation of the sample into numerous cryovials is often possible, each serving as the source of sperm for a future cycle of ICSI. Percutaneous approaches have been used as well but may limit the sperm quantity and quality obtained.

Azoospermia in the setting of impaired spermatogenesis: In the patient with nonobstructive azoospermia, microsurgical testis sperm extraction, also known as micro-TESE, can be employed in hopes of finding individual spermatozoa that can be used in conjunction with ICSI (as reviewed by Schlegel [88]). Certainly, prior genetic evaluation is mandatory with a karyotype and Y chromosomal microdeletion assay (as described above) prior to any operative intervention being carried out. If the patient has an *AZFa* or *AZFb* microdeletion, for example, no spermatozoa will be present as surgery will be fruitless, unnecessary, and inappropriate. Depending upon the etiology of the NOA, spermatozoa can be retrieved in 30–70% of patients but the details of the individual's circumstance can influence that significantly in both directions. Men with *AZFc* microdeletions, unknown genetic bases, prior cryptorchidism, prior chemotherapy, and prior inflammatory conditions are all candidates [29, 70]. Depending upon the circumstance, the actual TESE procedure may be performed prior to an ICSI cycle with the tissue cryopreserved if sperm are present or the TESE can be performed coincident with an ICSI cycle and oocyte harvesting. This decision is made based upon etiology (e.g., 47, XXY Klinefelter males are most often operated on at the time of ICSI in a combined approach) and other aspects of the couple's situation (e.g., has the couple chosen to have donor sperm back-up) [57, 58, 89]. As is true for just about any surgical procedure, the experience and expertise of the urologist is a critically important element in the success or no success equation. Interestingly, the babies born from 47, XXY men have all been 46, XY or 46, XX as it appears that the only spermatogonia that are capable of completing meiosis and generating haploid sperm are themselves, 46, XY [90]. So far, the data are encouraging that the use of testis sperm does not confer an increase in congenital anomalies in the offspring.

Conclusions

A proper evaluation in every male with reproductive compromise or failure is necessary prior to employing adjunctive advanced reproductive techniques or surgical sperm harvesting. Reversible causes may be found (e.g., anabolic steroid use or a clinically palpable varicocele) that, when "corrected," help the couple achieve pregnancy naturally, reduce the intensity of intervention to a simpler strategy, or maximize the success of ICSI. The genetic basis may help determine the path of treatment for a couple and inform them of risks to their offspring that need to be understood before embarking on therapy to achieve pregnancy. In well-educated hands, microsurgical reconstruction can be quite successful and help the couple avoid the rigors and intensity of an ICSI cycle while helping them become pregnant naturally. TESE has been a remarkable advance in the male fertility specialist's armamentarium and has allowed men with NOA to experience biological paternity.

References

1. AUA Best Practice Policy: Evaluation of the azoospermic male. *Fertil Steril.* Nov 2008;90(5 Suppl):S74-77.
2. Sigman M, Lipshultz L, Howards S. Office evaluation of the subfertile male. In: Lipshultz L, Howards S, Niederberger C, editors. Infertility in the male. 4th ed. New York: Cambridge University Press; 2009. p. 153–76.
3. McLachlan RI, Krausz C. Clinical evaluation of the infertile male: new options, new challenges. Asian J Androl. 2012;14(1):3–5.

4. Mulholland J, Mallidis C, Agbaje I, McClure N. Male diabetes mellitus and assisted reproduction treatment outcome. Reprod Biomed Online. 2010;22(2):215–9.
5. Handyside AH. Preimplantation genetic diagnosis after 20 years. Reprod Biomed Online. 2010;21(3):280–2.
6. Leigh MW, Pittman JE, Carson JL, et al. Clinical and genetic aspects of primary ciliary dyskinesia/Kartagener syndrome. Genet Med. 2009;11(7):473–87.
7. Canavese F, Mussa A, Manenti M, et al. Sperm count of young men surgically treated for cryptorchidism in the first and second year of life: fertility is better in children treated at a younger age. Eur J Pediatr Surg. 2009;19(6):388–91.
8. Chung E, Brock GB. Cryptorchidism and its impact on male fertility: a state of art review of current literature. Can Urol Assoc J. 2011;5(3):210–4.
9. Kolon TF, Patel RP, Huff DS. Cryptorchidism: diagnosis, treatment, and long-term prognosis. Urol Clin North Am. 2004;31(3):469–80. viii-ix.
10. Trsinar B, Muravec UR. Fertility potential after unilateral and bilateral orchidopexy for cryptorchidism. World J Urol. 2009;27(4):513–9.
11. Hadziselimovic F, Hadziselimovic NO, Demougin P, Oakeley EJ. Testicular gene expression in cryptorchid boys at risk of azoospermia. Sex Dev. 2011;5(2):49–59.
12. Agoulnik AI, Huang Z, Ferguson L. Spermatogenesis in cryptorchidism. Methods Mol Biol. 2012;825: 127–47.
13. Wood HM, Elder JS. Cryptorchidism and testicular cancer: separating fact from fiction. J Urol. 2009;181(2):452–61.
14. Anderson MJ, Dunn JK, Lipshultz LI, Coburn M. Semen quality and endocrine parameters after acute testicular torsion. J Urol. 1992;147(6):1545–50.
15. Arap MA, Vicentini FC, Cocuzza M, et al. Late hormonal levels, semen parameters, and presence of antisperm antibodies in patients treated for testicular torsion. J Androl. 2007;28(4):528–32.
16. Williamson RC. Torsion of the testis and allied conditions. Br J Surg. 1976;63(6):465–76.
17. Domingo C, Mirapeix RM, Encabo B, Roig J, Lopez D, Ruiz J. Clinical features and ultrastructure of primary ciliary dyskinesia and Young syndrome. Rev Clin Esp. 1997;197(2):100–3.
18. Kim ED, Winkel E, Orejuela F, Lipshultz LI. Pathological epididymal obstruction unrelated to vasectomy: results with microsurgical reconstruction. J Urol. 1998;160(6 Pt 1):2078–80.
19. Sheynkin YR, Hendin BN, Schlegel PN, Goldstein M. Microsurgical repair of iatrogenic injury to the vas deferens. J Urol. 1998;159(1):139–41.
20. Kolettis PN, Thomas Jr AJ. Vasoepididymostomy for vasectomy reversal: a critical assessment in the era of intracytoplasmic sperm injection. J Urol. 1997;158(2): 467–70.
21. Tanrikut C, Goldstein M. Obstructive azoospermia: a microsurgical success story. Semin Reprod Med. 2009;27(2):159–64.
22. Grey BR, Thompson A, Jenkins BL, Payne SR. UK practice regarding reversal of vasectomy 2001–2010: relevance to best contemporary patient management. BJU Int. 2012. doi:10.1111/j.1464-410X.2011.10853.x.
23. Elzanaty S, Dohle GR. Vasovasostomy and predictors of vasal patency: a systematic review. Scand J Urol Nephrol. 2012;46:241–6.
24. Brannigan RE. Vasectomy reversal: indications and outcomes. J Urol. 2012;187(2):385–6.
25. de Souza GL, Hallak J. Anabolic steroids and male infertility: a comprehensive review. BJU Int. 2011;108: 1860–5.
26. Dohle GR, Smit M, Weber RF. Androgens and male fertility. World J Urol. 2003;21(5):341–5.
27. Lombardo F, Sgro P, Salacone P, et al. Androgens and fertility. J Endocrinol Invest. 2005;28(3 Suppl):51–5.
28. Ko EY, Siddiqi K, Brannigan RE, Sabanegh Jr ES. Empirical medical therapy for idiopathic male infertility: a survey of the American Urological Association. J Urol. 2012;187(3):973–8.
29. Damani MN, Master V, Meng MV, Burgess C, Turek P, Oates RD. Postchemotherapy ejaculatory azoospermia: fatherhood with sperm from testis tissue with intracytoplasmic sperm injection. J Clin Oncol. 2002;20(4):930–6.
30. Chohan KR, Badawy SZ. Cigarette smoking impairs sperm bioenergetics. Int Braz J Urol. 2010;36(1): 60–5.
31. Collodel G, Capitani S, Pammolli A, Giannerini V, Geminiani M, Moretti E. Semen quality of male idiopathic infertile smokers and nonsmokers: an ultrastructural study. J Androl. 2010;31(2):108–13.
32. Gaur DS, Talekar MS, Pathak VP. Alcohol intake and cigarette smoking: impact of two major lifestyle factors on male fertility. Indian J Pathol Microbiol. 2010;53(1):35–40.
33. Huncharek M, Kupelnick B, Klassen H. Paternal smoking during pregnancy and the risk of childhood brain tumors: results of a meta-analysis. In Vivo. 2001;15(6):535–41.
34. Ji BT, Shu XO, Linet MS, et al. Paternal cigarette smoking and the risk of childhood cancer among offspring of nonsmoking mothers. J Natl Cancer Inst. 1997;89(3):238–44.
35. Milne E, Greenop KR, Scott RJ, et al. Parental prenatal smoking and risk of childhood acute lymphoblastic leukemia. Am J Epidemiol. 2012;175(1):43–53.
36. Santos EP, Lopez-Costa S, Chenlo P, et al. Impact of spontaneous smoking cessation on sperm quality: case report. Andrologia. 2011;43(6):431–5.
37. Braga DP, Halpern G, Figueira Rde C, Setti AS, Iaconelli Jr A, Borges Jr E. Food intake and social habits in male patients and its relationship to intracytoplasmic sperm injection outcomes. Fertil Steril. 2012;97(1):53–9.
38. Fariello RM, Pariz JR, Spaine DM, Cedenho AP, Bertolla RP, Fraietta R. Association between obesity and alteration of sperm DNA integrity and mitochondrial activity. BJU Int. 2012. doi:10.1111/j.1464-410X.2011.10813.x.
39. Relwani R, Berger D, Santoro N, et al. Semen parameters are unrelated to BMI but vary with SSRI use and prior urological surgery. Reprod Sci. 2011;18(4):391–7.

40. Sermondade N, Massin N, Boitrelle F, et al. Sperm parameters and male fertility after bariatric surgery: three case series. Reprod Biomed Online. 2012;24(2): 206–10.
41. Chipkevitch E, Nishimura RT, Tu DG, Galea-Rojas M. Clinical measurement of testicular volume in adolescents: comparison of the reliability of 5 methods. J Urol. 1996;156(6):2050–3.
42. Peng J, Yuan Y, Zhang Z, et al. Patency rates of microsurgical vasoepididymostomy for patients with idiopathic obstructive azoospermia: a prospective analysis of factors associated with patency–single-center experience. Urology. 2012;79(1):119–22.
43. Nagler H, Grotas A. Varicocele. In: Lipshultz L, Howards S, Niederberger C, editors. Infertility in the male. 4th ed. New York: Cambridge University Press; 2009. p. 331–61.
44. WHO. WHO laboratory manual for the examination and processing of human semen. 5th ed. Cambridge, England: Cambridge University Press; 2010.
45. Oates R. Evaluation of the azoospermic male. Asian J Androl. 2012;14(1):82–7.
46. Turner T. The epididymis and accessory sex organs. In: Lipshultz L, Howards S, Niederberger C, editors. Infertility in the male. 4th ed. New York: Cambridge University Press; 2009. p. 90–103.
47. Oates RD. Clinical evaluation of the infertile male with respect to genetic etiologies. Syst Biol Reprod Med. 2011;57(1–2):72–7.
48. Smith JF, Walsh TJ, Turek PJ. Ejaculatory duct obstruction. Urol Clin North Am. 2008;35(2):221–7. viii.
49. Hero M, Tommiska J, Vaaralahti K, et al. Circulating antimullerian hormone levels in boys decline during early puberty and correlate with inhibin B. Fertil Steril. 2012;97:1242–7.
50. Bonomi M, Libri DV, Guizzardi F, et al. New understandings of the genetic basis of isolated idiopathic central hypogonadism. Asian J Androl. 2012;14(1):49–56.
51. Madani AH, Falahatkar S, Heidarzadeh A, Roshan ZA, Sazgari E, Zareian M. Sensitivity and specificity of serum FSH and testis size in predicting the existence of spermatogenesis in azoospermic infertile men. Andrologia. 2011;25:1–5.
52. Young J. Approach to the male patient with congenital hypogonadotropic hypogonadism. J Clin Endocrinol Metab. 2012;97(3):707–18.
53. Harnisch B, Oates R. Genetic disorders related to male factor infertility and their adverse consequences. Semin Reprod Med. 2012;30:105–15.
54. Yu J, Chen Z, Ni Y, Li Z. CFTR mutations in men with congenital bilateral absence of the vas deferens (CBAVD): a systemic review and meta-analysis. Hum Reprod. 2012;27(1):25–35.
55. Harton GL, Tempest HG. Chromosomal disorders and male infertility. Asian J Androl. 2012;14(1):32–9.
56. Massart A, Lissens W, Tournaye H, Stouffs K. Genetic causes of spermatogenic failure. Asian J Androl. 2012;14(1):40–8.
57. Ramasamy R, Ricci JA, Palermo GD, Gosden LV, Rosenwaks Z, Schlegel PN. Successful fertility treatment for Klinefelter's syndrome. J Urol. 2009;182(3): 1108–13.
58. Bakircioglu ME, Ulug U, Erden HF, et al. Klinefelter syndrome: does it confer a bad prognosis in treatment of nonobstructive azoospermia? Fertil Steril. 2011;95(5):1696–9.
59. Harper JC, Sengupta SB. Preimplantation genetic diagnosis: state of the art 2011. Hum Genet. 2012;131(2):175–86.
60. Kuroda-Kawaguchi T, Skaletsky H, Brown LG, et al. The AZFc region of the Y chromosome features massive palindromes and uniform recurrent deletions in infertile men. Nat Genet. 2001;29(3):279–86.
61. Navarro-Costa P, Plancha CE, Goncalves J. Genetic dissection of the AZF regions of the human Y chromosome: thriller or filler for male (in)fertility? J Biomed Biotechnol. 2010;2010:936569.
62. Skaletsky H, Kuroda-Kawaguchi T, Minx PJ, et al. The male-specific region of the human Y chromosome is a mosaic of discrete sequence classes. Nature. 2003;423(6942):825–37.
63. Repping S, Skaletsky H, Lange J, et al. Recombination between palindromes P5 and P1 on the human Y chromosome causes massive deletions and spermatogenic failure. Am J Hum Genet. 2002;71(4):906–22.
64. Costa P, Goncalves R, Ferras C, et al. Identification of new breakpoints in AZFb and AZFc. Mol Hum Reprod. 2008;14(4):251–8.
65. Hopps CV, Mielnik A, Goldstein M, Palermo GD, Rosenwaks Z, Schlegel PN. Detection of sperm in men with Y chromosome microdeletions of the AZFa, AZFb and AZFc regions. Hum Reprod. 2003;18(8): 1660–5.
66. Patrat C, Bienvenu T, Janny L, et al. Clinical data and parenthood of 63 infertile and Y-microdeleted men. Fertil Steril. 2010;93(3):822–32.
67. Simoni M, Tuttelmann F, Gromoll J, Nieschlag E. Clinical consequences of microdeletions of the Y chromosome: the extended Munster experience. Reprod Biomed Online. 2008;16(2):289–303.
68. Stahl PJ, Masson P, Mielnik A, Marean MB, Schlegel PN, Paduch DA. A decade of experience emphasizes that testing for Y microdeletions is essential in American men with azoospermia and severe oligozoospermia. Fertil Steril. 2010;94(5):1753–6.
69. Gambera L, Governini L, De Leo V, et al. Successful multiple pregnancy achieved after transfer of frozen embryos obtained via intracytoplasmic sperm injection with testicular sperm from an AZFc-deleted man. Fertil Steril. 2010;94(6):2330.e1–3.
70. Mulhall JP, Reijo R, Alagappan R, et al. Azoospermic men with deletion of the DAZ gene cluster are capable of completing spermatogenesis: fertilization, normal embryonic development and pregnancy occur when retrieved testicular spermatozoa are used for intracytoplasmic sperm injection. Hum Reprod. 1997;12(3): 503–8.

71. Oates RD, Mulhall J, Burgess C, Cunningham D, Carson R. Fertilization and pregnancy using intentionally cryopreserved testicular tissue as the sperm source for intracytoplasmic sperm injection in 10 men with non-obstructive azoospermia. Hum Reprod. 1997;12(4):734–9.
72. Oates RD, Silber S, Brown LG, Page DC. Clinical characterization of 42 oligospermic or azoospermic men with microdeletion of the AZFc region of the Y chromosome, and of 18 children conceived via ICSI. Hum Reprod. 2002;17(11):2813–24.
73. Samli H, Samli MM, Yilmaz E, Imirzalioglu N. Clinical, andrological and genetic characteristics of patients with congenital bilateral absence of vas deferens (CBAVD). Arch Androl. 2006;52(6):471–7.
74. Lee JY, Dada R, Sabanegh E, Carpi A, Agarwal A. Role of genetics in azoospermia. Urology. 2010;77(3):598–601.
75. Bareil C, Guittard C, Altieri JP, Templin C, Claustres M, des Georges M. Comprehensive and rapid genotyping of mutations and haplotypes in congenital bilateral absence of the vas deferens and other cystic fibrosis transmembrane conductance regulator-related disorders. J Mol Diagn. 2007;9(5):582–8.
76. Grzegorczyk V, Rives N, Sibert L, Dominique S, Mace B. Management of male infertility due to congenital bilateral absence of vas deferens should not ignore the diagnosis of cystic fibrosis. Andrologia. 2012. doi:10.1111/j.1439-0272.2012.01288.x.
77. McCallum T, Milunsky J, Munarriz R, Carson R, Sadeghi-Nejad H, Oates R. Unilateral renal agenesis associated with congenital bilateral absence of the vas deferens: phenotypic findings and genetic considerations. Hum Reprod. 2001;16(2):282–8.
78. Miyaoka R, Esteves SC. A critical appraisal on the role of varicocele in male infertility. Adv Urol. 2012;2012:597495.
79. Schlegel PN, Goldstein M. Alternate indications for varicocele repair: non-obstructive azoospermia, pain, androgen deficiency and progressive testicular dysfunction. Fertil Steril. 2011;96(6):1288–93.
80. Abdel-Meguid TA. Predictors of sperm recovery and azoospermia relapse in men with nonobstructive azoospermia after varicocele repair. J Urol. 2012;187(1):222–6.
81. Fenig DM, Kattan MW, Mills JN, Gisbert M, Yu C, Lipshultz LI. Nomogram to preoperatively predict the probability of requiring epididymovasostomy during vasectomy reversal. J Urol. 2012;187(1):215–8.
82. Hsiao W, Goldstein M, Rosoff JS, et al. Nomograms to predict patency after microsurgical vasectomy reversal. J Urol. 2012;187(2):607–12.
83. van Dongen J, Tekle FB, van Roijen JH. Pregnancy rate after vasectomy reversal in a contemporary series: influence of smoking, semen quality and post-surgical use of assisted reproductive techniques. BJU Int. 2012;110:562–7.
84. Esteves SC, Miyaoka R, Agarwal A. Sperm retrieval techniques for assisted reproduction. Int Braz J Urol. 2011;37(5):570–83.
85. Oates RD, Lobel SM, Harris DH, Pang S, Burgess CM, Carson RS. Efficacy of intracytoplasmic sperm injection using intentionally cryopreserved epididymal spermatozoa. Hum Reprod. 1996;11(1):133–8.
86. Schroeder-Printzen I, Zumbe J, Bispink L, et al. Microsurgical epididymal sperm aspiration: aspirate analysis and straws available after cryopreservation in patients with non-reconstructable obstructive azoospermia. MESA/TESE Group Giessen. Hum Reprod. 2000;15(12):2531–5.
87. Van Peperstraten A, Proctor ML, Johnson NP, Philipson G. Techniques for surgical retrieval of sperm prior to intra-cytoplasmic sperm injection (ICSI) for azoospermia. Cochrane Database Syst Rev. 2008;(2):CD002807
88. Schlegel PN. Nonobstructive azoospermia: a revolutionary surgical approach and results. Semin Reprod Med. 2009;27(2):165–70.
89. Yarali H, Polat M, Bozdag G, et al. TESE-ICSI in patients with non-mosaic Klinefelter syndrome: a comparative study. Reprod Biomed Online. 2009;18(6):756–60.
90. Fullerton G, Hamilton M, Maheshwari A. Should non-mosaic Klinefelter syndrome men be labelled as infertile in 2009? Hum Reprod. 2010;25(3):588–97.

Ovulation Stimulation and Cycle Management in IVF

3

Ying C. Cheong, Elizabeth S. Ginsburg, and Nick S. Macklon

Introduction

The goal of ovarian stimulation is to induce ongoing development of multiple dominant follicles and to mature many oocytes to improve chances for conception. Ovarian stimulation enables the retrieval of many cumulus–oocyte complexes, and this allows for inefficiencies in subsequent oocyte maturation, fertilization in vitro, embryo culture, embryo selection for transfer, and implantation. However, in order to prevent premature luteinization and spontaneous ovulation, co-treatment with a GnRH agonist or antagonist is normally required.

Fresh embryo(s) can be transferred in the great majority of patients, and spare embryos may be cryopreserved to allow for subsequent chances of pregnancy without the need for repeated ovarian stimulation and oocyte retrieval. This paradigm has formed the basis of clinical practice since the early days of IVF. However, increased understanding of the intricacies of the follicular development and selection processes has been critical to many of the new developments in ovarian stimulation in clinical practice.

Y.C. Cheong, M.D.
Department of Obstetrics and Gynaecology, Princess Anne Hospital (MP815), University of Southampton, Coxford Road, Southampton SO16 5YA, UK
e-mail: y.cheong@soton.ac.uk

E.S. Ginsburg, M.D.
Division of Reproductive Endocrinology and Infertility, Department of Obstetrics and Gynecology, Brigham and Women's Hospital, Boston, MA 02115, USA
e-mail: eginsburg@partners.org

N.S. Macklon, M.D. (✉)
Division of Human Development and Health, Princess Anne Hospital, University of Southampton, Coxford Road, Southampton SO16 5YA, UK
e-mail: N.S.Macklon@soton.ac.uk

Preparations Used for Ovarian Stimulation

Gonadotropins

In the 1960s, human urinary preparations of LH and FSH (Human Menopausal Gonadotrophin, hMG) were used for ovarian stimulation. The initial preparations were very impure but by the early 1980s, improved purification techniques enabled the production of purified urinary FSH (uFSH) by the use of monoclonal antibodies. With the advent of recombinant DNA technology in the 1990s, pharmaceutical companies were able to produce large commercial quantities of human recombinant FSH (rFSH) thereby bypassing dependence on the variable supply of human postmenopausal urine and also addressing concerns about batch-to-batch consistencies. Because of its purity, rFSH can now be administered by protein weight rather than bioactivity, and the so-called "filled-by-mass" preparations are now in clinical use. The use of gonadotrophins has therefore developed over a number of decades from preparations with hMG (containing both LH and FSH bioactivity), followed by purified uFSH and more recently rFSH,

E.S. Ginsburg and C. Racowsky (eds.), *In Vitro Fertilization: A Comprehensive Guide*,
DOI 10.1007/978-1-4419-9848-4_3, © Springer Science+Business Media New York 2012

rLH, and rhCG. For a complete review of the development of gonadotropins in ovarian stimulation see Macklon et al. [1] and the American Society for Reproductive Medicine (ASRM) Educational Bulletin on this topic.

GnRH Analogs

Pituitary downregulation can be induced by the continued administration of GnRH which induces an initial stimulation of gonadotrophin release (the so-called flare effect) followed by a downregulation due to the clustering and internalization of the pituitary receptors. Without downregulation, a premature LH peak occurs in 20–25% of FSH or hMG stimulated cycles due to the positive feedback activity by high serum E_2 levels during the mid-follicular phase of the stimulation cycle [1]. In the 1980s, induced pituitary downregulation resulted in a significant reduction in the cancelation rate and improved the overall IVF outcome. Furthermore, the introduction of GnRH agonist (GnRHa) co-treatment facilitated scheduling of IVF and timing for oocyte retrieval.

Although GnRH antagonists (GnRHant) were developed soon after GnRHa, the low potency of the first two generations of drugs, and associated anaphylactic responses due to histamine release, delayed their clinical introduction until a third generation was shown to be safe and efficacious in IVF. Whilst the widely employed GnRHa long protocol requires a prolonged period of downregulation (usually 2 weeks) followed by high-dose FSH stimulation to induce multiple follicular growth, the immediate action of GnRHant means that it can be administered during the mid-to-late follicular phase to prevent premature luteinization. This avoids unpleasant "menopausal" side effects associated with pituitary downregulation, and allows the endogenous inter-cycle FSH rise to be utilized for follicle stimulation. The cyclic recruitment and the initial stages of dominant follicle selection can proceed within the natural cycle and the use of exogenous FSH for inducing multiple follicle growth can be restricted to the mid-to-late follicular phase, as in certain mild stimulation protocols [2]. Hence the overall length of stimulation is shorter than with conventional IVF. Other advantages of the GnRHant over agonist include the absence of the "flare effect" which may cause ovarian cyst formation and, in turn, lower oocyte quality, fertilization rate, number of oocytes retrieved and embryo quality [3].

Current Protocols in Ovarian Stimulation

GnRH Agonist Protocols

The long ovarian stimulation protocol combines the use of GnRHa with exogenous gonadotropin administration. This treatment regimen has remained popular since its introduction some 20 years ago. In the long protocol, the GnRHa is usually administered during the luteal phase in the preceding cycle and is continued until hCG administration (Fig. 3.1). In contrast, the so-called "short GnRH agonist protocol" or "flare" protocol delays administration of GnRHa until day 1–2 of the stimulation cycle, with the aim of utilizing the "flare" effect of the GnRHa as an additional initial stimulus for follicular recruitment. However, an early meta-analysis of studies comparing the long versus the short protocol for good prognosis patients revealed that although the long protocol required more gonadotrophins, it yielded more eggs and a higher pregnancy rate, and this perceived advantage served to restrict use of the antagonist [4]. Moreover, the long protocol was considered to be advantageous in that initiation of gonadotropin stimulation can be delayed, allowing scheduling of IVF cycles with no clear adverse effect on outcomes. However, the burden of treatment duration associated with this approach has been shown to be a significant cause of dropout from IVF treatment [5].

GnRH Antagonist Protocols

GnRHant protocols entered clinical practice after many years of refining of the GnRHa long protocol, with initial comparative studies indicating that a similar refinement of this new approach

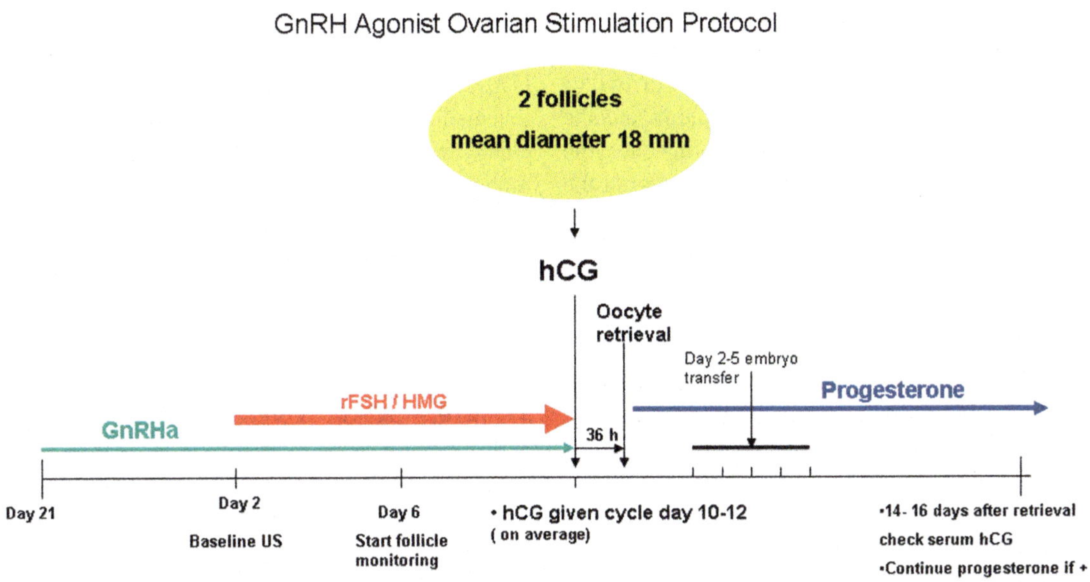

Fig. 3.1 Schematic diagram of the GnRH agonist (GnRHa), or "long" protocol

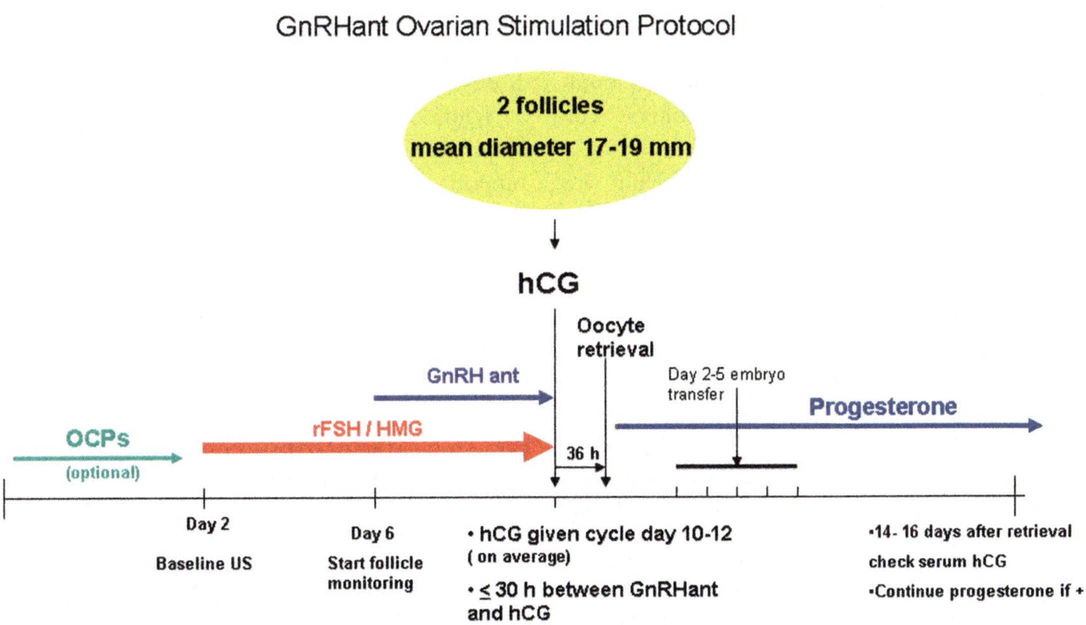

Fig. 3.2 Schematic diagram of the GnRH antagonist (GnRHant) protocol

was required. In the GnRHant protocol, ovarian stimulation with gonadotropins is begun on cycle day 2, and GnRHant administration is typically started on cycle day 6, when leading follicles are approximately 14 mm in diameter, and LH levels are increasing (Fig. 3.2). Oral contraceptive pills are often used as a lead-in prior to beginning the GnRHant cycle; indeed the early studies that lead to FDA approval of the GnRHant used OCPs. OCPs can be administered from 1 to 3 weeks, starting prior to menstrual cycle day 5 of the previous menstrual cycle, and can be helpful in "programming" the likely day of hCG triggering to assist in scheduling. It must be made clear to the patient that if she uses only a week or two of OCPs the endometrium may be quite thin and she may not have a withdrawal bleed; in this case, the baseline scan is performed the fourth day after the last OCP (as discussed later in the chapter). Other potential benefits are suppression of potential stimulation of a persistent corpus luteum cyst.

There are few well done RCTs of hormonal pre-treatment prior to GnRHant cycles. However, a meta-analysis reported that the number of oocytes and embryos, fertilization and ongoing pregnancy rates are comparable but dose of gonadotropins are higher and treatment is effectively prolonged [6]. There is therefore no apparent medical indication for pretreatment of OCPs in GnRHant cycles.

GnRHa Versus GnRHant Protocols

The first meta-analysis that was published, comparing outcomes following co-treatment with antagonist versus agonist (involving five multicenter RCTs), concluded that the GnRHant was as efficient as GnRHa for preventing a premature LH surge. However, clinical pregnancy rates were shown to be lower in the GnRHa group. Although the reported 5% lower clinical pregnancy rate was thought to be of marginal clinical significance, these studies were not powered to show superiority of one product over the other; the data generated a significant amount of concern which resulted in a lower acceptance of GnRHant in ovarian stimulation in IVF [7]. Data from the German national IVF registry suggested that in reporting programs, this regimen was only used in patients with a poorer prognosis—those who were older and who had undergone more unsuccessful IVF cycles [8].

Recent systematic reviews which have included data from studies using more refined protocols have shown no differences in the live birth rate [9, 10]. The nonsignificant difference in the live birth rate should not be unexpected, because no clear difference between the two analogs has been demonstrated in terms of quality of either embryo [11, 12] or endometrium [13]. It has been proposed that early studies also revealed the presence of a "learning curve" associated with adoption of GnRH antagonist regimens, which could account for the relatively poor performance of the antagonist protocol in the early years. More recent randomized studies comparing the agonist and antagonist protocol have shown no significant differences in pregnancy outcomes in GnRHant despite fewer oocytes being obtained at retrieval than following a GnRHa protocol.

In addition to the markedly reduced burden of treatment, GnRHant protocols result in a lower risk of developing OHSS associated with hospital admission [10]. Moreover, the use of GnRHant in a stimulation cycle offers the possibility of replacing hCG used for triggering final oocyte maturation with a single bolus of GnRHa [14]. This approach, which has been shown to effectively eliminate the risk of developing severe OHSS, is discussed later in this chapter.

While more may still be learned regarding the optimal protocol for GnRHant, current evidence supports the use of this protocol [14] particularly for patients who are expected to be normal responders: i.e., patients with 5–9 antral follicles per ovary, age <35 years, no PCOS, normal menstrual cycle, no history of poor responses and no pelvic pathology.

Which Gonadotropin Preparation: Urinary or Recombinant?

Preparations of gonadotrophins available for ovarian stimulation were initially urinary hMG (containing both LH and FSH bioactivity, with a "75 IU" vial containing 75 IU of FSH and 75 IU of LH activity), followed by highly purified hMG (HP-hMG), purified urinary FSH (FSH-P), highly purified FSH (FSH-HP) and more recently, rFSH and rLH. Several randomized controlled trials (RCTs) comparing IVF outcomes in patients treated with hMG versus rFSH during the long GnRHa protocol have been summarized in the most recent Cochrane systematic review and meta-analyses [15]. Of the 28 trials with live birth data, 11 trials compared rFSH versus hMG/HP-hMG, 5 trials compared rFSH with FSH-P and 13 trials compared rFSH with FSH-HP. There were significantly fewer live births after rFSH as compared to HMG (OR 0.84, 95% CI 0.72–0.99; 11 trials, $N=3197$), implying that for a live birth rate of 25%, use of rFSH instead would be expected to result in a live birth rate between 19 and 25%. There was no evidence of a statistically significant difference in live birth between rFSH and FSH-P (5 trials, $N=1430$; OR 1.26, 95% CI 0.96–1.64; I2 of 0%;) and between rFSH and FSH-HP (13 trials, $N=2712$; OR 1.03, 95% CI 0.86–1.22; I2 of 0%). The pooled data comparing rFSH versus all urinary products (HMG/HP-HMP/FSH-P/FSH-HP) showed no evidence of a statistically significant difference in the likelihood of live births or pregnancies ongoing beyond 20 weeks (28 trials, $N=7339$; OR 0.97, 95% CI 0.87–1.08). This latest review also showed no evidence of a difference in the OHSS rate (32 trials, 7740 couples, OR 1.18, 95% CI 0.86–1.61).

Only two RCTs have thus far evaluated IVF outcome stimulated with hMG versus rFSH in GnRHant cycles [16, 17]. In one study ($n=280$ women), the number of oocytes retrieved was significantly reduced in patients treated with hMG compared with those treated with rFSH (11.3 ± 6.0 versus 14.4 ± 8.1 oocytes; mean ± SD). However, live birth rates were not significantly different between patients randomized to receive hMG versus those randomized to receive rFSH (34.3% versus 31.4%, respectively, 95% CI: −8.1 to +13.7). In the more recent MEGASET (Menopur in GnRH antagonist cycle with single embryo transfer) study, again there was no difference in the ongoing pregnancy rate shown by intention to treat analysis (OR 2.2; 95% CI: −4.2 to 8.6).

Of continuing concern is the further consideration that urinary derived gonadotropins may pose the theoretical risk of transmission of prion proteins. Although the risk is now considered very low, and transmission has never been documented, it has influenced policy regarding the use of urinary versus recombinant gonadotropins in certain countries.

Exogenous LH During Ovarian Stimulation?

Studies treating women with hypogonadotropic hypogonadism with recombinant gonadotropins lacking LH activity demonstrated that LH is not required for follicular development to the pre-ovulatory stage [18]. However, the debate continues regarding the benefits of LH for oocyte maturation and quality. LH activity can be provided in the form of: (i) hMG (as urinary-derived LH activity), (ii) rLH, (iii) hCG, and (iv) rhCG. A recent meta-analysis assessed the benefits of the addition of rLH to rFSH during ovarian stimulation in IVF cycles [19]. No statistically significant differences in live birth rates were observed between patients who received rLH and those who did not. Based on these data, the addition of rLH during the follicular phase does not seem to increase the probability of pregnancy in patients treated with rFSH and GnRH analogs for the general population undergoing IVF. However, a Cochrane systematic review suggested that certain subgroups of patients with very low endogenous LH activity may benefit from the addition of LH [20].

It has been suggested that LH-induced androgen production prior to ovarian stimulation might lead to an increased follicular recruitment as intra-ovarian follicular androgens can promote the aromatase activity of antral follicles [21]. The potential role of LH activity in this context during early folliculogenesis was investigated in a recently published RCT [22]. In this randomized study, 146 women were treated in a long course high-dose GnRHa triptorelin acetate (Decapeptyl, Ferring Inc, Lausanne Switzerland, 4.2 mg s.c.) protocol and were randomized to receive rLH (Luveris, Serono Inc, Rockland MA; 300 IU/day) for a fixed 7 days, or no rLH treatment. This was followed by a standard rFSH stimulation regime (Gonal-F, 150 IU/day). The LH treatment was associated with increased number of small antral follicles prior to FSH stimulation ($P=0.007$), and an increased yield of normally fertilized (2 PN) embryos ($P=0.03$) but no difference in the ongoing pregnancy rate. Although more studies are required, at present rLH pretreatment of patients undergoing ovarian stimulation with the use of GnRH agonists and rFSH does not seem to increase the probability of ongoing pregnancy.

Endogenous LH During Ovarian Stimulation

In recent years, several groups have focused on the potential significance of late follicular phase LH levels for clinical IVF outcome. Based on classical principles, both LH and FSH are required for adequate ovarian estrogen biosynthesis and follicle development. Theca-cell derived androgen production (under LH control) is mandatory as a substrate for the conversion to estrogens by FSH-induced aromatase activity in the granulosa cells. It has been shown that during the mid-to-late follicular phase, FSH induces LH/hCG receptor expression in granulosa cells of large follicles [23]. A number of studies have indicated that excessively suppressed late follicular phase LH may be detrimental to IVF outcome. In a meta-analysis of six studies which evaluated the association between endogenous LH levels during ovarian stimulation and the likelihood of ongoing pregnancy in normo-ovulatory patients treated for IVF with GnRH analogs, there was no evidence that low LH levels on day 8 of stimulation reduced ongoing pregnancy rates [24].

hCG Supplementation During Ovarian Stimulation

The demonstration of expression of LH receptors by follicles in the late follicular phase has led to a number of investigators advocating the substitution of FSH with the administration of hCG during the mid-to-late follicular phase of ovarian stimulation for IVF [25–28]. In one study, hCG (200–300 IU) was administered concurrently with a discontinued or reduced dosage of FSH (75 IU) when the leading follicle reached approximately 12–14 mm in diameter. Final oocyte maturation was then triggered when the follicles reached 18 mm. Although these studies did not show any differences in clinical pregnancy rate with and without hCG supplementation, the total dose of rFSH required for ovarian stimulation was significantly decreased in the low-dose hCG group. Evidence thus far suggests that hCG could partially or completely substitute the role of FSH during mid-to-late stages of the follicular phase in an ovarian stimulation cycle, without compromising pregnancy rates and leading to a significant reduction in the cost of IVF cycles.

Follicular Monitoring During Ovarian Stimulation

The Baseline Ultrasound

A baseline transvaginal ultrasound is typically performed in all ovarian stimulation cycles to ensure not only that there are no large cysts on baseline that could potentially undergo significant enlargement in response to gonadotropin stimulation, but also that small baseline simple cysts are not counted as developing follicles during stimulation. At Brigham and Women's Hospital (BWH) ovarian stimulation is not started if there is a simple cyst >5 cm or a complex cyst >3 cm, unless the patient has a known history of endometriosis. If a simple cyst >5 cm is present, it is aspirated and the fluid sent for cytologic evaluation prior to stimulation starting. Complex cysts ≥3 cm in maximal diameter, which are persistent, undergo cystectomy prior to start of ovarian stimulation, to ensure that there is no chance of ovarian malignancy. At the Complete Fertility Centre (CFC) evidence of a functional ovarian cyst such as thickened endometrium or a high estradiol level is a further indication to delay ovarian stimulation until the cyst has resolved.

Baseline Blood Testing

In GnRHa cycles, baseline estradiol and progesterone are often evaluated to ensure pituitary downregulation. The desired results depend on the assays used; at BWH the estradiol must be <50 pg/mL and the progesterone <1.0 ng/mL for downregulation to be confirmed. Alternatively, at the CFC, a thin endometrium evident at baseline scan at least 2 weeks after commencing GnRHa treatment and following menstrual bleeding is taken to confirm pituitary downregulation.

Follicle Monitoring

In most ART programs, unless a patient has a history of rapid or exuberant response, ovarian stimulation is begun the day of the baseline ultrasound with blood testing, and continued for 4 days prior to the patient returning for testing. From that point on, at the BWH, estradiol measurements and ultrasound monitoring are performed, expecting follicular growth at 1–2 mm in mean diameter per day. Follicles are measured by placing calipers at right angles to each other in the longest follicular diameter first, and then at right angles to that. A mean of the two measurements is then taken. Generally testing to monitor the response is performed every 2 days, although less frequently in women with slow responses and daily in patients with high responses who require decreases in gonadotropin dosing. In cycles using only FSH as the follicle stimulation agent, particularly when GnRHa is used, estradiol levels will typically be lower than 100 pg/mature follicle. When LH is supplemented, the estradiol:follicle ratio is typically higher due to LH stimulation of ovarian theca cell androgen production. The added of value of routine estradiol monitoring in addition to ultrasound has been questioned in recent literature, and is not employed at the CFC unless the trajectory of follicle development is abnormal, or there is concern of developing hyperstimulation.

Adjusting Ovarian Stimulation Dosing Medications

There are no data to support increasing gonadotropin dosing during follicle monitoring, or after day 6 testing begins. It is tempting to increase dosing when faced with a few follicles, or a stimulation that appears to be moving excessively slowly. However, as oocyte recruitment is complete by cycle day 5; there is no evidence to support an improvement in outcomes [29]. In contrast, withholding or lowering gonadotropins during stimulation withdraws support to developing follicles and appears to reduce continued follicular recruitment and, in high responders, OHSS risk (see avoiding OHSS section)

Decision Making Regarding the Ovulatory Trigger

There is a great deal of inter-program variation, and even variation within programs, as to which ovulatory trigger to use, and at what point during ovarian stimulation to trigger. At the Complete Fertility Centre, hCG or GnRHa triggering is used when at least two follicles have a mean diameter of at least 17 mm. At BWH, two follicles with a mean diameter of 18 mm and an estradiol of >500 pg/mL are typically the goal (except when letrozole is used during stimulation as it maintains a low estradiol—see Chap. 13.) In a randomized trial, no difference in pregnancy rates were observed when hCG was administered a day later than the standard when at least three follicles with >16 mm mean diameter were present [30]. In a recent study, it was demonstrated that either delaying hCG or bringing it forward by 1 day had no impact on outcomes [31]. The flexibility this implies means that scheduling to avoid weekend retrievals is possible when co-treating with GnRH antagonist.

However, if a patient has a greater than expected response, hCG or GnRHa triggering may be done at smaller follicle diameters, in the hopes of reducing OHSS risk by triggering prior to recruitment of more follicles, albeit with an anticipated reduction in the average percentage of mature oocytes retrieved.

Contemporary Concepts in Ovarian Stimulation

The objectives of ovarian stimulation in ART are evolving, with more focus being placed on quality of the patient's experience. Whilst the end point of traditional IVF was previously "pregnancy at any cost," there is a shift in modern ART towards achieving the optimal balance between treatment burden and effectiveness. The following section will highlight some of the new emerging approaches to ART, particularly regarding the trend towards milder stimulations used in Europe versus the more aggressive stimulations performed in the United States.

A European Approach: Milder Treatment Regimens

Increasing recognition of the detrimental effects of conventional profound stimulation regimens has led to a trend in Europe toward changes in the paradigm for ovarian stimulation in IVF. Milder regimens are being adopted as they reduce patient burden, risk of hyperstimulation and costs, and as the need for fewer embryos as single embryo transfer becomes more accepted in clinical practice. Moreover, possible additional benefits on embryo and endometrial quality are cited [32].

Key to the development of milder stimulation protocols has been the introduction of GnRHant, which allows for the initiation of the IVF treatment cycle in a normal menstrual cycle with an undisturbed recruitment of a cohort of follicles during the early follicular phase. This approach enables the endogenous inter-cycle FSH rise to be utilized rather than suppressed, resulting in a reduction of gonadotropins required. The treatment cycles are thus shorter and not associated with hypoestrogenic side effects related to GnRHa downregulation and reduced cancelation rates [33]. Cost analysis studies have also suggested these cycles to be overall cheaper and more cost effective [34].

Traditional IVF stimulation regimes are associated with aggressive use of gonadotrophins to stimulate the development of a large number of follicles. These regimens are often complex, expensive, extend over a prolonged period of time and require intensive monitoring. In recent years, it has become apparent that milder approaches aimed at generating the "optimum" rather than "maximum" number of oocytes are of benefit.

A retrospective analysis of 7,422 women who underwent oocyte retrieval after long protocol IVF (GnRHa) showed that overall the highest pregnancy rates per embryo transfer and per started cycle were observed when 13 oocytes were obtained (31 and 28% respectively) [35]. In a larger study of 400,135 IVF cycles performed in the United Kingdom from 1991 to 2008, the median number of oocytes obtained was 9, the overall live birth rate per cycle was 21.8%, and there was a strong association between the number of oocytes obtained and live birth rate. Live birth rate increased with oocyte yield up to 15, plateaued between 15 and 20, and declined after 40. Hence, using large doses of gonadotrophins to stimulate the development of more than 15 oocytes does not increase the pregnancy rate and may, in fact, increase patient discomfort, side effects and serious complications such as OHSS. Moreover, several randomized controlled trials have failed to demonstrate improvements in outcome when higher doses of FSH are used, even in poor response patients [36–39]. In a recent meta-analysis of studies comparing starting doses between 100 and 225 IU, 150 IU was found to provide the best balance of oocyte numbers versus risk of OHSS [40]. There is also evidence that ovarian stimulation and excessive response may be detrimental to oocyte and embryo quality. Furthermore, profound stimulation also has a detrimental effect on luteal phase endocrinology and in turn potentially impacts endometrial receptivity [41, 42].

Despite the increasingly recognized benefits of mild stimulation for some patients, one of the concerns for some IVF practitioners is that such a regimen has a lower oocyte yield and thus poorer pregnancy rates. A recent meta-analysis combining three studies with a total of 592 first treatment cycles, showed that the mild stimulation protocol resulted in a significant reduction of retrieved oocytes compared with conventional ovarian stimulation (median 6 versus 9, respectively; $P<0.001$) [43]. Optimal embryo implantation rates were observed with five oocytes retrieved following mild stimulation (31%) versus ten oocytes following conventional stimulation (29%) ($P=0.045$). It would appear that in this study the modest number of oocytes obtained after mild ovarian stimulation was not a reflection of poor ovarian response and the authors claimed that "the fear of reducing the number of oocytes retrieved following mild ovarian stimulation appears to be unjustified." Milder stimulation regimens have been shown to produce proportionally more chromosomally normal embryos. The increased chromosomal abnormalities observed after conventional IVF are mainly due to an increased incidence of mitotic segregation errors resulting in chromosomal mosaicism [44].

It can be argued that the older patient with reduced ovarian reserve should be stimulated harder in order to achieve a higher egg yield to enable enhanced embryo selection which may potentially translate into a higher live birth rate. Several observational studies have suggested that "minimal stimulation of the older patient" has a high cancelation rate and a low pregnancy rate [45, 46]; one study including 250 cycles of "minimal stimulation" IVF found that 39.6% of cycles never underwent embryo transfer, compared to a cancelation rate of 13.7% for standard IVF. If embryo transfer was performed, ongoing pregnancy rates were 27.2% and 34.3%, respectively [45] and a further study of a series of 7,244 infertile women undergoing 20,244 cycles had a 22% rate of no retrieval, although the authors showed that if oocytes were obtained and fertilized, and transfers were performed, pregnancy rates were consistent with patient age [46]. However, it is crucial to note that these studies are observational and none are randomized or controlled. Decreased ovarian reserve, whether in the younger or older patient, despite the stimulation regimen, is associated with a lower delivery rate per initiated cycle.

"Minimal Stimulation" and Natural Cycle IVF

Key to an understanding of what constitutes "minimal stimulation" and "natural cycle," are clarifications of what constitutes a modified natural cycle versus "minimal" or "mild"stimulation. The recent definitions proposed by the International Society for Mild Approaches in Assisted Reproduction (ISMAAR) [47] are helpful in this regard: Natural and modified natural cycles aim to achieve monofollicular development, whereas the "minimal" stimulation protocols, exemplified by clomiphene citrate or letrozole use, target 2–3 follicles. The "mild" protocols involving either low-dose or late-start gonadotropin regimes are focused on producing 6–8 oocytes.

The use of natural cycle and "minimal" stimulation protocols has been re-gaining some support in recent US clinical practice. However, it is important to acknowledge that true natural cycle IVF does not employ any ovulation induction medications, is associated with a high spontaneous ovulation rate, a high rate of obtaining no oocytes, and low pregnancy and delivery rates [48]. Given the time and cost involved with monitoring a natural cycle, and the expected low delivery rate per cycle, it is not currently considered to be a cost effective therapy for the patient in most settings.

A US Approach to Ovarian Stimulation: BWH Experience

A concern related to universal adoption of mild stimulation stems from studies suggesting that, particularly in older patients, it is beneficial to have a larger number of embryos as this affords the opportunity for improved embryo selection. It can be argued that the older patient with reduced ovarian reserve should be stimulated with higher doses of gonadotropins in order to attempt to achieve a higher egg yield, better embryo selection which potentially translates into a higher live birth rate. Low dose stimulation in women with decreased ovarian reserve is unlikely to result in production of more than a few eggs and/ or embryos [45]. Thus, using a regimen with a high cancelation rate, and low pregnancy rate in older women who have a closing reproductive window would seem to be questionable.

For the young patient, transfer of one or two embryos can still result in reasonable pregnancy rates, though it is clear that decreased ovarian reserve is associated with lower delivery rates per initiated cycle even in young patients [49]. In women of advanced maternal age, i.e. 40 or older, the increase in the proportion of oocytes with age-related chromosomal abnormality results in embryos with lower implantation, pregnancy and delivery rates. Experience at BWH has shown that patients in this age group who had five or more embryos transferred had significantly increased pregnancy and live birth rates, and significantly decreased miscarriage rates with no difference in the multiple birth rate compared with those patients with less than five embryos transferred [50]. Additionally, a SART data study showed that pregnancy, delivery, and multiple birth rates increased when up to three embryos were transferred in 38-year-olds and four in 39-year-olds but over this number only multiple birth rates increased. In women ≥40, both delivery rates and multiple rates increased with increasing numbers of transferred. Multivariate analysis confirmed the statistically significant effect of age, number of oocytes retrieved, and embryo cryopreservation on delivery and multiple rates [51].

Practice in Europe differs markedly; the number of embryos transferred is dictated by legislation in some European countries; for example, in the UK, transfer of three embryos is only permitted in women over 40 (see Chap. 15 for a more extensive discussion). The trend from the three to two embryo transfer practice was influenced by a study showing that transferring more than two embryos increased the multiple pregnancy rate without significantly impacting the pregnancy rate [52]. However, pregnancy rates were higher when 5–6 as compared to 3–4 eggs fertilized. This indicates the importance of using an ovarian stimulation protocol that will result in retrieval of enough eggs to allow for embryo selection.

Reducing the Burden of IVF Treatment

As covered in Chap. 16, the stress associated with IVF can be severe, and is often cited as the reason for couples electing not to proceed with treatment after initial failure [5]. The introduction of a long-acting FSH preparation that reduces the number of injections required during an IVF treatment cycle reduces the burden of ovarian stimulation. Corifollitropin α is a recombinant fusion protein composed of FSH and the carboxy terminal peptide (CTP) of the hCG β-subunit which has a two-fold longer elimination half-life and an almost fourfold extended time interval to peak serum concentration than rFSH preparations. This allows a single injection of corifollitropin α to initiate and sustain multiple follicular growth for up to 7 days. Furthermore, after its injection, peak FSH activity is reached in 2 days compared to that of rFSH in 4–5 days. A recent multicentre "double-blind double dummy" randomized controlled study comparing corifollitropin α and rFSHin a GnRH antagonist protocol reported no difference in the pregnancy rate of the corifollitropin α treatment group compared to the rFSH treatment group [53]. This preparation will become available for the treatment of women with an antral follicle count (AFC) of less than 20, who are co-treated with GnRHant, as data from GnRHa co-treatment studies remains sparse. A recent uncontrolled phase III study found that the cumulative ongoing pregnancy rate after three cycles of corifollitropin α, including frozen-thawed embryo transfer cycles and spontaneous pregnancies, was 61% (95% CI: 56–65%)[54], consistent with expected outcomes in the literature using other preparations (see Chap. 1, Fig. 9).

Clomiphene citrate starting day 2–3 of the menstrual cycle for 5 days and followed by gonadotropins, or concurrently with low-dose gonadotropins has also been shown to reduce the cost of ovarian stimulation in IVF in good prognosis patients, albeit with pregnancy rates that appear somewhat lower than with standard regimens [55, 56].

Luteal Phase Support

For many years progesterone has been administered for luteal phase support during IVF cycles. The mechanisms underlying the abnormal luteal phase after ovarian stimulation have long been debated. It has been proposed that luteal support is necessary in GnRHa cycles because endogenous progesterone is decreased due to GnRH downregulation and to disruption of mural granulosa cells at oocyte retrieval [1–4]. However, recent studies have demonstrated that the key mechanism causing suppression of gonadotropin and thus progesterone in the luteal phase is the high level of negative feedback to the pituitary caused by supraphysiological sex steroid levels at the end of the follicular phase [1]. Concerns remain however that the oocyte retrieval itself, which results in removal of mural granulosa cells as well as the oocyte and coronal complex, could theoretically result in suboptimal ovarian progesterone secretion, and thereby cause a detrimental effect on development of a secretory endometrium that is in phase with the developing embryo.

A Cochrane review restricted to randomized trials concluded that pregnancy rates in IVF are indeed higher after progesterone supplementation compared to no supplementation or placebo. HCG administered for luteal support also led to a higher pregnancy rate than no treatment or placebo, but also, and not surprisingly, it resulted in a high rate of OHSS due to the long half-life of hCG and its stimulatory effect on follicular VEG-F production.

There is no consensus about whether intramuscular progesterone results in higher pregnancy rates than does intravaginal progesterone. However, there is good evidence that oral progesterone undergoes extensive hepatic metabolism and therefore has poor bioavailability [57].

Randomized trials required by the FDA to bring new products to market are powered to show equivalence, and not superiority between a new product and an established one. Older data support vaginal progesterone suppositories 200 mg pv tid being comparable to intramuscular progesterone 50 mg IM qd for luteal support [58]. A retrospective, multivariate analysis compared IM progesterone 50 mg per day starting the day after oocyte retrieval to crinone gel 8% (Serono Inc, Rockland MA) and found a lower live birth rate after crinone: 24.5% versus 39.4%, OR 2.00, 95% CI 1.10–3.70 [59]. The authors theorized that as the nonpregnant patients using crinone bled several days earlier than the patients on IM progesterone, this might be due to high drug delivery between the vaginal mucosa and the endometrium, advancing the endometruim too rapidly. To test this possibility, a prospective randomized trial was then performed using crinone 8% starting 2 days (rather than 1 day) following the oocyte retrieval and compared this to IM progesterone (50 mg) starting the day following oocyte retrieval. This study found equivalent pregnancy rates between patients randomized to crinone and those randomized to IMP: 45.2% for Crinone versus 42.2% for IMP, OR 1.1, 95% CI 0.8–1.7 [59]. *Indeed* early evidence suggests that the timing of progesterone administration may be of importance; a prospective randomized trial assigned 282 IVF patients to 12.5 mg IM progesterone starting the day prior to oocyte retrieval, or 25 mg starting the day of oocyte retrieval. The clinical pregnancy rate was 12.9% in the first group and 24.6% in the second [60]. Administration of progesterone before oocyte retrieval negatively impacts the implantation rate. No formulation was clearly better than any other [61]. Patients prefer vaginal progesterone formulations for ease of use, and reduction of systemic absorption [62].

In summary, there is considerable heterogeneity concerning progesterone utilization between IVF programs, with no clear benefit from any specific regimen. At Brigham & Women's Hospital, patients start Crinone 8% once per day starting 2 days after oocyte retrieval, or IM progesterone 50 mg starting the day after oocyte retrieval. Both are continued until the tenth week of gestation when the luteal placental shift should be complete. Many centers continue luteal support for a similar period. However, two randomized controlled trials comparing treatment for 2 weeks with prolonged treatment have shown no significant impact on pregnancy rates [30, 63]. It is important to counsel patients using vaginal progesterone that it is messy and that vaginal discharge will persist until after the progesterone is discontinued. Patients using IM progesterone must be carefully taught IM injection technique to ensure that they do not hit a major nerve, such as the sciatic, and to watch for signs of allergy or infection at the injection sites.

Ovarian Hyperstimulation Syndrome

The most important and sometimes life-threatening complication of IVF treatment remains the risk of developing severe ovarian hyperstimulation syndrome (OHSS). Mild hyperstimulation may be difficult to differentiate from ovaries still enlarged status post oocyte retrieval, but in the literature has been defined as ovarian enlargement up to 5 cm without ascites. Moderate ovarian hyperstimulation has been defined as ovarian enlargement with ovaries >5 to <10 cm in diameter, and severe hyperstimulation defined as ovarian enlargement (ovaries >10 cm) with ascites or pleural effusions, significant hemoconcentration (hematocrit >50), and/ or elevated liver transaminases [64, 65].

OHSS is moderated by vascular endothelial growth factor secreted from the ovaries in response to hCG. The syndrome typically appears 7–10 days following oocyte retrieval, but can occur earlier. Patients with severe OHSS typically present with abdominal distension, weight gain due to intraperitoneal fluid accumulation, and if ascites is tense, shortness of breath and pain when walking.

Treatment of Ovarian Hyperstimulation Syndrome

Patients with mild and moderate OHSS should be monitored, and remain in contact with the clinic to ensure that their condition is not worsening. Pelvic rest is sometimes recommended to avoid potential trauma to enlarged ovaries with distended capsules during intercourse. Treatment of severe OHSS is largely supportive but should be prompt for patients with weight gain of >2 lbs in a day or decreased urine output or shortness of breath; hemoconcentration can lead to intravascular coagulation and pulmonary embolism in rare cases. Care must be taken to avoid intravascular fluid depletion, so patients must be encouraged to drink solute-rich fluids such as Gatorade; if hemoconcentration becomes severe, hospitalization for intravenous fluids and thromboprophylaxis is prudent, and plasma expansion with albumin may be helpful. Though not commonly employed, diuretics may be used after intravenous fluids are replaced, but serum chemistries must be followed to avoid hyponatremia and hyperkalemia, and worsening intravascular depletion avoided. If patients are uncomfortable, but hemodynamically stable, outpatient paracentesis is easy to perform with ultrasound guidance in the outpatient setting, either transvaginally or transabdominally [66]. Transvaginally, an oocyte retrieval needle may be used; abdominally, at BWH we generally use a thoracentesis kit; a large bore angiocatheter may also be used. It is safe to remove as much fluid as will drain; using intravenous line tubing connecting the paracentesis needle to negative pressure bottles facilitates removal of fluid. Ascites is exudative, so it is common to see a low serum albumin in patients with significant ascites. In the absence of pregnancy, symptoms generally abate within a week. In pregnant patients, however, the production of hCG 7–10 days post oocyte retrieval often increases symptoms and in severe cases ascites may persist for several weeks before spontaneously resolving.

Avoiding OHSS; GnRHa Trigger in GnRHant Cycles

It is clearly best to avoid OHSS risk altogether. Less aggressive stimulation protocols provide the opportunity to reduce the rate of this complication [67]. However, occasionally it can arise even when milder regimens are used. The introduction of GnRHant has enabled the use of GnRHa for triggering oocyte maturation by inducing an endogenous LH surge. This more physiological approach promises to reduce the risk of OHSS known to be associated with the administration of hCG to trigger final oocyte maturation. The GnRH agonist displaces the GnRH antagonist from the receptor and initiates a "flare up effect" seen typically in the use of GnRH long protocol. Moreover, the luteal phase steroid concentrations may approximate more closely to the physiological range with possible benefits for improving endometrial receptivity [68]. Initial studies showed the resultant LH peak to be short lived [69] raising concerns that the early luteal phase may be inadequately supported by this regimen. A recent systematic review compared the effectiveness of a GnRHa with HCG for triggering final oocyte maturation in IVF and ICSI patients undergoing controlled ovarian hyperstimulation in a GnRHant protocol followed by embryo transfer; 11 RCTs ($n=1055$) were identified. Eight studies assessed fresh IVF cycles and three studies assessed donor-recipient cycles. In the fresh cycles, GnRHa was less effective than hCG in terms of the live birth rate per randomized woman (OR 0.44, 95% CI 0.29–0.68; 4 RCTs). Moderate to severe OHSS incidence per randomized woman was significantly lower in the GnRH agonist group compared to the hCG group (OR 0.10, 95% CI 0.01–0.82; 5 RCTs). In donor recipient cycles, there was no evidence of a statistical difference in the live birth rate per randomized woman (OR 0.92, 95% CI 0.53–1.61; 1 RCT) [70]. The decreased clinical pregnancy rate observed was likely due to a luteal phase defect and poorer endometrial function despite luteal phase support with progesterone and estradiol due to the shorter half-life (24–36 h) and lower amplitude of the GnRH a induced endogenous LH surge compared to that of a natural cycle (48 h) [71]. This was supported by good birth rates in the frozen–thawed embryo replacement cycles in the cycles where GnRHa has been used as a trigger for oocyte maturation [72]. More recent studies have addressed how best to support the luteal phase when GnRHa is used as a trigger. Several studies have examined the role of using hCG concurrently with GnRHa as the ovulation trigger compared to hCG (10,000 IU) alone. A small dose of hCG (1,500 IU) has been used as a supplementary dose after GnRHa administration as a trigger for final oocyte maturation [73]. Whilst both groups showed similar miscarriage, ongoing pregnancy and delivery rates when compared to 10,000 hCG in ovulation induction cycles, no OHSS cases were seen in the GnRHa group. Several dosing schedules may be used for GnRHa triggering of final oocyte maturation. Using a single dose of 20–40 units of leuprolide acetate (1–2 mg) 36 h prior to oocyte retrieval appears reliable.

Luteal Phase Support with Use of the GnRHa Trigger

Current evidence seems to support the fact that the luteal phase in IVF cycles, with final oocyte maturation triggered by GnRHa, can be rescued by the use of LH activity, resulting in reproductive outcome comparable to that of hCG triggered final oocyte maturation. Given the risks of exacerbating the effects of ovarian hyperstimulation in the event of a successful implantation, the alternative strategy will be to "freeze all" the embryos and perform a frozen embryo transfer in the subsequent cycle, although this may have cost implications for the patients, depending on local health care context.

Other Approaches to Avoiding OHSS

Other approaches, which may help reduce the risk of developing severe OHSS, include the use of adjuvant therapies such as the dopamine agonist cabergoline. This treatment (0.5 mg daily) normally given daily for 8 days from the day of hCG administration is thought to act by reducing VEGF production [74]. Initial clinical studies indicated that cabergoline can reduce the rate of OHSS compared with placebo [75]. In a meta-analysis of four studies, the incidence but not the severity of OHSS was found to be reduced by the drug, without reducing pregnancy rates [76].

Towards Individualized Protocols

In assisted conception, unsuccessful treatment cycles are often due to a suboptimal individual response to treatment. Hence there has been great interest in identifying factors which enable the optimal individual dose to be determined for each patient.

Fine-tuning of the FSH dosage can be achieved by adding specific patient markers such as smoking status, ovarian ultrasound features, and age into a scoring system. This system was shown to improve pregnancy outcome compared with fixed dosing [77]. With regard to whether and how the dose should be increased for poor responders and decreased with overresponders is still unclear.

Managing the High Responder

Although PCOS is considered to be a major risk for OHSS, a meta-analysis of women with PCOS undergoing IVF suggested only a trend towards higher OHSS rate [78]. This is likely due to the fact that young women with excellent ovarian reserve may also be at high risk of exuberant responses to stimulation accompanied by OHSS. Similarly, increasing the dosages for women who are deemed poor responders (obese, older women and previous failed response) is not well supported by research evidence. In a randomized, placebo-controlled trial of 120 PCO patients at high risk of OHSS, the use of 500 mg metformin three times a day during ovarian stimulation resulted in a reduced number of small <10 mm follicles and OHSS risk (0.28 CI: 0.11–0.67) [79].

The CONSORT study utilizes a dosing algorithm that individualizes rFSH doses (starting from 37.5 IU rFSH) according to patient characteristics (basal FSH, body mass index, age and antral follicle count) [80]. Overall, a median of 9.0 oocytes were retrieved (8.5, 8.0, 10.0, 12.0, and 8.0 in the 75, 112.5, 150, 187.5, and 225 IU groups, respectively). Clinical pregnancy rates/cycle started were 31.3, 31.1, 35.3, 50.0 and 20.0%, respectively (overall, 34.2%). Two patients had severe OHSS. The authors concluded that individualized dosing in increments of 37.5 IU of rFSH to achieve a good rate of oocyte retrieval and pregnancy is possible through the use of the CONSORT dosing algorithm.

Ovarian Reserve Testing and Gonadotropin Dosing

Recently, there has been increased interest in the use of anti-Mullerian hormone (AMH) to help predict dosing regimens. Seifer et al. [81] first reported that a higher AMH level on day 3 was associated with a greater number of oocytes retrieved. Since then, a number of retrospective and prospective studies have demonstrated similar findings [82–84]. A recent meta-analysis [85] of 13 studies reporting on AMH and 17 on antral follicle counts (AFC) showed that in terms of predicting poor response and nonpregnancy, there was no significant difference in terms of the predictive value of AMH over ACF. The advantage of AMH over any menstrual cycle dependent predictor marker is its low inter- and intra-cycle variability. La Marca et al. [86] first demonstrated that AMH measured during any time of the menstrual cycle predicted a reasonable response for ovarian stimulation cycles. More recent work by the same author showed that in a cohort of 389 women, AMH and age permitted the identification of live birth with a sensitivity of 79% and specificity of 44% [87]. Hence, whilst serum AMH measurements may be effective in predicting response, they have not been shown to effectively predict the likelihood of achieving pregnancy after ART. Moreover, it is important to note that with extremely low-serum AMH levels, moderate, but reasonable pregnancy and live birth rates are still possible. A recent study examined 128 women with mean (±SD) age of 40.8±4.1 years who underwent a total of 254 IVF cycles where the mean (±SD) AMH of 0.2±0.1 ng/ml. Twenty clinical pregnancies were recorded (7.9% per cycle start [95% confidence interval (CI): 4.9–11.9%]; 15.6% cumulative [CI: 9.8–23.1%]) [88]. Hence, extremely low levels of AMH should not be used as a sole deciding factor to withhold treatment.

Given that the use of AMH can predict response, albeit not outcome, one line of treatment strategy has emerged whereby AMH alone (excluding age or BMI of patient) is utilized to provide individualized treatment. Nelson et al. [84] demonstrated that aggressive dosing of patients who have AMH <5pmol/l (i.e., <0.7 pg/mL) is safe whilst that of the normally suggested 150 IU FSH dosage for women with an AMH >15 pmol/l (2.1 pg/mL) led to a high incidence of OHSS. This dosing regimen was associated with reduced treatment burden, cycle cancelation and a trend towards more cycle efficacy. However, these data derive from a nonrandomized study, and future well-designed studies will be required to confirm the cost/benefit and clinical efficacy of such a regimen. There may also be substantial benefit combining AMH testing with protocols in mild stimulation treatment strategies as described by Popovic-Todorovic et al. [77], so that ovarian stimulation regimes can be tailor made for patients according to their needs.

A US Approach to the "Poor Responder"

The approach to treating women who are expected to produce only a few follicles during IVF stimulation depends, to a certain extent, on physician preferences and on how many embryos are felt to be ideal to optimize pregnancy rates. As previously mentioned, most US practitioners prefer to produce supernumerary embryos, in the hope that during the culture process "survival of the fittest" will be demonstrated, with a cohort of the embryos growing optimally and allowing for embryo selection and cryopreservation.

There is no clear consensus as to what criteria constitute a "poor responder." A patient who develops fewer than six follicles on a standard long GnRHa protocol using 300–450 IU FSH per day, or 300–375 IU per day on a GnRHant protocol is likely to have decreased ovarian reserve based on criteria used in many IVF programs, and is perhaps reasonably labeled as such. ESHRE has defined the poor responder as a patient with decreased ovarian reserve testing or poor responses to maximal ovulation induction dosing [89].

The literature is replete with a multitude of protocols designed to maximize follicular recruitment, and minimize ovarian suppression, in an effort to enable such patients to successfully undergo oocyte retrieval and embryo transfer. A review of 19 studies of poor responders demonstrated that (1) pregnancy rates are lower in this patient group; (2) prognosis is far better in young versus old poor responders, with pregnancy rates of 13–25% compared to 1.5–12.7% respectively; and (3) that pregnancy rates were reduced when 1 versus 4 oocytes were obtained (0–7% versus 11.5–18.6% [90].

It is clear from a Cochrane review that in poor responders, the long GnRHa protocol is more likely to result in both cycle cancelation and fewer eggs despite utilization of more gonadotropins, than GnRHant protocols or protocols in which the GnRHa is stopped at the time ovulation induction begins [91]. There was no evidence that increasing FSH dose beyond 450 IU improves outcomes.

When poor response is previously encountered during a long GnRHa protocol, the likelihood of obtaining oocytes may be better with either the GnRHant protocol and its variations, such as the estrogen "priming protocol" or a microdose GnRHa protocol. In the "microdose lupron protocol," oral contraceptives are generally used for a short course of 7–14 days followed by aggressive stimulation with at least 450 IU per day FSH, and twice daily dosing of diluted GnRHa throughout stimulation (see Table 3.1, Fig. 3.3). In the luteal estradiol/ GnRHant protocol, or "estrogen priming protocol," an estradiol transdermal patch (0.1 mg) or oral estradiol, is administered starting approximately 10 days following the prior cycle LH surge, as well as a few days of GnRHant; this is done to theoretically synchronize the follicular cohort and prevent recruitment of a corpus luteum cyst, and suppress circulating FSH, increasing induction of FSH receptors in follicles to be recruited (Fig. 3.4). In one study of 186 young poor responders less than 35 years old, ongoing pregnancy rates per initiated cycle were 37% versus 25% respectively [92]. This has been confirmed in a small randomized trial in 54 poor responders [93]. Letrozole and gonadotropins have also been used, with letrozole 2.5–5.0 mg employed generally starting cycle day 2 for 5 days, with gonadotropins used from the start of letrozole, or after letrozole is discontinued [94, 95].

At present there is little evidence to support one "poor responder" protocol over another. Ovarian stimulation protocols used at the Complete Fertility Centre Southampton, UK (Table 3.2) and Brigham and Women's Hospital (Table 3.1), demonstrate inter-practice variations. Patients must be treated as individuals, so that if the preferred ovarian stimulation method is unsuccessful, discussion of alternative protocols with the patient, including the lack of definitive evidence that one is superior to the other, should be undertaken.

Table 3.1 Brigham and Women's Hospital ovarian stimulation guidelines for IVF/ICSI cycles

Estimated ovarian response	Age	GnRH Antagonist	GnRH Agonist	Gonadotropin starting dose
		Start antagonist when lead follicle 14 mm or stimulation day 6	*Long protocol*: start agonist approximately 1 week after LH surge or after documentation of ovulatory progesterone until menses or minimum of 10 days	Dose as below or based on prior response [unclear if doses >450 IU per day increase oocyte yield] Doses over 300 IU per day or protocols using hMG given in divided doses (twice per day)
Normal responder	≤39	OCPb starting cycle days 1–4 for 2–3 weeks if indicated	*Long protocol* with full strength leuprolide acetate 0.5–0.25 mg with stimulation start	187–225 IU/day
	≥40	OCPs × 7–14 days	*Long protocol* with diluted leuprolide acetate 0.05–0.025 mg with stimulation start	300–450 IU/day
Poor responder	Any	No OCPs *Estrogen priming protocol*: start antagonist and 0.1 mg transdermal estradiol patch 10 days after LH surge. Change patch every other day. Menstrual cycle day 2 stop patch and antagonist and start stimulation; restart antagonist as standard	*Long protocol* with diluted leuprolide acetate 0.05–0.025 mg with stimulation start or "*Microdose*" *leuprolide acetate*: Menstrual cycle day 1 start 7–10 days OCPs. Day 2 of menstrual bleed following pills or by day 4 after OCP ends, start 0.05 mg leuprolide acetate bid until hCG. Gonadotropin stimulation starts day 2 of leuprolide acetate	450–600 IU/day hMG/FSH mixed protocol
High responder	Any	OCP × 3 weeks	Long protocol with full strength leuprolide acetate 0.5–0.25 mg with stimulation start or 1.0–0.5 mg with stimulation start Overlap lupron with last week of OCP	75–150 IU/day

AMH: Low <0.9, Normal: ≥1.0–3.0, High: >3.0 pg/mL
AFC: Low <6, Normal 6–11, High ≥12
FSH: Low >10, Normal <10 mIU/mL. Note: Elevated FSH reflects decreased ovarian reserve and low response; due to suppression of FSH by estradiol, a very low FSH (e.g. <4) is not predictive of high response

[a]Ovarian reserve test results by expected response: Dosing is by AMH if AMH is discrepant with FSH or AFC results

[b]OCP used is always a low dose combination oral contraceptive

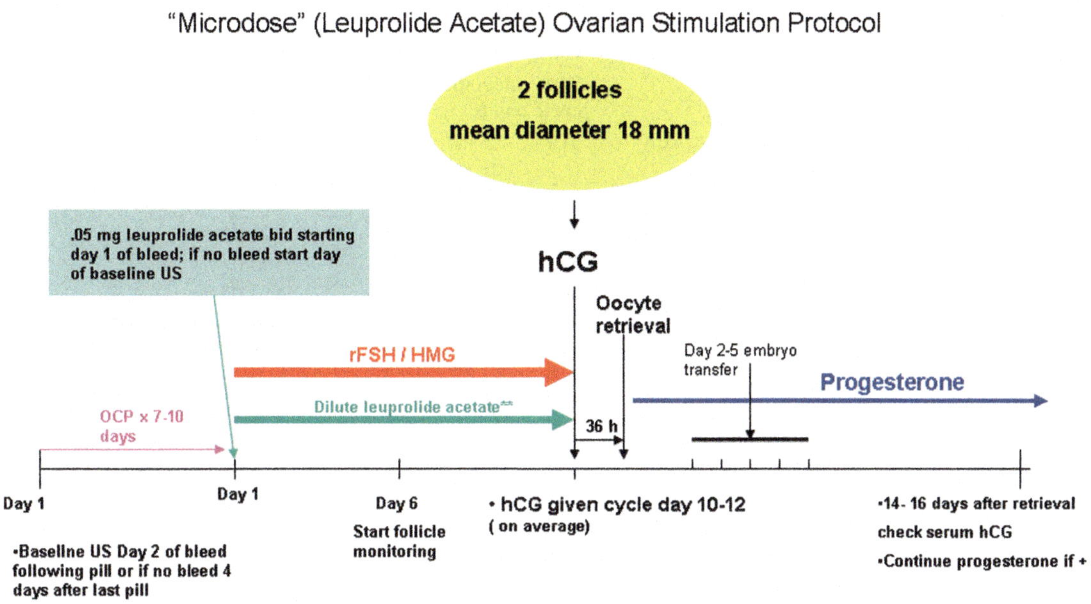

Fig. 3.3 Schematic diagram of the "microdose" or "microflare" protocol

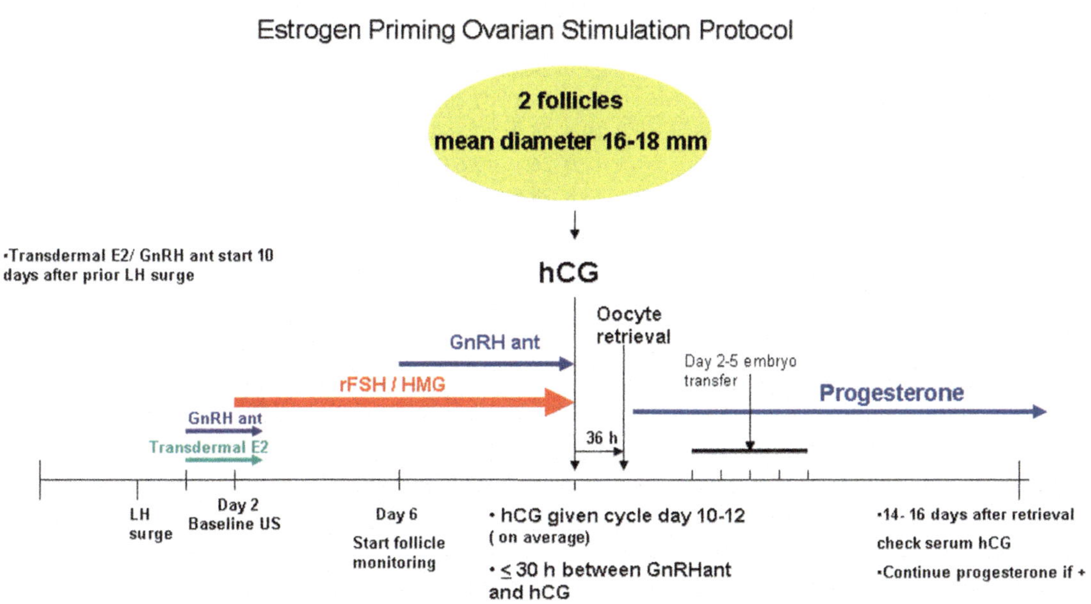

Fig. 3.4 Schematic diagram of the estrogen priming protocol

Table 3.2 Complete Fertility Centre, Southampton UK, IVF ovarian stimulation protocol

	Age	GnRH ant	GnRH a	rFSH Starting Dose/day[a]
		Start antagonist cycle day 6		Start rFSH cycle day 2
AMH ≥ 15 pmol/L (>2.1 ng/mL) AFC ≥ 15	Any	Yes	No	112.5–150 IU
AMH 7–15 pmol/L (1.0–2.1 ng/mL)	<37	Yes	No	150 IU
	38–39	Yes	No	225 IU
	40–42	Yes	No	300 IU
AFC 6–15	Any	Yes	No	150 IU
AFC ≤ 6 AMH < 7 pmol/L (<1.0 ng/mL)	Any	Yes		300 IU (first cycle) 450 IU (second cycle)
Endometriosis patients and patients with dyssychronous prior ovulation induction (1–2 follicles at 18 mm mean diameter, with rest of follicles 13–14 mm)	Any	No	yes	Consider GnRH agonist cycle and dose as with GnRH antagonist cycles, according to age, AMH/AFC

No OCP lead-in employed
[a]Urinary products e.g. HMG considered after first cycle if poor response
[b]If AMH level is not available dosing is based on AFC performed at baseline ultrasound

Table 3.3 Cumulative live birth rates per woman from linkage between SART cycles within Massachusetts (n = 14,265 women)

Cycle No.	Total cycles at each level (n)	Live births (n)	Live birth/cycle (%)	95% CI	Cumulative live births (n)	Cumulative live birth rate/woman (%)	95% CI
1	14,265	4,331	30.4	29.6–31.1	4,331	30.4	29.7–31.1
2	7,125	1,848	25.8	24.8–26.9	6,179	43.3	42.5–44.1
3	3,550	825	23.2	21.9–24.6	7,004	49.1	48.3–49.9
4	1,685	396	23.5	21.5–25.5	7,400	51.9	51.1–52.7
5	752	169	22.5	19.5–25.5	7,569	53.1	52.3–53.9
6	316	68	21.5	17.0–26.1	7,637	53.5	52.6–54.4
7	118	25	21.2	13.8–28.6	7,662	53.7	52.9–54.5
8	47	10	21.3	9.6–33.0	7,672	53.8	53.0–54.6
9–11	21	3	14.3	0.0–29.3	7,675	53.8	53.0–54.6

Adapted from Stern Fertil Steril 2010

Counseling About Oocyte Donation

One of the most difficult discussions to have with a patient is one in which moving on to donor oocyte is recommended. There are no strict criteria to guide a physician as to when to advise a patient to move on to donor egg, versus to continuing to attempt conception with one or two follicles. Clearly as maternal age advances, the chances of a single oocyte resulting in delivery become lower. Pregnancy rates in IVF decrease slowly with successive attempts. In patients <35, 35–37, 38–40 and 41–42 the likelihood of live-birth on the fourth IVF attempt in the Massachusetts' population is still 30, 21.2, 14.2, 9.4, and 5.0% respectively (Table 3.3). After four cycles, cumulative live birth rates per age were over 60% in women <35 but less than 9% in women >43 (Fig. 3.5) [96]. In a life table analysis performed by a large single US center, the delivery rate in the sixth IVF attempt in patients proceeding with six autologous cycles without a prior delivery was 13% [97]. It is difficult to determine which patients should be encouraged in continued attempts to conceive with their own oocytes and which should not. ASRM guidelines suggest that if program statistics show that the likelihood of delivery is less than 5% (very poor),

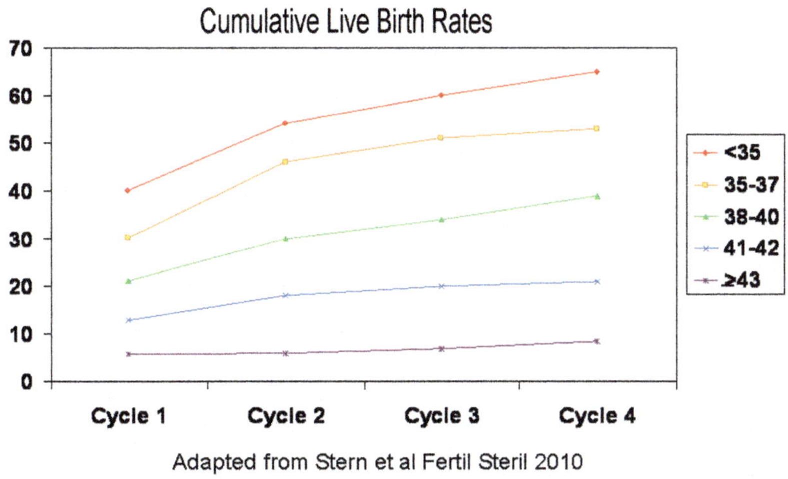

Fig. 3.5 Cumulative live birth rates after four IVF/ICSI cycles using autologous oocytes, from the Massachusetts SART data linkage study

that continued treatment should be discouraged and if less than 1% should be considered futile and not undertaken [98]. Each program must determine from their own experience and thorough patient counseling when "enough is enough" and the patient should be encouraged to move to alternative methods of having or completing her family. At BWH criteria include patient age and the ability to produce embryos deemed of sufficient number and morphology.

Conclusions

Advancement in modern medicine now provides an opportunity for patient treatments to be more individualized. In women with normal ovarian reserve, a mild stimulation regimen with GnRH antagonist regimen has an equivalent live birth rate to a conventional IVF stimulation regimen, and has advantages of tolerability and safety. Though not uniformly accepted, protocols for women with decreased ovarian reserve may increase the likelihood of undergoing successful oocyte retrieval and embryo transfer. Attention to all aspects of ovarian stimulation including ovulatory triggering and luteal support is important. In addition, patient education regarding ovarian stimulation treatment decisions is necessary in order for her to having the best possible experience. Despite impressive development in ovarian stimulation preparations and regimens, the principal determinant of outcome from ovarian stimulation remains the patient and her age and ovarian reserve.

References

1. Macklon NS, Stouffer RL, Giudice LC, Fauser BC. The science behind 25 years of ovarian stimulation for in vitro fertilization. Endocr Rev. 2006;27:170–207.
2. Macklon NS, Fauser BC. Mild stimulation in in vitro fertilization. Ann N Y Acad Sci. 2003;997:105–11.
3. Qublan HS, Amarin Z, Tahat YA, Smadi AZ, Kilani M. Ovarian cyst formation following GnRH agonist administration in IVF cycles: incidence and impact. Hum Reprod. 2006;21:640–4.
4. Daya S. Gonadotropin releasing hormone agonist protocols for pituitary desensitization in in vitro fertilization and gamete intrafallopian transfer cycles. Cochrane Database Syst Rev. 2000:CD001299.
5. Verberg MF, Eijkemans MJ, Heijnen EM, Broekmans FJ, de Klerk C, Fauser BC, Macklon NS. Why do couples drop-out from IVF treatment? A prospective cohort study. Hum Reprod. 2008;23:2050–5.
6. Griesinger G, Venetis CA, Marx T, Diedrich K, Tarlatzis BC, Kolibianakis EM. Oral contraceptive pill pretreatment in ovarian stimulation with GnRH antagonists for IVF: a systematic review and meta-analysis. Fertil Steril. 2008;90:1055–63.
7. Al-Inany HG, Abou-Setta AM, Aboulghar MA, Mansour RT, Serour GI. Efficacy and safety of human menopausal gonadotrophins versus recombinant FSH: a meta-analysis. Reprod Biomed Online. 2008;16:81–8.

8. Griesinger G, Felberbaum R, Diedrich K. GnRH antagonists in ovarian stimulation: a treatment regimen of clinicians' second choice? Data from the German national IVF registry. Hum Reprod. 2005;20:2373–5.
9. Kolibianakis EM, Collins J, Tarlatzis BC, Devroey P, Diedrich K, Griesinger G. Among patients treated for IVF with gonadotrophins and GnRH analogues, is the probability of live birth dependent on the type of analogue used? A systematic review and meta-analysis. Hum Reprod Update. 2006; 12:651–71.
10. Al-Inany HG, Youssef MA, Aboulghar M, Broekmans F, Sterrenburg M, Smit J, Abou-Setta AM. Gonadotrophin-releasing hormone antagonists for assisted reproductive technology. Cochrane Database Syst Rev. 2011:CD001750.
11. Kol S. Embryo implantation and GnRH antagonists: GnRH antagonists in ART: lower embryo implantation? Hum Reprod. 2000;15:1881–2.
12. Zikopoulos K, Kolibianakis EM, Camus M, Tournaye H, Van den Abbeel E, Joris H, Van Steirteghem A, Devroey P. Duration of gonadotropin-releasing hormone antagonist administration does not affect the outcome of subsequent frozen-thawed cycles. Fertil Steril. 2004;81:473–5.
13. Simon C, Oberye J, Bellver J, Vidal C, Bosch E, Horcajadas JA, Murphy C, Adams S, Riesewijk A, Mannaerts B, Pellicer A. Similar endometrial development in oocyte donors treated with either high- or standard-dose GnRH antagonist compared to treatment with a GnRH agonist or in natural cycles. Hum Reprod. 2005;20:3318–27.
14. Devroey P, Aboulghar M, Garcia-Velasco J, Griesinger G, Humaidan P, Kolibianakis E, Ledger W, Tomas C, Fauser BC. Improving the patient's experience of IVF/ICSI: a proposal for an ovarian stimulation protocol with GnRH antagonist co-treatment. Hum Reprod. 2009;24:764–74.
15. van Wely M, Kwan I, Burt AL, Thomas J, Vail A, Van der Veen F, Al-Inany HG. Recombinant versus urinary gonadotrophin for ovarian stimulation in assisted reproductive technology cycles. Cochrane Database Syst Rev. 2011:CD005354
16. Bosch E, Vidal C, Labarta E, Simon C, Remohi J, Pellicer A. Highly purified hMG versus recombinant FSH in ovarian hyperstimulation with GnRH antagonists—a randomized study. Hum Reprod. 2008;23:2346–51.
17. Devroey P, Pellicer A, Nyboe Andersen A, Arce JC. A randomized assessor-blind trial comparing highly purified hMG and recombinant FSH in a GnRH antagonist cycle with compulsory single-blastocyst transfer. Fertil Steril. 2012;97:561–71.
18. Schoot DC, Coelingh Bennink HJ, Mannaerts BM, Lamberts SW, Bouchard P, Fauser BC. Human recombinant follicle-stimulating hormone induces growth of preovulatory follicles without concomitant increase in androgen and estrogen biosynthesis in a woman with isolated gonadotropin deficiency. J Clin Endocrinol Metab. 1992;74:1471–3.
19. Kolibianakis EM, Schultze-Mosgau A, Schroer A, van Steirteghem A, Devroey P, Diedrich K, Griesinger G. A lower ongoing pregnancy rate can be expected when GnRH agonist is used for triggering final oocyte maturation instead of HCG in patients undergoing IVF with GnRH antagonists. Hum Reprod. 2005;20:2887–92.
20. Mochtar MH, Van der V, Ziech M, van Wely M. Recombinant Luteinizing Hormone (rLH) for controlled ovarian hyperstimulation in assisted reproductive cycles. Cochrane Database Syst Rev. 2007:CD005070.
21. Hillier SG. Current concepts of the roles of follicle stimulating hormone and luteinizing hormone in folliculogenesis. Hum Reprod. 1994;9:188–91.
22. Durnerin CI, Erb K, Fleming R, Hillier H, Hillier SG, Howles CM, Hugues JN, Lass A, Lyall H, Rasmussen P, Thong J, Traynor I, Westergaard L, Yates R. Effects of recombinant LH treatment on folliculogenesis and responsiveness to FSH stimulation. Hum Reprod. 2008;23:421–6.
23. Hillier SG, Zeleznik AJ, Ross GT. Independence of steroidogenic capacity and luteinizing hormone receptor induction in developing granulosa cells. Endocrinology. 1978;102:937–46.
24. Kolibianakis EM, Collins J, Tarlatzis B, Papanikolaou E, Devroey P. Are endogenous LH levels during ovarian stimulation for IVF using GnRH analogues associated with the probability of ongoing pregnancy? A systematic review. Hum Reprod Update. 2006;12:3–12.
25. Koichi K, Yukiko N, Shima K, Sachiko S. Efficacy of low-dose human chorionic gonadotropin (hCG) in a GnRH antagonist protocol. J Assist Reprod Genet. 2006;23:223–8.
26. Gomes MK, Vieira CS, Moura MD, Manetta LA, Leite SP, Reis RM, Ferriani RA. Controlled ovarian stimulation with exclusive FSH followed by stimulation with hCG alone, FSH alone or hMG. Eur J Obstet Gynecol Reprod Biol. 2007;130:99–106.
27. Filicori M, Cognigni GE, Samara A, Melappioni S, Perri T, Cantelli B, Parmegiani L, Pelusi G, DeAloysio D. The use of LH activity to drive folliculogenesis: exploring uncharted territories in ovulation induction. Hum Reprod Update. 2002;8:543–57.
28. Filicori M, Cognigni GE, Taraborrelli S, Parmegiani L, Bernardi S, Ciampaglia W. Intracytoplasmic sperm injection pregnancy after low-dose human chorionic gonadotropin alone to support ovarian folliculogenesis. Fertil Steril. 2002;78:414–6.
29. Hock DL, Louie H, Shelden RM, Ananth CV, Kemmann E. The need to step up the gonadotropin dosage in the stimulation phase of IVF treatment predicts a poor outcome. J Assist Reprod Genet. 1998;15:427–30.
30. Kyrou D, Kolibianakis EM, Fatemi HM, Tarlatzis BC, Tournaye H, Devroey P. Is earlier administration of human chorionic gonadotropin (hCG) associated with the probability of pregnancy in cycles stimulated with recombinant follicle-stimulating hormone and gonadotropin-releasing hormone (GnRH) antagonists? A

prospective randomized trial. Fertil Steril. 2011;96:1112–5.
31. Tremellen KP, Lane M. Avoidance of weekend oocyte retrievals during GnRH antagonist treatment by simple advancement or delay of hCG administration does not adversely affect IVF live birth outcomes. Hum Reprod. 2010;25:1219–24.
32. Fauser BC, Nargund G, Andersen AN, Norman R, Tarlatzis B, Boivin J, Ledger W. Mild ovarian stimulation for IVF: 10 years later. Hum Reprod. 2010;25:2678–84.
33. Hohmann FP, Macklon NS, Fauser BC. A randomized comparison of two ovarian stimulation protocols with gonadotropin-releasing hormone (GnRH) antagonist cotreatment for in vitro fertilization commencing recombinant follicle-stimulating hormone on cycle day 2 or 5 with the standard long GnRH agonist protocol. J Clin Endocrinol Metab. 2003;88:166–73.
34. Ledger W, Wiebinga C, Anderson P, Irwin D, Holman A, Lloyd A. Costs and outcomes associated with IVF using recombinant FSH. Reprod Biomed Online. 2009;19:337–42.
35. van der Gaast MH, Eijkemans MJ, van der Net JB, de Boer EJ, Burger CW, van Leeuwen FE, Fauser BC, Macklon NS. Optimum number of oocytes for a successful first IVF treatment cycle. Reprod Biomed Online. 2006;13:476–80.
36. Hoomans EH, Andersen AN, Loft A, Leerentveld RA, van Kamp AA, Zech H. A prospective, randomized clinical trial comparing 150 IU recombinant follicle stimulating hormone (Puregon((R))) and 225 IU highly purified urinary follicle stimulating hormone (Metrodin-HP((R))) in a fixed-dose regimen in women undergoing ovarian stimulation. Hum Reprod. 1999;14:2442–7.
37. Out HJ, Braat DD, Lintsen BM, Gurgan T, Bukulmez O, Gokmen O, Keles G, Caballero P, Gonzalez JM, Fabregues F, Balasch J, Roulier R. Increasing the daily dose of recombinant follicle stimulating hormone (Puregon) does not compensate for the age-related decline in retrievable oocytes after ovarian stimulation. Hum Reprod. 2000;15:29–35.
38. Out HJ, David I, Ron-El R, Friedler S, Shalev E, Geslevich J, Dor J, Shulman A, Ben-Rafael Z, Fisch B, Dirnfeld M. A randomized, double-blind clinical trial using fixed daily doses of 100 or 200 IU of recombinant FSH in ICSI cycles. Hum Reprod. 2001;16:1104–9.
39. Yong PY, Brett S, Baird DT, Thong KJ. A prospective randomized clinical trial comparing 150 IU and 225 IU of recombinant follicle-stimulating hormone (Gonal-F*) in a fixed-dose regimen for controlled ovarian stimulation in in vitro fertilization treatment. Fertil Steril. 2003;79:308–15.
40. Sterrenburg MD, Veltman-Verhulst SM, Eijkemans MJ, Hughes EG, Macklon NS, Broekmans FJ, Fauser BC. Clinical outcomes in relation to the daily dose of recombinant follicle-stimulating hormone for ovarian stimulation in in vitro fertilization in presumed normal responders younger than 39 years: a meta-analysis. Hum Reprod Update. 2011;17:184–96.
41. Macklon NS, Fauser BC. Progress in ovarian stimulation. Ann Endocrinol (Paris). 1999;60:137–42.
42. Macklon NS, Fauser BC. Impact of ovarian hyperstimulation on the luteal phase. J Reprod Fertil Suppl. 2000;55:101–8.
43. Verberg MF, Eijkemans MJ, Macklon NS, Heijnen EM, Baart EB, Hohmann FP, Fauser BC, Broekmans FJ. The clinical significance of the retrieval of a low number of oocytes following mild ovarian stimulation for IVF: a meta-analysis. Hum Reprod Update. 2009;15:5–12.
44. Baart EB, Martini E, van den Berg I, Macklon NS, Galjaard RJ, Fauser BC, Van Opstal D. Preimplantation genetic screening reveals a high incidence of aneuploidy and mosaicism in embryos from young women undergoing IVF. Hum Reprod. 2006;21:223–33.
45. Aanesen A, Nygren KG, Nylund L. Modified natural cycle IVF and mild IVF: a 10 year Swedish experience. Reprod Biomed Online. 2010;20:156–62.
46. Kato K, Takehara Y, Segawa T, Kawachiya S, Okuno T, Kobayashi T, Bodri D, Kato O. Minimal ovarian stimulation combined with elective single embryo transfer policy: age-specific results of a large, single-centre, Japanese cohort. Reprod Biol Endocrinol. 2012;10:35.
47. Nargund G, Fauser BC, Macklon NS, Ombelet W, Nygren K, Frydman R. The ISMAAR proposal on terminology for ovarian stimulation for IVF. Hum Reprod. 2007;22:2801–4.
48. Claman P, Domingo M, Garner P, Leader A, Spence JE. Natural cycle in vitro fertilization-embryo transfer at the University of Ottawa: an inefficient therapy for tubal infertility. Fertil Steril. 1993;60:298–302.
49. Yanushpolsky EH, Hurwitz S, Tikh E, Racowsky C. Predictive usefulness of cycle day 10 follicle-stimulating hormone level in a clomiphene citrate challenge test for in vitro fertilization outcome in women younger than 40 years of age. Fertil Steril. 2003;80:111–5.
50. Combelles CM, Orasanu B, Ginsburg ES, Racowsky C. Optimum number of embryos to transfer in women more than 40 years of age undergoing treatment with assisted reproductive technologies. Fertil Steril. 2005;84:1637–42.
51. Stern JE, Goldman MB, Hatasaka H, MacKenzie TA, Surrey ES, Racowsky C. Optimizing the number of cleavage stage embryos to transfer on day 3 in women 38 years of age and older: a Society for Assisted Reproductive Technology database study. Fertil Steril. 2009;91:767–76.
52. Templeton A, Morris JK. Reducing the risk of multiple births by transfer of two embryos after in vitro fertilization. N Engl J Med. 1998;339:573–7.
53. Devroey P, Boostanfar R, Koper NP, Mannaerts BM, Ijzerman-Boon PC, Fauser BC. A double-blind, non-inferiority RCT comparing corifollitropin alfa and recombinant FSH during the first seven days of ovarian stimulation using a GnRH antagonist protocol. Hum Reprod. 2009;24:3063–72.
54. Norman RJ, Zegers-Hochschild F, Salle BS, Elbers J, Heijnen E, Marintcheva-Petrova M, Mannaerts B.

Repeated ovarian stimulation with corifollitropin alfa in patients in a GnRH antagonist protocol: no concern for immunogenicity. Hum Reprod. 2011;26:2200–8.

55. Karimzadeh MA, Ahmadi S, Oskouian H, Rahmani E. Comparison of mild stimulation and conventional stimulation in ART outcome. Arch Gynecol Obstet. 2010;281:741–6.
56. Aleyamma TK, Kamath MS, Muthukumar K, Mangalaraj AM, George K. Affordable ART: a different perspective. Hum Reprod. 2011;26:3312–8.
57. Nahoul K, Dehennin L, Jondet M, Roger M. Profiles of plasma estrogens, progesterone and their metabolites after oral or vaginal administration of estradiol or progesterone. Maturitas. 1993;16:185–202.
58. Smitz J, Devroey P, Faguer B, Bourgain C, Camus M, Van Steirteghem AC. A randomized prospective study comparing supplementation of the luteal phase and early pregnancy by natural progesterone administered by intramuscular or vaginal route. Rev Fr Gynecol Obstet. 1992;87:507–16.
59. Propst AM, Hill JA, Ginsburg ES, Hurwitz S, Politch J, Yanushpolsky EH. A randomized study comparing Crinone 8% and intramuscular progesterone supplementation in in vitro fertilization-embryo transfer cycles. Fertil Steril. 2001;76:1144–9.
60. Sohn SH, Penzias AS, Emmi AM, Dubey AK, Layman LC, Reindollar RH, DeCherney AH. Administration of progesterone before oocyte retrieval negatively affects the implantation rate. Fertil Steril. 1999;71:11–4.
61. van der Linden M, Buckingham K, Farquhar C, Kremer JA, Metwally M. Luteal phase support for assisted reproduction cycles. Cochrane Database Syst Rev. 2011:CD009154.
62. Yanushpolsky E, Hurwitz S, Greenberg L, Racowsky C, Hornstein M. Crinone vaginal gel is equally effective and better tolerated than intramuscular progesterone for luteal phase support in in vitro fertilization-embryo transfer cycles: a prospective randomized study. Fertil Steril. 2010;94:2596–9.
63. Nyboe Andersen A, Popovic-Todorovic B, Schmidt KT, Loft A, Lindhard A, Hojgaard A, Ziebe S, Hald F, Hauge B, Toft B. Progesterone supplementation during early gestations after IVF or ICSI has no effect on the delivery rates: a randomized controlled trial. Hum Reprod. 2002;17:357–61.
64. Golan A, Weissman A. Symposium: Update on prediction and management of OHSS. A modern classification of OHSS. Reprod Biomed Online. 2009;19:28–32.
65. Bulletin E. Ovarian hyperstimulation syndrome. Fertil Steril. 2008;90:S188–93.
66. Shmorgun D, Claman P. The diagnosis and management of ovarian hyperstimulation syndrome. J Obstet Gynaecol. 2011;33:1156–62.
67. Devroey P, Polyzos NP, Blockeel C. An OHSS-Free Clinic by segmentation of IVF treatment. Hum Reprod. 2011;26:2593–7.
68. Simon C, Garcia Velasco JJ, Valbuena D, Peinado JA, Moreno C, Remohi J, Pellicer A. Increasing uterine receptivity by decreasing estradiol levels during the preimplantation period in high responders with the use of a follicle-stimulating hormone step-down regimen. Fertil Steril. 1998;70:234–9.
69. Fauser BC, de Jong D, Olivennes F, Wramsby H, Tay C, Itskovitz-Eldor J, van Hooren HG. Endocrine profiles after triggering of final oocyte maturation with GnRH agonist after cotreatment with the GnRH antagonist ganirelix during ovarian hyperstimulation for in vitro fertilization. J Clin Endocrinol Metab. 2002;87:709–15.
70. Youssef MA, Al-Inany HG, Aboulghar M, Mansour R, Abou-Setta AM. Recombinant versus urinary human chorionic gonadotrophin for final oocyte maturation triggering in IVF and ICSI cycles. Cochrane Database Syst Rev. 2011:CD003719.
71. Itskovitz J, Boldes R, Levron J, Erlik Y, Kahana L, Brandes JM. Induction of preovulatory luteinizing hormone surge and prevention of ovarian hyperstimulation syndrome by gonadotropin-releasing hormone agonist. Fertil Steril. 1991;56:213–20.
72. Griesinger G, von Otte S, Schroer A, Ludwig AK, Diedrich K, Al-Hasani S, Schultze-Mosgau A. Elective cryopreservation of all pronuclear oocytes after GnRH agonist triggering of final oocyte maturation in patients at risk of developing OHSS: a prospective, observational proof-of-concept study. Hum Reprod. 2007;22:1348–52.
73. Humaidan P. Luteal phase rescue in high-risk OHSS patients by GnRHa triggering in combination with low-dose HCG: a pilot study. Reprod Biomed Online. 2009;18:630–4.
74. Pellicer A, Albert C, Mercader A, Bonilla-Musoles F, Remohi J, Simon C. The pathogenesis of ovarian hyperstimulation syndrome: in vivo studies investigating the role of interleukin-1beta, interleukin-6, and vascular endothelial growth factor. Fertil Steril. 1999;71:482–9.
75. Alvarez C, Marti-Bonmati L, Novella-Maestre E, Sanz R, Gomez R, Fernandez-Sanchez M, Simon C, Pellicer A. Dopamine agonist cabergoline reduces hemoconcentration and ascites in hyperstimulated women undergoing assisted reproduction. J Clin Endocrinol Metab. 2007;92:2931–7.
76. Youssef MA, van Wely M, Hassan MA, Al-Inany HG, Mochtar M, Khattab S, van der Veen F. Can dopamine agonists reduce the incidence and severity of OHSS in IVF/ICSI treatment cycles? A systematic review and meta-analysis. Hum Reprod Update. 2010;16:459–66.
77. Popovic-Todorovic B, Loft A, Bredkjaeer HE, Bangsboll S, Nielsen IK, Andersen AN. A prospective randomized clinical trial comparing an individual dose of recombinant FSH based on predictive factors versus a 'standard' dose of 150 IU/day in 'standard' patients undergoing IVF/ICSI treatment. Hum Reprod. 2003;18:2275–82.
78. Aboulghar MA, Mansour RT. Ovarian hyperstimulation syndrome: classifications and critical analysis of preventive measures. Hum Reprod Update. 2003;9:275–89.

79. Palomba S, Falbo A, Carrillo L, Villani MT, Orio F, Russo T, Di Cello A, Cappiello F, Capasso S, Tolino A, Colao A, Mastrantonio P, La Sala GB, Zullo F, Cittadini E. Metformin reduces risk of ovarian hyperstimulation syndrome in patients with polycystic ovary syndrome during gonadotropin-stimulated in vitro fertilization cycles: a randomized, controlled trial. Fertil Steril. 2011;96(1384–1390):e1384.
80. Olivennes F, Howies CM, Borini A, Germond M, Trew G, Wikland M, Zegers-Hochschild F, Saunders H, Alam V. Individualizing FSH dose for assisted reproduction using a novel algorithm: the CONSORT study. Reprod Biomed Online. 2011;22 Suppl 1:S73–82.
81. Seifer DB, MacLaughlin DT, Christian BP, Feng B, Shelden RM. Early follicular serum mullerian-inhibiting substance levels are associated with ovarian response during assisted reproductive technology cycles. Fertility and sterility 2002;77:468–471.
82. Nardo LG, Gelbaya TA, Wilkinson H, Roberts SA, Yates A, Pemberton P, Laing I. Circulating basal anti-Mullerian hormone levels as predictor of ovarian response in women undergoing ovarian stimulation for in vitro fertilization. Fertil Steril. 2009;92: 1586–93.
83. Muttukrishna S, McGarrigle H, Wakim R, Khadum I, Ranieri DM, Serhal P. Antral follicle count, anti-mullerian hormone and inhibin B: predictors of ovarian response in assisted reproductive technology? BJOG. 2005;112:1384–90.
84. Nelson SM, Yates RW, Lyall H, Jamieson M, Traynor I, Gaudoin M, Mitchell P, Ambrose P, Fleming R. Anti-Mullerian hormone-based approach to controlled ovarian stimulation for assisted conception. Hum Reprod. 2009;24:867–75.
85. Broer SL, Mol BW, Hendriks D, Broekmans FJ. The role of anti-Mullerian hormone in prediction of outcome after IVF: comparison with the antral follicle count. Fertil Steril. 2009;91:705–14.
86. La Marca A, Broekmans FJ, Volpe A, Fauser BC, Macklon NS. Anti-Mullerian hormone (AMH): what do we still need to know? Hum Reprod. 2009;24:2264–75.
87. La Marca A, Nelson SM, Sighinolfi G, Manno M, Baraldi E, Roli L, Xella S, Marsella T, Tagliasacchi D, D'Amico R, Volpe A. Anti-Mullerian hormone-based prediction model for a live birth in assisted reproduction. Reprod Biomed Online. 2011;22:341–9.
88. Weghofer A, Dietrich W, Barad DH, Gleicher N. Live birth chances in women with extremely low-serum anti-Mullerian hormone levels. Hum Reprod. 2011;26:1905–9.
89. Ferraretti AP, La Marca A, Fauser BC, Tarlatzis B, Nargund G, Gianaroli L. ESHRE consensus on the definition of 'poor response' to ovarian stimulation for in vitro fertilization: the Bologna criteria. Hum Reprod. 2011;26:1616–24.
90. Oudendijk JF, Yarde F, Eijkemans MJ, Broekmans FJ, Broer SL. The poor responder in IVF: is the prognosis always poor? A systematic review. Hum Reprod Update. 2012;18:1–11.
91. Pandian Z, McTavish AR, Aucott L, Hamilton MP, Bhattacharya S. Interventions for 'poor responders' to controlled ovarian hyper stimulation (COH) in in-vitro fertilisation (IVF). Cochrane Database Syst Rev. 2010:CD004379.
92. Shastri SM, Barbieri E, Kligman I, Schoyer KD, Davis OK, Rosenwaks Z. Stimulation of the young poor responder: comparison of the luteal estradiol/gonadotropin-releasing hormone antagonist priming protocol versus oral contraceptive microdose leuprolide. Fertil Steril. 2011;95:592–5.
93. DiLuigi AJ, Engmann L, Schmidt DW, Benadiva CA, Nulsen JC. A randomized trial of microdose leuprolide acetate protocol versus luteal phase ganirelix protocol in predicted poor responders. Fertil Steril. 2011;95:2531–3.
94. Schoolcraft WB, Surrey ES, Minjarez DA, Stevens JM, Gardner DK. Management of poor responders: can outcomes be improved with a novel gonadotropin-releasing hormone antagonist/letrozole protocol? Fertil Steril. 2008;89:151–6.
95. Elassar A, Engmann L, Nulsen J, Benadiva C. Letrozole and gonadotropins versus luteal estradiol and gonadotropin-releasing hormone antagonist protocol in women with a prior low response to ovarian stimulation. Fertil Steril. 2011;95:2330–4.
96. Stern JE, Brown MB, Luke B, Wantman E, Lederman A, Missmer SA, Hornstein MD. Calculating cumulative live-birth rates from linked cycles of assisted reproductive technology (ART): data from the Massachusetts SART CORS. Fertil Steril. 2010;94:1334–40.
97. Malizia BA, Hacker MR, Penzias AS. Cumulative live-birth rates after in vitro fertilization. N Engl J Med. 2009;360:236–43.
98. Medicine TECotASoR. Fertility treatment when the prognosis is very poor or futile. Fertil Steril. 2009;92:1194–7.

4 Oocyte Retrieval and Embryo Transfer

Sara E. Barton and Elizabeth S. Ginsburg

Oocyte Retrieval

History of Oocyte Retrieval

Drs. Steptoe and Edwards reported the first IVF success in 1978 with the birth of Louise Brown. Louise Brown's mother, Lesley Brown, had undergone laparoscopy to retrieve an oocyte from a single ovarian follicle without ovarian stimulation. Since that time, great advances have been made in IVF, including dramatic changes in the mode of oocyte recovery. Current IVF typically involves the retrieval of multiple oocytes from the ovaries which have been stimulated with medication containing FSH. Oocyte retrieval has shifted to an ultrasound-guided transvaginal procedure where a needle is passed through the vaginal wall and into the ovary, and follicular fluid and oocytes are aspirated via negative pressure generated from a suction apparatus. In modern IVF, oocyte retrieval is undertaken in the outpatient setting and has been shown to be very safe and highly effective at retrieving oocytes.

Prior studies have documented the relative ease and safety of ultrasound-guided oocyte retrieval as compared to the early laparoscopic approach for IVF [1–3]. Furthermore, laparoscopic retrieval has been shown to result in lower rates of mature oocyte recovery and lower oocyte fertilization rates than ultrasound guided abdominal and vaginal retrieval [2]. Early use of ultrasound guided follicular aspiration used a transabdominal–transvesical approach [4, 5]. This procedure was reported to be associated with frequent urinary tract infections and hematuria [5]. Subsequent studies have shown both patient and clinician preference for transvaginal ultrasound over abdominal ultrasound for visualizing pelvic organs and for follicular monitoring and aspiration [6–8]. Therefore, transvaginal ultrasound-guided aspiration has become the standard of care in women undergoing oocyte retrieval during IVF. The first description of this procedure was published by Wikland and colleagues in 1985 and in more detail shortly thereafter leading to rapid adoption of an ultrasound guided transvaginal approach [9, 10].

Anesthesia for Oocyte Retrieval

For ultrasound guided transvaginal oocyte retrieval, the patient is brought to the operating room where analgesia or anesthesia is employed.

S.E. Barton, M.D. • E.S. Ginsburg, M.D. (✉)
Division of Reproductive Endocrinology and Infertility, Department of Obstetrics and Gynecology, Brigham and Women's Hospital, Boston, MA 02115, USA
e-mail: sbarton@partners.org; eginsburg@partners.org

E.S. Ginsburg and C. Racowsky (eds.), *In Vitro Fertilization: A Comprehensive Guide*, DOI 10.1007/978-1-4419-9848-4_4,

Typically, either conscious sedation with opiates and benzodiazepines or a general anesthetic with intravenous propofol (AstraZeneca, London, United Kingdom) is used. Endotrachael tube intubation is rarely required [11]. Some centers prefer sedation, as this does not require an anesthesiologist on-site. Propofol has the advantage of rapid onset and recovery and less postoperative nausea and vomiting. However, the requirement for specifically trained administrators limits its use in some centers [12]. Others centers also offer neuraxial anesthesia such as spinal anesthesia with lidocaine and narcotics [13] or injection of local anesthesia in the cervix and vaginal wall [12]. A survey of SART affiliated ART centers reported conscious sedation was by far the most commonly employed analgesic agents (95% of centers). However, this study included propofol in the conscious sedation group although this medication is often considered a general anesthetic due to the depressed level of consciousness achieved [11]. In addition, these data were published over a decade ago and have not been repeated, so these statistics may not be representative of current practice.

Local anesthesia with use of a paracervical block has been described, usually in poor resource settings. In a survey study of women undergoing oocyte retrievals with paracervical blocks, 43% of women described the procedure as either "very painful" or "painful," but 98% of them would undergo the procedure again without anxiety. 28% of these women required intraoperative administration of additional analgesia with an unspecified sedative highlighting that local anesthetic alone may be inadequate for many women [14]. In cases where multiple vaginal and ovarian punctures are required, local analgesia is likely to be poorly tolerated. Studies aiming to examine the toxicity of general analgesic agents and their effects on pregnancy rates have been performed. Propofol does not appear to have a negative impact on pregnancy rates [15] or on embryo quality [16] when compared with paracervical block. Concerns have been raised about the toxicity of inhaled nitrous agents on oocyte quality and embryo development and a negative impact on pregnancy rates [17, 18].

Oocyte Retrieval Technique

After administration of the chosen anesthetic agent, if a paracervical block is not used alone, the patient is placed in the dorsal lithotomy position and a sterile speculum is inserted into the vagina. The sterile operating room table, vaginal ultrasound probe with needle guide attached, and prepared tubes containing culture media in a warming unit have been previously prepared (Fig. 4.1). The vagina is rinsed with saline, or betadine. If betadine is used the vagina should then be copiously rinsed with saline due to the risk of toxicity to oocytes if betadine were to become in contact with oocytes during retrieval. The speculum is then removed and a transvaginal ultrasound probe with a needle guide attached is inserted into the vagina. A retrieval needle (17-gauge is common, though 16, 18 and 19-gauge needles are also available) is passed through the vaginal wall and into the follicles under ultrasound guidance. Surrounding structures such as the iliac vessels, bowel, and bladder can easily be seen and avoided. A vacuum pump is activated and follicular fluid and oocytes, are aspirated into warmed tubes containing culture media. The tubes are then placed in a tube warming rack in the adjacent embryology laboratory. Ultimately, the contents of the tubes are poured into culture plates and the oocytes are identified [19]. Generally, all follicles regardless of size that are visualized on ultrasound that can be safely entered are aspirated. It may be helpful to have Doppler capability on the ultrasound machine. In some cases of peritoneal disease patients may have collections of peritoneal fluid which can be differentiated from venous lakes or veins using the Doppler flow mode, and avoided during oocyte retrieval. The retrieval also provides an opportunity to visualize the endometrial stripe and confirm a normal thickness (≥7 mm). If a mass is seen within the endometrium, Doppler can be used to determine whether there is a feeding blood vessel and likely polyp, or merely an endometrial fold.

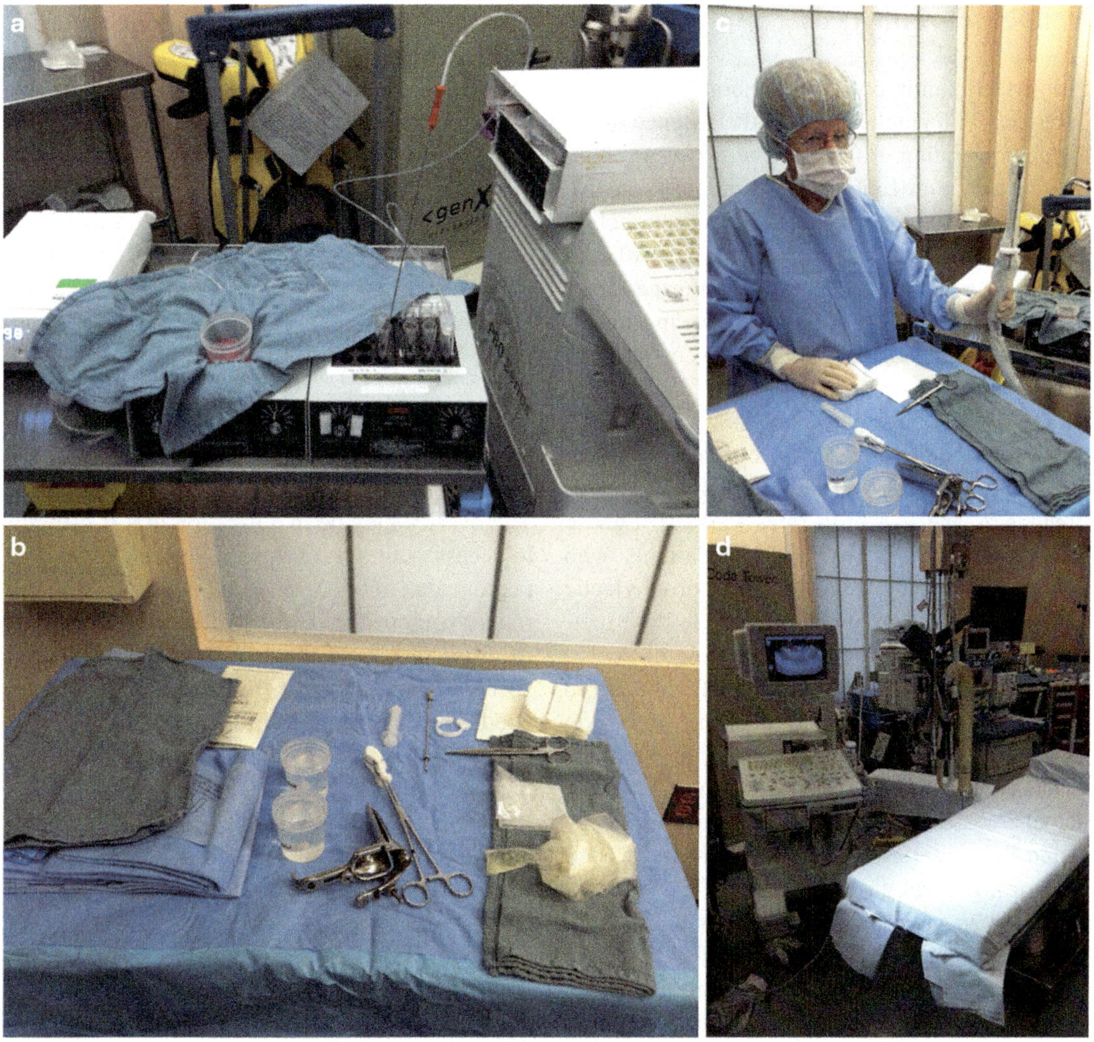

Fig. 4.1 Equipment list: (**a**) Vacuum pump, vacuum tubing, retrieval needle and tubing, tubing with culture media, tube warmer; (**b**) sterile speculum, sterile gloves, sterile drapes, sterile ultrasound probe cover, ultrasound probe needle guide; (**c**) transvaginal ultrasound probe with sterile cover and needle guide attached; (**d**) Ultrasound machine and operating room table with stirrups for lithotomy position

Follicular Flushing

The number of embryos obtained in IVF is directly related to the number of oocytes retrieved. In an attempt to increase oocyte yield in IVF, follicular flushing after follicular aspiration has been advocated. Early studies showed a potential benefit of this procedure, which involves using a double lumen retrieval needle and flushing culture media into follicles during aspiration and then reaspirating the flushed fluid [20]. However, subsequent randomized trials have failed to show benefit. A recent Cochrane review of randomized trials concluded there is no benefit to follicular flushing in terms of oocyte yield, clinical pregnancy rates, or live birth rates [21]. Additionally, procedure times are noted to be longer and more anesthetic is required when flushing is performed [22]. Given this, we do not advocate follicular flushing.

Antibiotic Prophylaxis

Prophylactic antibiotics are generally employed in clinical IVF practice despite the absence of trials demonstrating a benefit in terms of a reduction of pelvic infections, or an increase in live birth rate. As the incidence of pelvic infection after oocyte retrieval is rare, clinical trials of adequate power are difficult to perform. Furthermore, pelvic infections can be severe requiring hospitalization and parenteral antibiotics or surgical treatment of abscesses [23, 24].

There is evidence that positive microbial cultures from the tip of the embryo transfer catheter are associated with a reduction in implantation, pregnancy, and live birth rates [25–27]. Egbase and colleagues reported on 430 patients who underwent oocyte retrieval with prophylactic antibiotics using a regimen of a single-dose metronidazole and ceftriaxone at the time of oocyte retrieval 48 h prior to transfer. Mock embryo transfer was performed at the time of oocyte retrieval, and the catheter tips for both the mock transfer and the catheter used on the day of the actual transfer were cultured for bacteria. They found only 69.9% of mock transfers were positive for microbial growth, but noted a significant reduction in microbial growth after administration of antibiotics. In fact, 78.1% of the subjects that had positive cultures from the mock catheter used at the egg retrieval had embryo transfer catheter tips that were culture negative after receiving antibiotics at the time of the oocyte retrieval. They concluded that routine prophylactic antibiotics are warranted at the time of oocyte retrieval due to the association with microbes on the transfer catheter and poor IVF outcomes [28]. Doxycycline, although commonly used as prophylaxis for oocyte retrievals, has not been shown in clinical studies to reduce bacterial cultures obtained from the vagina or to improve implantation and pregnancy rates [27].

In conclusion, evidence suggests that antibiotics administered at the time of retrieval may decrease bacterial contamination present at embryo transfer. There is no clear evidence that routine antibiotics are warranted to prevent pelvic infection, but given the rarity of this complication, an adequately powered trial would be difficult to perform. Since vaginal preparations containing bacteriostatic solutions such as betadine are not employed due to concerns regarding the effect of these solutions on oocytes, it is reasonable to consider antibiotic prophylaxis. There is no clear evidence which antibiotic to use, but it seems prudent to target vaginal flora with antibiotics used routinely in other gynecologic procedures.

Oocyte Retrieval in Cases with Abnormal Anatomy

The ovaries may be in a location that is difficult to access with a transvaginal approach. A small percentage of oocyte retrievals will require transmyometrial passage of the retrieval needle in order to access the follicles. Limited retrospective data indicate that when the retrieval needle passes through the uterine muscle there does not seem to be a detrimental effect on pregnancy rates [29].

Greater difficulties arise when the ovaries cannot be accessed at all through the vagina due to anatomic position. This may occur with enlarged uteri due to fibroids, ovarian transposition prior to pelvic or spinal radiation, pelvic adhesions, or Müllerian anomalies, for example. Historically, if the ovaries could not be accessed vaginally for oocyte retrieval, laparoscopy with general endotracheal tube anesthesia was performed, or these patients were not considered candidates for IVF. However, case reports have been described of successful oocyte retrieval during IVF in cases of Müllerian agenesis or ovarian transposition via ultrasound guided transabdominal oocyte retrieval [30–32]. Recently, a retrospective case-control study of 69 women who underwent ultrasound guided transabdominal oocyte retrieval was published (Fig. 4.2). In this series, all cases had one or both ovaries inaccessible through the vagina. The most commonly cited causes were enlarged uteri from fibroids or adenomyosis causing ovarian displacement high in the abdomen, prior ovarian transposition prior to radiation therapy for malignancy, Müllerian anomalies, and mor-

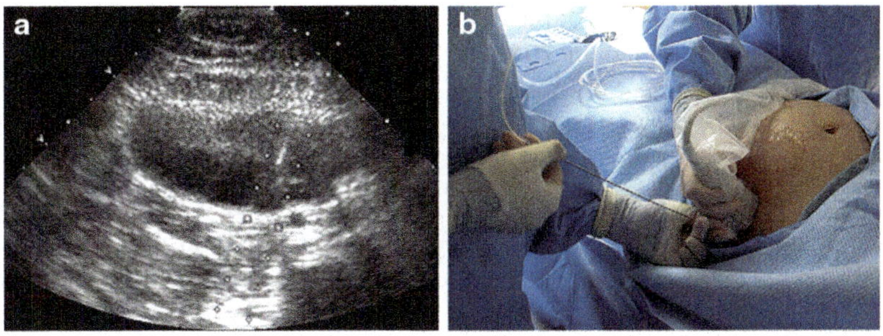

Fig. 4.2 (**a**) Ultrasound image showing the use of the needle guide (*dotted lines*) during transabdominal oocyte retrieval. (**b**) Operative setup during transabdominal oocyte retrieval in a case when the ovaries could not be accessed vaginally [33]

bid obesity. General anesthesia with propofol (not requiring endotracheal intubation) or spinal anesthesia was used in equal proportion to those patients undergoing standard transvaginal retrievals. There were no significant differences in the number of mature oocytes retrieved, damaged oocytes, fertilization rates, or clinical and ongoing pregnancy rates. One infectious complication in the transabdominal retrieval group occurred in a patient with obesity (BMI 38). She presented 2 days after retrieval with abdominal pain and fever, but abdominal imaging with CT scanning did not show a pelvic abscess. However, given her recent procedure, she was presumed to have a pelvic infection that was treated conservatively with antibiotics. This study demonstrates that transabdominal oocyte retrieval is a safe and efficacious alternative when transvaginal retrieval is not possible [33].

Complications of Oocyte Retrieval

In general, the risks of oocyte retrieval are those associated with any surgical procedure. Bleeding from the puncture sites in the vagina or ovaries, intra-abdominal infection, damage to surrounding organs or blood vessels from inadvertent needle puncture, and complications related to anesthesia are all associated risks. The risks associated with transvaginal guided oocyte retrieval appear to very low in prospective studies, and are certainly less than risks attributable to laparoscopy in general [23, 34, 35].

There is generally minimal blood loss attributable to oocyte retrieval. Studies have reported median blood loss of <100 mL and no significant decrease in hemoglobin concentrations before and after oocyte retrieval [36]. Other studies have highlighted the overall safety of this procedure. A large prospective study of over 1,000 cases to assess complications related to ultrasound-guided transvaginal retrieval was published by Ludwig and colleagues [35]. Complications reported in this study included complications related to anesthesia, vaginal bleeding requiring tamponade or vaginal suture, intra-abdominal bleeding or infection, hospitalization related to pain, and injury to surrounding organs. Overall pain scores related to the procedure were also assessed. There were no complications related to anesthesia (95% had general anesthesia and 5% had sedation with midazolam). 2.8% required compression or tamponade for vaginal bleeding, but none required a vaginal suture for bleeding. No cases of intra-abdominal bleeding or pelvic infection were noted. Only 0.7% of patients were admitted for pain attributed to the oocyte retrieval after presenting to the emergency department. One case of ureteral injury was noted which was repaired with a ureteral stent, but no bowel complications were seen. Overall the procedure was well tolerated. Pain scores were reported prospectively 2 h after the procedure and on the day of embryo transfer. Moderate to severe pain was noted in 20% of subjects 2 h after the procedure and 9.8% on the day of embryo transfer. Not surprisingly, pain was directly correlated with the number of oocytes retrieved [35].

Bennett and colleagues reported on all oocyte retrievals performed in a large IVF practice over a 4-year period and similarly found a low rate of complications. They noted a higher incidence of bleeding in this series at 8.6%, but all were managed with either pressure or placement of a vaginal suture. In one case, emergency laparotomy was required for intra-abdominal bleeding from an ovarian puncture site. Clinically diagnosed infections requiring antibiotics occurred in 0.6%, and half of those (0.3% of all oocyte retrievals) had pelvic abscesses noted on imaging. Prior pelvic surgery or peritoneal damage did not seem to be associated with infectious risk in this study [23]. In our experience in the rare cases that intra-abdominal bleeding occurs, patients experience much greater than expected abdominal pain-post retrieval. Ultrasound shows intraperitoneal fluid and/or clot. In greater than 20 years of practice in our large academic center, all cases of bleeding in our practice were treated supportively, with observation, serial hematocrits and if needed, transfusion.

Summary and Conclusions

In conclusion, oocyte retrieval is a generally safe and well-tolerated procedure that is most often accomplished in the outpatient setting with conscious sedation and rarely requires general endotracheal intubation. Oocyte retrieval is typically performed transvaginally with ultrasound guidance, but in cases of abnormal anatomy, ultrasound guided transabdominal retrieval is an option which avoids the need for laparoscopy in nearly all cases. In common practice prophylactic antibiotics are administered intravenously prior to the procedure, and complications such as clinically significant bleeding or infection are remarkably unusual.

Embryo Transfer

Overview of Embryo Transfer

Embryo transfer is the final technical step in the process of IVF, and proper technique is crucial. Ovarian stimulation protocols and laboratory techniques have improved dramatically since the inception of IVF, and it is now recognized that embryo transfer is an important determinant of IVF success and may be a rate-limiting step in an IVF program's pregnancy rates. It is important to maintain an ongoing quality assurance program in any ART program, as research has shown there can be significant differences in pregnancy rates between individual providers [37], even when only those transfers that had high-quality embryos are included. One study found a range of pregnancy rates from 17 to 54.3% in the same ART program [38].

In general, embryo transfer is a minor procedure that is well tolerated and does not require analgesia. In cases of very difficult transfer or poor patient tolerance which significantly impacts the ease of transfer, anxiolytics or anesthesia can be considered. In our program, if patients have a history of a difficult transfer causing them significant anxiety or discomfort we offer oral benzodiazepines 30–60 min prior to the transfer, for example Valium 10 mg. In cases where extreme difficulty has been encountered in the past or the patient cannot tolerate the procedure even with benzodiazepine pretreatment, we occasionally use general intravenous anesthesia with propofol, requiring an anesthesiologist.

The goal of the embryo transfer is to deposit the embryo(s) in the mid-portion of the uterine body for subsequent implantation. The patient is placed in the dorsal lithotomy position, and speculum is placed into the vagina until the cervix is in view, and centered in the speculum if possible. The cervix is prepared with either saline solution or culture media, and excess cervical mucous is aspirated with a syringe or wiped with sterile cotton swabs. Betadine solution is not recommended due to concerns of toxicity of these solutions to embryos. Some centers perform a mock transfer with an empty transfer catheter at the time of embryo transfer prior to loading the embryos into another transfer catheter to ensure that the cervical canal can be successfully navigated; we advocate also performing a mock transfer in a prior cycle as explained below. Next, the embryos are loaded into a soft transfer catheter by a member of the embryology team, and brought out to the clinician. The clinician passes the catheter through the cervix and into the uterine body where the embryos are deposited. The catheter is then withdrawn from the cervix and immediately flushed by the embryologist to confirm that none of the embryos are retained. If embryos are found to have been retained in the catheter, they are immediately reloaded and retransferred [39].

Studies on a number of technical factors relating to embryo transfer have been published. Results from these studies have often been conflicting; however, there is mounting evidence to guide good transfer technique. In this section, emphasis will be placed on the aspects of embryo transfer technique, which, evidence shows, affect IVF outcome.

Cervical Preparation

At the time of transfer, cervical mucus is aspirated to prevent the cervical mucus from plugging the catheter tip and interfering with embryo deposition or to avoid cervical mucus sticking to embryos and displacing them from their point of deposition as the catheter is withdrawn. The mucus should be gently removed from the exterior cervix with a sterile cotton swab soaked in saline or transfer medium. This is followed by aspiration of the cervical canal with a sterile syringe or IV catheter with a syringe attached to it. (We use an insulin syringe at our center). Clinical trials evaluating the effect of removal of cervical mucus on pregnancy rates have been inconsistent, but some have shown a benefit [40] and none have shown detriment [41]; therefore, we advocate performing this step prior to transfer.

In addition to aspiration of cervical mucus, it has been speculated that bacterial contamination may adversely affect implantation. Egbase et al. cultured catheter tips after transfer and found that pregnancy rates were lower in those with positive microbial cultures [25]. However, antibiotics at the time of embryo transfer have not been shown to increase clinical pregnancy or live birth rates, and are not routinely employed. In a prospective, blinded, randomized-controlled trial, subjects were allocated to receiving co-amoxiclav (amoxicillin with clavulanic acid) on the day before and the day of embryo transfer versus no antibiotics. Bacterial contamination at the catheter tip and clinical pregnancy rates were compared. Despite a reduction in bacterial contamination, no benefit on pregnancy rates was noted. The authors conclude that their results do not support the routine administration of antibiotics at embryo transfer [42]. In patients using vaginal progesterone for luteal support in stimulated cycles (see Chap. 3) or complete endometrial support as in cryopreserved embryo transfer cycles, oocyte donation, or gestational carrier cycles (see Chaps. 10 and 11 on oocyte donation and gestational carrier for uterine preparation protocols) we remove only the progesterone product from the external os to prevent it from entering the transfer catheter.

Mock (Trial) Transfers

Strong evidence supports performing a mock embryo transfer at some point either prior to or during ovarian stimulation in IVF. Mansour et al. demonstrated in a randomized trial that when a mock transfer is performed there are significantly fewer difficult transfers encountered, and higher implantation and pregnancy rates. In this study, 335 women were randomized to mock transfer prior to IVF stimulation start or no mock transfer. In those who underwent the mock procedure, no difficult transfers were encountered versus 29.8% difficult transfers in the control group. Pregnancy rates were 22.8 versus 13.1% in the mock and no mock groups respectively [43]. The mock transfer allows measurement of the length of the uterine cavity from the fundus to the external cervical os, notes the position of the uterus and cervix, records the type of catheter used to successfully navigate the cervical canal, whether a bend of the catheter and/or extension of the internal catheter was necessary, and notes the type of speculum allowing good visualization of the cervix. Taken together, information gained in the mock transfer allows the clinician to avoid difficult transfers and to be better prepared if difficulty is encountered.

There are no strong data that the timing of mock transfer affects implantation or pregnancy rates, despite concerns that a mock transfer close to the time of the actual transfer may cause endometrial injury and negatively impact pregnancy rates. Katariya and colleagues published a retrospective study comparing women who underwent mock transfer prior to the start of ovarian stimulation in IVF to those undergoing mock transfer at oocyte retrieval 3–5 days prior to actual transfer. There were no significant differences in implantation or clinical pregnancy rates (47.6% versus 48.4%, OR 0.97 95% CI 0.58–1.61). The mean cavity length was noted to be slightly shorter when measured prior to the start of stimulation. The authors suggest this may indicate the measurement changes due to changes in uterine position from large stimulated ovaries. However, given no statistical difference was seen between groups, they conclude the timing of mock transfer does not affect IVF outcome [44]. It is important to note that this study was retrospective, and although the study groups appeared similar, they did not control for prior cycle information available or prior transfer attempts, a factor that is likely to affect pregnancy rates. It is reassuring, however, that no detriment was observed when doing a mock transfer close to the time of actual transfer. Others have described only performing a mock transfer immediately prior to the actual transfer. Acceptable pregnancy and implantation rates were reported after this strategy in a case series, but the interpretation of these data is limited as no comparison group was used [45]. In addition, this tactic would reveal patients with severe cervical stenosis only at the time of transfer, which would not prepare the clinician for alternative techniques as noted below.

Approach to Cervical Stenosis

A benefit of performing the mock transfer prior to the start of ovarian stimulation is identification of patients with cervical stenosis who may benefit from a cervical dilation procedure prior to IVF to aid in embryo transfer. Multiple techniques have been described to alleviate cervical stenosis if it is identified. Much of the data in this regard is in the form of case series or case-control studies, but the results of these studies provide some evidence for their use. Cervical dilation can be accomplished with mechanical dilation, osmotic dilators (Laminaria), or placement of a Malecot catheter (CR Bard Inc., Covington, GA) following mechanical dilatation.

Mechanical dilation with Hegar dilators was described in a group of 57 patients with prior transfers rated as difficult, none of whom had conceived in prior IVF attempts. Cervical dilation to size 7 Hegar was performed at the initial IVF visit, an average of 14 days prior to the embryo transfer. In 70.2% of the women who had the dilation, the embryo transfer was rated as easy after dilation, and the pregnancy rate was 31.6% [46]. In a study by Prapas et al., 288 women with a history of two prior failed IVF attempts and prior embryo transfers classified as difficult were randomly assigned to cervical dilation to size 9 Hegar 1–3 months prior to starting IVF stimulation or no dilation. Implantation rate, pregnancy rate, and live birth rate were significantly higher in the cervical dilation group. No increase in preterm delivery or spontaneous abortion was seen. Furthermore, 95% of the transfers were classified as easy after the cervical dilation [47]. Care should be taken to allow adequate interval between dilation and embryo transfer, as other studies have shown very low pregnancy rates when dilation was done at the time of oocyte retrieval, only 48 h before embryo transfer in one study [48].

An alternate method of managing cervical stenosis is dilatation followed by placement of a

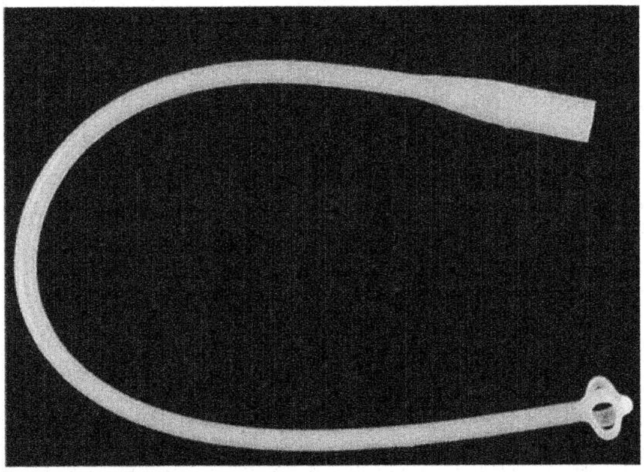

Fig. 4.3 Picture of the Malecot catheter which can be used to alleviate cervical stenosis in cases of difficult embryo transfer. The mushroom tip end is inserted through the internal os after hysteroscopy and the distal end is cut so that it can be retrieved in the office through the external os without protruding out of the vagina to minimize patient discomfort [49]

Malecot catheter which is used preferentially at our center. In this technique, a rubber Malecot catheter size 16–22 French with a mushroom tip (Fig. 4.3) is inserted into the uterus after cervical dilatation and hysteroscopy in the operating room. If an endocervical ridge is encountered it is shaved flush with the endocervical canal. Generally this requires resection of only 1–3 mm of tissue. The catheter is trimmed 2–4 cm past the external os so that it is within the vagina and is kept in place for 7–10 days. Antibiotic prophylaxis with doxycycline 100 mg two times daily is used while the catheter is in place; the catheter is then easily removed in the office with minimal patient discomfort. This technique was described in a prospective case series of 36 patients with cervical stenosis. The catheter was left in place on average for 10 days, and in 32 of 36 patients the subsequent procedures requiring entry into the uterine cavity were easier. All catheters were removed in the office, with only one requiring any form of analgesia due to the necessity of an IUD hook to remove the catheter as it had been cut too short and migrated into the endometrial cavity. No infections occurred; however, three patients had to have the catheter removed after only 3 days due to uterine cramping [49]. Overall, we find this procedure effective and well tolerated. Case reports and case series of additional methods including operative hysteroscopy with shaving of a cervical ridge at the internal os [50] and placement of osmotic dilators including Dilapan-S rods or laminaria [51, 52] have been described.

Embryo Transfer Catheter Choice

Ideally, the embryo transfer catheter is soft enough to avoid endometrial trauma while being able to navigate the cervical canal without difficulty. There have been many studies aimed at comparing catheter types, and some guiding principles have emerged. Soft catheters are preferred over firm, more rigid catheters [53]. A meta-analysis of all published trials comparing soft to rigid catheters showed a benefit on pregnancy rates, even when only randomized prospective trials were included [54]. This is likely due to the fact that rigid catheters may more easily disrupt the endometrium and cause bleeding, and blood on the catheter tip has been associated with lower pregnancy rates [55]. In addition, passage through the internal os with a rigid catheter may cause more prostaglandin release and uterine cramping, which has been associated with decreased implantation and pregnancy rates. In a prospective study of 209 women undergoing IVF embryo transfer, the frequency of uterine contractions was measured for 5 min immediately prior to the embryo transfer by digital ultrasound recordings. Pregnancy rates were negatively correlated with the frequency of uterine contractions in a dose related fashion [56]. No significant difference in pregnancy rates between different soft-tipped catheters such as those manufactured by Cook (K-Jets-7019-SIVF; Cook IVF, Eight Miles Plains, Queensland, Australia) and Wallace (Classic Embryo Replacement Catheter; Smiths Medical, Hythe, Kent, U.K.) have been noted in prospective trials [57]. It is reasonable to base selection of the soft catheter on the experience of the physician(s) in the practice after trialing several different models.

Eco-dense catheters such as the Sureview catheter (Wallace Sureview ultrasound embryo replacement catheter; Smiths Medical, Hythe, Kent, U.K.) have been developed to help with visualization of the catheter on ultrasound during embryo transfer. This allows the clinician to more easily confirm deposition of embryos in the desired location. The Sureview catheter was compared to a standard Wallace catheter in a prospective randomized trial. It was noted that the catheter was consistently seen better on ultrasound with the Sureview, but implantation and pregnancy rates did not differ [58]. As these catheters are often significantly more costly, one strategy is to reserve the use of eco-dense catheters in cases with a difficult mock transfer or distorted anatomy when confirmation of catheter placement is essential.

Catheter Loading and Embryo Deposition

Embryos are loaded into the catheter by the embryologist after confirming both patient and embryo identities. Two techniques have been commonly described for embryo loading, "air-fluid" and "fluid only" techniques. In the air-fluid method two columns of air surround the fluid media containing embryos; in the fluid only method the syringe and entire catheter is filled with medium and the embryo-containing media is aspirated without being bracketed by air. A review of two randomized trials failed to detect any differences in live birth or pregnancy rates between the two methods [59]. In our program embryos are loaded using the air-fluid method in which air bubbles are created on both sides of the droplet containing the embryos [60], with the embryos being delivered in a 10–15 μL volume of medium. Others describe a continuous fluid column of 30 μL attached to an airtight 1 mL syringe [61]. It should be noted that if there is no air in the catheter, the echodense spot will not be seen coming from the catheter tip when ultrasound guidance is used. The volume of media used for transfer has been shown to affect pregnancy rates, with volumes less than 10 μL negatively impacting pregnancy rates [62] and volumes greater than 60 μL being associated with both ectopic pregnancies and embryo expulsion to the vagina or cervix [63].

Somewhat alarming studies have shown high rates of embryos either adherent to the outside of the transfer catheter with mucous or embryos that have been expelled into the cervix or vagina. In one study, microscopic examination of the embryo catheter and flushing of the vagina and cervix with media followed by microscopic inspection of the media showed that 17.4% of embryos had not been deposited during the transfer [64]. In response, several techniques have been tested that may be of benefit. The first is the removal of cervical mucus as mentioned above [65]. In addition, the injection of air into the catheter used for the embryo transfer immediately after transfer has been advocated. In a recent prospective, randomized, controlled trial of 110 women undergoing IVF women were divided into two groups. One group received standard embryo transfer by loading the embryos with the 3-drop technique and the other received the addition of 0.2 mL of air pushed into the catheter with an insulin syringe immediately after the embryos were released, without removing the transfer catheter. The implantation and pregnancy rates were significantly higher in the group that received the additional air injection [66]. Finally, others have tested gentle pressure of the cervix prior to injection by loosening the screw on the speculum and letting the blades rest on the cervix. In a randomized trial of 639 women, those receiving the cervical pressure immediately prior to depressing the plunger of the syringe, expelling the embryos and maintaining pressure for 5–7 min had a higher implantation (33.3% versus 23.5%, OR 1.54; 95% CI 1.26–1.89) and pregnancy rates (67% versus 47.8%, OR 1.39; 95% CI 1.11–1.74) [67].

Additional evidence suggests that the time interval between embryo loading into the transfer catheter and embryo deposition is an important factor in the pregnancy rate. Matorras and colleagues published a large retrospective study associating the loading to deposition interval with pregnancy rates. They found a significant reduction in pregnancy rates with a longer interval, even in transfers that were classified as easy.

The highest pregnancy rate was in the <30 second (s) interval at 40.0%, an interval of 31–60 s had a pregnancy rate of 33.3%, 61–120 s had a pregnancy rate of 32.0%, and >120 s had a pregnancy rate of 19.4% (p=0.03) [68]. The study highlights that an efficient and easy transfer are important to achieve good outcomes in IVF.

Depth of Transfer

The depth in the uterus for optimal deposition has been examined in several studies. Deposition of embryos <10 mm from the uterine fundus has been associated with ectopic pregnancy [69], and several studies have indicated that deposition in the low to mid-uterus is preferred. Coroleu et al. performed a randomized trial comparing 180 sequential transfers randomized to 10, 15, or 20 mm from the endometrial edge at the fundus as visualized on ultrasound during the transfer. Implantation rates were significantly higher in the 15 mm or 20 mm transfer groups (31.3% and 33.3% respectively) compared to the 10 mm group (20.6%) [70]. Others have advocated for a "fixed" depth of transfer instead of determining transfer depth by mock transfer or ultrasound guidance. A retrospective review of over 4,000 IVF cycles in which the first half were done by cavity measurement and the second half by a fixed transfer distance of 6.0 cm from the external cervical os found an increase in the pregnancy rate over the study time period. They attributed this increase primarily due to a change in transfer technique to a fixed distance [71]. This study did not, however, account for other practice changes over the study time period that may have contributed to improvement in pregnancy rates. Some patients have elongated cervical canals and this distance may lead to cervical deposition of embryos, or very short cavities in cases where multiple cervical surgeries such as cone biopsies have been performed, risking fundal deposition or ectopic pregnancy, respectively. In summary, available prospective and retrospective evidence suggests that transfer at the low to mid-uterine fundal region at least 15 mm is preferable over high fundal transfer. If a mock measurement is not available, ultrasound guidance should be used and the embryo(s) deposited to the mid-uterine fundal region [70, 72, 73].

Ultrasound Guidance

Considerable effort has been directed to clarify the role of ultrasound in facilitating embryo transfer. The advantage of ultrasound guidance is that it may help guide the clinician in navigating the cervical canal and performing a less traumatic transfer. In addition, the depth of embryo deposition can be visualized when the air bubbles in the catheter are released, ensuring deposition in the desired location in the uterine body (Fig. 4.4). As studies have suggested length discrepancies between a mock transfer and measurement on the day of actual embryo transfer after ovarian stimulation, this reassurance is welcome. The disadvantage of using ultrasound is that it requires the patient to have a full bladder for adequate visualization which can lead to discomfort, and it requires an assistant operator skilled in ultrasound. It may also increase the time of embryo transfer. Additionally, ultrasound guidance in overweight or obese patients may not be feasible. A full bladder in patients with severely retroflexed uteri may in fact render the transfer more difficult; in such cases a mock transfer prior to the cycle and transfer with an empty bladder with deposition of the embryos 1.5 cm from the fundus may be preferable.

A recent Cochrane review of 17 randomized, controlled trials comparing ultrasound guided transfers to those done by previous mock measurements found an increase in ongoing clinical pregnancy rates when ultrasound was employed (OR 1.38, 95% CI 1.16–1.64). The authors comment that the overall study quality was poor with inadequate randomization and statistical techniques [74]. Other meta-analyses have come to similar conclusions in favor of ultrasound guidance [75]. *If feasible, it is therefore reasonable to perform ultrasound guided embryo transfers.* Despite the suggestion of improved ongoing pregnancy rates, some centers still rely on mock measurements with good success.

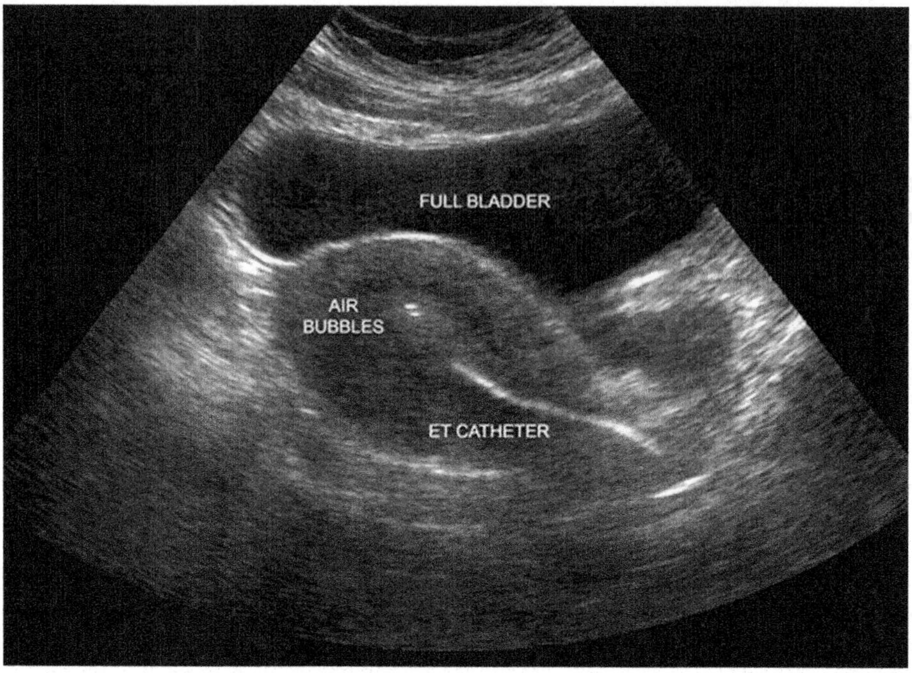

Fig. 4.4 Ultrasound image taken during an embryo transfer showing the eco-dense catheter tip depositing the embryos in the mid-fundal region of the uterus. A full bladder is useful to aid in visualization of the uterus with transabdominal ultrasound [39]

Difficult Transfers

Multiple studies have shown that transfers rated by the clinician as difficult result in lower pregnancy rates [43, 76, 77]. One large retrospective study of 4,800 embryo transfers employed a multivariate analysis and found higher pregnancy rates (OR 1.7, 95% CI 1.3–2.2) when transfers were classified as easy or intermediate as opposed to difficult, [77]. Typical descriptions of a difficult embryo transfer would include comments such as the transfer was time consuming, required changing to a rigid catheter, required the use of a tenaculum on the cervix, or required cervical dilation.

In addition to the aforementioned strategies to avoid difficult transfers (i.e., mock transfers, Malecot placement, ultrasound guidance), other techniques have been tested. One option that appears promising to avoid difficult transfers, is retaining the outer sheath of the catheter just past the internal os after the mock transfer and feeding the inner flexible catheter through the retained sheath. This is commonly referred to as afterloading. Neithardt and colleagues reported a retrospective series comparing the afterloading technique to "direct" transfer without afterloading. The implantation rate did not statistically differ, but the clinical pregnancy rate was noted to be higher in the afterloading group (59.4% versus 34.9%, $p=0.06$) [78]. This study is problematic in that they did not specify how providers decided which technique to use, or if one provider was responsible for all the afterloading procedures. It is known that pregnancy rates can vary between providers in the same program, and this alone could have accounted for the difference in pregnancy rates. It is however, a commonly adopted practice in cases where the mock transfer was noted to be difficult in order to minimize endometrial trauma and the time that the embryos are in the catheter and out of the incubator.

Other scenarios can also pose challenges to embryo transfer such as extreme uterine ante or retroflexion. We have found that placement of a vicryl suture on the anterior lip of the cervix at the time of oocyte retrieval can be useful. We typically place a 0 vicryl suture cut so that the tail is longer than the vaginal length. The excess suture is tucked into the vagina until embryo transfer, where it can be pulled gently to apply traction on the cervix and straighten the cervical canal. Patients generally do not feel cramping when this is done. This procedure allows cervical traction, straightening the utero-cervical junction and aids embryo transfer without requiring tenaculum placement at the time of transfer which can stimulate uterine contractions. After the transfer the suture tails are cut short and the stitch in the cervix is allowed to dissolve. An additional challenge that exists with a retroverted or retroflexed uterus is that abdominal ultrasound is less useful. Furthermore, the full bladder required to allow for proper uterine visualization can make the retroversion more pronounced. In these cases, a prior mock with "mapping" of the cervical canal is essential because the transfer must be done by feel and the depth of transfer is based on the prior measurement.

In cases where trans-cervical transfer is not possible due to refractory cervical stenosis, alternate methods have been described. Kato reported a case series of 104 cases with cervical stenosis that underwent transmyometrial transfer with vaginal ultrasound probe and a needle with a removable stylet. The stylet is used to position the needle and the transfer catheter is passed through the needle and into the uterus [79]. Alternatively, zygote intrafallopian tube (ZIFT) transfer can be done via laparoscopy. These techniques should be reserved for cases in which transcervical transfer is anatomically impossible or extremely difficult.

Removing the Catheter

After the embryos are deposited, pressure on the plunger should be maintained until the catheter is completely withdrawn from the cervix in order to avoid creating negative pressure. Studies have aimed to clarify if there is benefit to a time delay prior to withdrawal in an attempt to allow the embryos to move away from the catheter tip and avoid being dragged out of the spot of deposition. In a randomized trial of 100 women, no statistical benefit from seen between a 30-s delay and immediate withdrawal of the catheter. This study, however, did not report an appropriate power analysis in the trial, and there was a trend to improved pregnancy rates with the 30 s delay (60.8% in the immediate withdrawal and 69.4% in the 30-s delay group) [80]. Generally in our practice, we wait 30–60 s after deposition and then slowly withdraw the catheter.

Retained Embryos

Occasionally, inspection of the catheter by the embryologist after the transfer will reveal embryos which have stuck to the internal lumen of the catheter, often in cervical mucus. In this situation, the embryos should be immediately reloaded into the catheter and redeposited. If the catheter is coated internally with mucus the embryo(s) should be loaded into a fresh catheter. Early studies suggested lower pregnancy rates when embryos were retained [81], but these results have not been substantiated in subsequent studies [82]. Even though the pregnancy rate may not be affected, retained embryos can be a source of anxiety and distress for the patient, and therefore removal of cervical mucus in an attempt to minimize the risk of retained embryos is recommended as noted above.

Post Transfer Patient Activity

Traditionally, some period of bed rest or limited mobility was prescribed after embryo transfer. Indeed, some years ago many IVF programs would transport patients to the transfer procedure room in a stretcher and several hours of bed rest was carried out in the recovery room, followed by 24 h of bed rest at home. No support exists for such practices. In fact, prospective randomized trials comparing implantation and pregnancy rates between 1 and 24 h of bed rest and 30 min of bed rest versus immediate ambulation found no difference in pregnancy rates (21.5% versus 18.2%) and a lower implantation rate in the 24 h bed rest

Table 4.1 ASRM and SART recommended limits on the number of embryos to transfer. Favorable prognosis is defined as first cycle of IVF, good embryo quality, excess embryos available for cryopreservation, or previous successful IVF cycle (2009)

	Age			
Prognosis	<35 years	35–37 years	38–40 years	41–42 years
Cleavage-stage embryos				
Favorable	1–2	2	3	5
All others	2	3	4	5
Blastocysts				
Favorable	1	2	2	3
All others	2	2	3	3

group [83, 84]. Another prospective study in which patients were allowed to select immediate ambulation or a short period of bed rest similarly showed no benefit to bed rest with pregnancy rates being 24.6% and 21.3% respectively [85]. Therefore, most centers allow immediate ambulation or only a short period (less than 30 min) of rest prior to ambulation. Similarly, limited evidence suggests that intercourse around the time of embryo transfer does not negatively impact pregnancy rates. A multicenter randomized trial of 478 IVF cycles where participants were randomized to abstinence or intercourse found similar pregnancy rates of 21.2% and 23.6% respectively [86].

Number of Embryos to Transfer

Ideally, reproductive medicine providers would have the ability to select the most competent embryo and perform single embryo transfer in all patients, while maintaining an acceptable pregnancy rate. Unfortunately, this is currently not a reality. Strategies to screen embryos prior to transfer including aneuploidy screening with fluorescent in situ hybridization have not lead to increased pregnancy rates [87]. Currently, many programs culture embryos to the blastocyst stage to aid in embryo selection. Available data to date suggests that in good prognosis patients, culturing embryos to the blastocyst stage improves pregnancy rates [88] and minimizes high-order multiple rates [89]. Ongoing efforts to find the ideal technique for preimplantation genetic screening for anueploidy are ongoing [90].

The practice committee of the American Society for Reproductive Medicine (ASRM) and the Society for Assisted Reproductive Technology (SART) have published guidelines on the number of embryos to transfer in ART [91]. ESHRE has also published guidelines for good laboratory practice in IVF, strongly supporting a practice of single embryo transfer and discouraging the transfer of more than two embryos [92]. ASRM guidelines emphasize that treatment plans should be individualized and include patient age and embryo quality. They also encourage programs to generate internal data regarding pregnancy rates and multiple rates and regularly adjust algorithms for the number of embryos to transfer to optimize success and minimize complications. Table 4.1 summarizes these recommendations. It should be kept in mind that these are general recommendations, and patient preferences, the individual success of the program, ability for cryopreservation, embryo quality, and patient history may alter these recommendations. In addition, in some countries the number of embryos which may be cultured and/or transferred is under governmental regulation and local IVF practitioners must be cognizant of these laws.

Complications of Embryo Transfer: Ectopic Pregnancy

Patients undergoing embryo transfer may be at an increased risk for ectopic pregnancy—implantation at a site other than the endometrium of the uterine cavity, when compared to spontaneously conceived pregnancies. Studies examining the risk of ectopic pregnancy after ART have been inconsistent with the rate of ectopic pregnancy reported between 2.1 and 8.6% [93]. Retrospective studies of patient and cycle characteristics have attempted to identify risk factors in women undergoing ART to identify those who may be at higher risk. Tubal factor infertility has consistently been shown to be significantly associated with an increased risk for ectopic pregnancy [94, 95]. Additionally, zygote intrafallopian transfer (ZIFT) significantly increases the risk of ectopic pregnancy [95]. More recent data from the Society for Assisted Reproductive Technologies have reported an ectopic pregnancy risk after ART that is similar to the background risk in the population at between 1 and 2% (1.7% for IVF and 1.4% for ICSI). Those undergoing ZIFT remained at elevated risk for ectopic pregnancy (4.3%) [96]. An elevated risk of heterotopic pregnancy, defined as the simultaneous intrauterine and extrauterine implantation, has also been reported. The reported risk of heterotopic pregnancy after ART has ranged from 1.5 per 1,000 to 1 in 100, which greatly exceeds the background rate of 1 in 30,000 [97–100].

It is recommended that early pregnancy monitoring after ART follow strict protocols to identify potential abnormal early gestations and allow for early intervention of ectopic pregnancies with the goal of minimizing complications. Serial quantitative hCG monitoring every 2 days for 2–3 measurements is generally performed with the first value obtained between 10 and 16 days after the egg retrieval. The early rate of hCG rise in successful pregnancies has been well described [101]. The first ultrasound after ART is done to document intrauterine pregnancy location and rule out ectopic or heterotopic pregnancy and is generally performed between 5 and 6 weeks of gestational age. A repeat ultrasound to confirm ongoing embryo development and fetal heart rate should be performed 2–3 weeks later. Generally, a fetal heart rate of 100 or greater should be seen by 6 weeks of gestation [102].

In the ART population where pregnancy is highly desired, interventions such as endometrial curettage or presumed medical management of early ectopic pregnancy should only be undertaken when the suspicion for ectopic pregnancy is very high. Recent studies have documented that the initial rate of rise of hCG in healthy pregnancies may be lower than previously described and advocate multiple (more than 2) hCG data points prior to any intervention that may disrupt an intrauterine pregnancy in the asymptomatic patient with a pregnancy of undetermined location [103]. In clinical practice, hCG rises of ≤50% are followed with serial hCG and ultrasounds; if persistently low or abnormal rises are confirmed the patient is counseled regarding the risk of ectopic pregnancy and alerted to potential symptoms. Intervention is undertaken when hCG rises have been low over two measurements (or more) or are plateauing in the absence of ultrasound documentation of an intrauterine gestation. Declining hCGs can be managed expectantly with the patient alerted to signs and symptoms of ectopic pregnancy. Management of ectopic pregnancy when symptoms such as pain or intraperitoneal bleeding are present is surgical (salpingectomy or salpingostomy). Medical management with methotrexate is appropriate in patients with plateaued or increasing hCGs that are pain free and whose ectopic pregnancy is not large [104]. Established clinical protocols have been published and systematic reviews have compared the efficacy of various treatment protocols [105].

In the case of heterotopic pregnancy, systemic methotrexate cannot be used due to the risk of teratogenicity and/or disruption of the intrauterine gestation. Case reports of local surgical excision and KCl injection into the ectopic gestation have been reported in heterotopic pregnancies with the intrauterine pregnancy leading to a live birth [106, 107]. Ectopic pregnancies of unusual location such as cesarean scar or cervical implantations may also require additional therapies beyond methotrexate such as KCL injection into the gestational sac [108].

Summary and Conclusions

In conclusion, embryo transfer technique significantly impacts IVF success. Attention to careful and systematic technique can avoid difficult or traumatic transfers, which are associated with lower pregnancy rates. Evidence supports the performance of a mock transfer, use of soft-tipped catheter, transferring embryos in the mid-portion of the uterus, and using ultrasound guidance if any difficulty is anticipated or the uterine measurement is uncertain. Other techniques described above such as injection of air post-transfer, afterloading, and removal of cervical mucus may also provide benefit. Activity after embryo transfer appears to have no demonstrable on IVF outcome. In cases where a difficult transfer is anticipated, preparation in advance is helpful.

References

1. Deutinger J, Reinthaller A, Csaicsich P, Riss P, Fischl F, Bernaschek G, Muller-Tyl E. Follicular aspiration for in vitro fertilization: sonographically guided transvaginal versus laparoscopic approach. Eur J Obstet Gynecol Reprod Biol. 1987;26:127–33.
2. Seifer DB, Collins RL, Paushter DM, George CR, Quigley MM. Follicular aspiration: a comparison of an ultrasonic endovaginal transducer with fixed needle guide and other retrieval methods. Fertil Steril. 1988;49:462–7.
3. Lavy G, Restrepo-Candelo H, Diamond M, Shapiro B, Grunfeld L, Decherney AH. Laparoscopic and transvaginal ova recovery: the effect on ova quality. Fertil Steril. 1988;49:1002–6.
4. Fateh M, Ben-Rafael Z, Blasco L, Tureck RW, Meloni F, Mastroianni Jr L. Comparison of ultrasonographic transurethral and laparoscopic guided oocytes retrieval. Fertil Steril. 1986;46:653–6.
5. Ashkenazi J, Ben David M, Feldberg D, Shelef M, Dicker D, Goldman JA. Abdominal complications following ultrasonically guided percutaneous transvesical collection of oocytes for in vitro fertilization. J In Vitro Fert Embryo Transf. 1987;4:316–8.
6. Lavy G, Diamond MP, Nero F, Schark K, Decherney AH. Transvaginal and transabdominal ultrasound for monitoring of follicular development in an in vitro fertilization and embryo transfer program: patient response. J In Vitro Fert Embryo Transf. 1987;4:293–5.
7. O'Shea RT, Forbes KL, Scopacasa L, Jones WR. Comparison of transabdominal and transvaginal pelvic ultrasonography for ovarian follicle assessment in in vitro fertilisation. Gynecol Obstet Invest. 1988; 26:52–5.
8. Blumenfeld Z, Yoffe N, Bronshtein M. Transvaginal sonography in infertility and assisted reproduction. Obstet Gynecol Surv. 1991;46:36–49.
9. Wikland M, Enk L, Hamberger L. Transvesical and transvaginal approaches for the aspiration of follicles by use of ultrasound. Ann N Y Acad Sci. 1985;442: 182–94.
10. Wikland M, Enk L, Hammarberg K, Nilsson L. Use of a vaginal transducer for oocyte retrieval in an IVF/ET program. J Clin Ultrasound. 1987;15:245–51.
11. Ditkoff EC, Plumb J, Selick A, Sauer MV. Anesthesia practices in the United States common to in vitro fertilization (IVF) centers. J Assist Reprod Genet. 1997;14:145–7.
12. Vlahos NF, Giannakikou I, Vlachos A, Vitoratos N. Analgesia and anesthesia for assisted reproductive technologies. Int J Gynaecol Obstet. 2009;105:201–5.
13. Martin R, Tsen LC, Tzeng G, Hornstein MD, Datta S. Anesthesia for in vitro fertilization: the addition of fentanyl to 1.5% lidocaine. Anesth Analg. 1999;88:523–6.
14. Hammarberg K, Wikland M, Nilsson L, Enk L. Patients' experience of transvaginal follicle aspiration under local anesthesia. Ann N Y Acad Sci. 1988;541:134–7.
15. Christiaens F, Janssenswillen C, van Steirteghem AC, Devroey P, Verborgh C, Camu F. Comparison of assisted reproductive technology performance after oocyte retrieval under general anaesthesia (propofol) versus paracervical local anaesthetic block: a case-controlled study. Hum Reprod. 1998;13:2456–60.
16. Ben-Shlomo I, Moskovich R, Golan J, Eyali V, Tabak A, Shalev E. The effect of propofol anaesthesia on oocyte fertilization and early embryo quality. Hum Reprod. 2000;15:2197–9.
17. Gonen O, Shulman A, Ghetler Y, Shapiro A, Judeiken R, Beyth Y, Ben-Nun I. The impact of different types of anesthesia on in vitro fertilization-embryo transfer treatment outcome. J Assist Reprod Genet. 1995;12: 678–82.
18. Matt DW, Steingold KA, Dastvan CM, James CA, Dunwiddie W. Effects of sera from patients given various anesthetics on preimplantation mouse embryo development in vitro. J In Vitro Fert Embryo Transf. 1991;8:191–7.
19. Yuzpe AA, Brown SE, Casper RF, Nisker J, Graves G, Shatford L. Transvaginal, ultrasound-guided oocyte retrieval for in vitro fertilization. J Reprod Med. 1989;34:937–42.
20. Waterstone JJ, Parsons JH. A prospective study to investigate the value of flushing follicles during transvaginal ultrasound-directed follicle aspiration. Fertil Steril. 1992;57:221–3.
21. Wongtra-Ngan S, Vutyavanich T, Brown J. Follicular flushing during oocyte retrieval in assisted reproductive techniques. Cochrane Database Syst Rev. 2010:CD004634.
22. Tan SL, Waterstone J, Wren M, Parsons J. A prospective randomized study comparing aspiration only with aspiration and flushing for transvaginal ultrasound-directed oocyte recovery. Fertil Steril. 1992;58: 356–60.

23. Bennett SJ, Waterstone JJ, Cheng WC, Parsons J. Complications of transvaginal ultrasound-directed follicle aspiration: a review of 2670 consecutive procedures. J Assist Reprod Genet. 1993;10:72–7.
24. Kelada E, Ghani R. Bilateral ovarian abscesses following transvaginal oocyte retrieval for IVF: a case report and review of literature. J Assist Reprod Genet. 2007;24:143–5.
25. Egbase PE, Al-Sharhan M, Al-Othman S, Al-Mutawa M, Udo EE, Grudzinskas JG. Incidence of microbial growth from the tip of the embryo transfer catheter after embryo transfer in relation to clinical pregnancy rate following in-vitro fertilization and embryo transfer. Hum Reprod. 1996;11:1687–9.
26. Fanchin R, Harmas A, Benaoudia F, Lundkvist U, Olivennes F, Frydman R. Microbial flora of the cervix assessed at the time of embryo transfer adversely affects in vitro fertilization outcome. Fertil Steril. 1998;70:866–70.
27. Moore DE, Soules MR, Klein NA, Fujimoto VY, Agnew KJ, Eschenbach DA. Bacteria in the transfer catheter tip influence the live-birth rate after in vitro fertilization. Fertil Steril. 2000;74:1118–24.
28. Egbase PE, Udo EE, Al-Sharhan M, Grudzinskas JG. Prophylactic antibiotics and endocervical microbial inoculation of the endometrium at embryo transfer. Lancet. 1999;354:651–2.
29. Davis LB, Ginsburg ES. Transmyometrial oocyte retrieval and pregnancy rates. Fertil Steril. 2004;81: 320–2.
30. Damario MA. Transabdominal-transperitoneal ultrasound-guided oocyte retrieval in a patient with Mullerian agenesis. Fertil Steril. 2002;78:189–91.
31. Wood EG, Batzer FR, Corson SL. Ovarian response to gonadotrophins, optimal method for oocyte retrieval and pregnancy outcome in patients with vaginal agenesis. Hum Reprod. 1999;14:1178–81.
32. Steigrad S, Hacker NF, Kolb B. In vitro fertilization surrogate pregnancy in a patient who underwent radical hysterectomy followed by ovarian transposition, lower abdominal wall radiotherapy, and chemotherapy. Fertil Steril. 2005;83:1547–9.
33. Barton SE, Politch JA, Benson CB, Ginsburg ES, Gargiulo AR. Transabdominal follicular aspiration for oocyte retrieval in patients with ovaries inaccessible by transvaginal ultrasound. Fertil Steril. 2011;95: 1773–6.
34. Bergh T, Lundkvist O. Clinical complications during in-vitro fertilization treatment. Hum Reprod. 1992;7:625–6.
35. Ludwig AK, Glawatz M, Griesinger G, Diedrich K, Ludwig M. Perioperative and post-operative complications of transvaginal ultrasound-guided oocyte retrieval: prospective study of >1000 oocyte retrievals. Hum Reprod. 2006;21:3235–40.
36. Ragni G, Scarduelli C, Calanna G, Santi G, Benaglia L, Somigliana E. Blood loss during transvaginal oocyte retrieval. Gynecol Obstet Invest. 2009;67:32–5.
37. Karande VC, Morris R, Chapman C, Rinehart J, Gleicher N. Impact of the "physician factor" on pregnancy rates in a large assisted reproductive technology program: do too many cooks spoil the broth? Fertil Steril. 1999;71:1001–9.
38. Hearns-Stokes RM, Miller BT, Scott L, Creuss D, Chakraborty PK, Segars JH. Pregnancy rates after embryo transfer depend on the provider at embryo transfer. Fertil Steril. 2000;74:80–6.
39. Mains L, van Voorhis BJ. Optimizing the technique of embryo transfer. Fertil Steril. 2010;94:785–90.
40. Eskandar MA, Abou-Setta AM, El-Amin M, Almushait MA, Sobande AA. Removal of cervical mucus prior to embryo transfer improves pregnancy rates in women undergoing assisted reproduction. Reprod Biomed Online. 2007;14:308–13.
41. Visschers BA, Bots RS, Peeters MF, Mol BW, van Dessel HJ. Removal of cervical mucus: effect on pregnancy rates in IVF/ICSI. Reprod Biomed Online. 2007;15:310–5.
42. Brook N, Khalaf Y, Coomarasamy A, Edgeworth J, Braude P. A randomized controlled trial of prophylactic antibiotics (co-amoxiclav) prior to embryo transfer. Hum Reprod. 2006;21:2911–5.
43. Mansour R, Aboulghar M, Serour G. Dummy embryo transfer: a technique that minimizes the problems of embryo transfer and improves the pregnancy rate in human in vitro fertilization. Fertil Steril. 1990;54: 678–81.
44. Katariya KO, Bates GW, Robinson RD, Arthur NJ, Propst AM. Does the timing of mock embryo transfer affect in vitro fertilization implantation and pregnancy rates? Fertil Steril. 2007;88:1462–4.
45. Sharif K, Afnan M, Lenton W. Mock embryo transfer with a full bladder immediately before the real transfer for in-vitro fertilization treatment: the Birmingham experience of 113 cases. Hum Reprod. 1995;10:1715–8.
46. Abusheikha N, Lass A, Akagbosu F, Brinsden P. How useful is cervical dilatation in patients with cervical stenosis who are participating in an in vitro fertilization-embryo transfer program? The bourn hall experience. Fertil Steril. 1999;72:610–2.
47. Prapas N, Prapas Y, Panagiotidis Y, Prapa S, Vanderzwalmen P, Makedos G. Cervical dilatation has a positive impact on the outcome of IVF in randomly assigned cases having two previous difficult embryo transfers. Hum Reprod. 2004;19:1791–5.
48. Groutz A, Lessing JB, Wolf Y, Yovel I, Azem F, Amit A. Cervical dilatation during ovum pick-up in patients with cervical stenosis: effect on pregnancy outcome in an in vitro fertilization-embryo transfer program. Fertil Steril. 1997;67:909–11.
49. Yanushpolsky EH, Ginsburg ES, Fox JH, Stewart EA. Transcervical placement of a Malecot catheter after hysteroscopic evaluation provides for easier entry into the endometrial cavity for women with histories of difficult intrauterine inseminations and/or embryo transfers: a prospective case series. Fertil Steril. 2000;73:402–5.
50. Pabuccu R, Ceyhan ST, Onalan G, Goktolga U, Ercan CM, Selam B. Successful treatment of cervical

stenosis with hysteroscopic canalization before embryo transfer in patients undergoing IVF: a case series. J Minim Invasive Gynecol. 2005;12:436–8.
51. Serhal P, Ranieri DM, Khadum I, Wakim RA. Cervical dilatation with hygroscopic rods prior to ovarian stimulation facilitates embryo transfer. Hum Reprod. 2003;18:2618–20.
52. Glatstein IZ, Pang SC, McShane PM. Successful pregnancies with the use of laminaria tents before embryo transfer for refractory cervical stenosis. Fertil Steril. 1997;67:1172–4.
53. Choe JK, Nazari A, Check JH, Summers-Chase D, Swenson K. Marked improvement in clinical pregnancy rates following in vitro fertilization-embryo transfer seen when transfer technique and catheter were changed. Clin Exp Obstet Gynecol. 2001;28: 223–4.
54. Abou-Setta AM, Al-Inany HG, Mansour RT, Serour GI, Aboulghar MA. Soft versus firm embryo transfer catheters for assisted reproduction: a systematic review and meta-analysis. Hum Reprod. 2005;20:3114–21.
55. Goudas VT, Hammitt DG, Damario MA, Session DR, Singh AP, Dumesic DA. Blood on the embryo transfer catheter is associated with decreased rates of embryo implantation and clinical pregnancy with the use of in vitro fertilization-embryo transfer. Fertil Steril. 1998;70:878–82.
56. Fanchin R, Righini C, Olivennes F, Taylor S, de Ziegler D, Frydman R. Uterine contractions at the time of embryo transfer alter pregnancy rates after in-vitro fertilization. Hum Reprod. 1998;13:1968–74.
57. Saldeen P, Abou-Setta AM, Bergh T, Sundstrom P, Holte J. A prospective randomized controlled trial comparing two embryo transfer catheters in an ART program. Fertil Steril. 2008;90:599–603.
58. Allahbadia GN, Kadam K, Gandhi G, Arora S, Valliappan JB, Joshi A, Allahbadia S, Wolman I. Embryo transfer using the SureView catheter-beacon in the womb. Fertil Steril. 2010;93:344–50.
59. Abou-Setta AM. Air fluid versus fluid-only models of embryo catheter loading: a systematic review and meta-analysis. Reprod Biomed Online. 2007;14:80–4.
60. Moreno V, Balasch J, Vidal E, Calafell JM, Cívico S, Vanrell JA. Air in the transfer catheter does not affect the success of embryo transfer. Fertil Steril. 2004;81:1366–70.
61. Schoolcraft WB, Surrey ES, Gardner DK. Embryo transfer: techniques and variables affecting success. Fertil Steril. 2001;76:863–70.
62. Ebner T, Yaman C, Moser M, Sommergruber M, Pölz W, Tews G. The ineffective loading process of the embryo transfer catheter alters implantation and pregnancy rates. Fertil Steril. 2001;76:630–2.
63. Marcus SF, Brinsden PR. Analysis of the incidence and risk factors associated with ectopic pregnancy following in-vitro fertilization and embryo transfer. Hum Reprod. 1995;10:199–203.
64. Poindexter 3rd AN, Thompson DJ, Gibbons WE, Findley WE, Dodson MG, Young RL. Residual embryos in failed embryo transfer. Fertil Steril. 1986;46:262–7.
65. Mansour RT, Aboulghar MA, Serour GI, Amin YM. Dummy embryo transfer using methylene blue dye. Hum Reprod. 1994;9:1257–9.
66. Madani T, Ashrafi M, Jahangiri N, Abadi AB, Lankarani N. Improvement of pregnancy rate by modification of embryo transfer technique: a randomized clinical trial. Fertil Steril. 2010;94:2424–6.
67. Mansour R. Minimizing embryo expulsion after embryo transfer: a randomized controlled study. Hum Reprod. 2005;20:170–4.
68. Matorras R, Mendoza R, Exposito A, Rodriguez-Escudero FJ. Influence of the time interval between embryo catheter loading and discharging on the success of IVF. Hum Reprod. 2004;19:2027–30.
69. Nazari A, Askari HA, Check JH, O'Shaughnessy A. Embryo transfer technique as a cause of ectopic pregnancy in in vitro fertilization. Fertil Steril. 1993;60:919–21.
70. Coroleu B, Barri PN, Carreras O, Martinez F, Parriego M, Hereter L, Parera N, Veiga A, Balasch J. The influence of the depth of embryo replacement into the uterine cavity on implantation rates after IVF: a controlled, ultrasound-guided study. Hum Reprod. 2002;17:341–6.
71. van de Pas MM, Weima S, Looman CW, Broekmans FJ. The use of fixed distance embryo transfer after IVF/ICSI equalizes the success rates among physicians. Hum Reprod. 2003;18:774–80.
72. Pope CS, Cook EKD, Arny M, Novak A, Grow DR. Influence of embryo transfer depth on in vitro fertilization and embryo transfer outcomes. Fertil Steril. 2004;81:51–8.
73. Frankfurter D, Trimarchi JB, Silva CP, Keefe DL. Middle to lower uterine segment embryo transfer improves implantation and pregnancy rates compared with fundal embryo transfer. Fertil Steril. 2004;81: 1273–7.
74. Brown J, Buckingham K, Abou-Setta AM, Buckett W. Ultrasound versus 'clinical touch' for catheter guidance during embryo transfer in women. Cochrane Database Syst Rev. 2010:CD006107.
75. Abou-Setta AM, Mansour RT, Al-Inany HG, Aboulghar MM, Aboulghar MA, Serour GI. Among women undergoing embryo transfer, is the probability of pregnancy and live birth improved with ultrasound guidance over clinical touch alone? A systemic review and meta-analysis of prospective randomized trials. Fertil Steril. 2007;88:333–41.
76. Lass A, Abusheikha N, Brinsden P, Kovacs GT. The effect of a difficult embryo transfer on the outcome of IVF. Hum Reprod. 1999;14:2417.
77. Tomas C, Tikkinen K, Tuomivaara L, Tapanainen JS, Martikainen H. The degree of difficulty of embryo transfer is an independent factor for predicting pregnancy. Hum Reprod. 2002;17:2632–5.
78. Neithardt AB, Segars JH, Hennessy S, James AN, McKeeby JL. Embryo afterloading: a refinement in

embryo transfer technique that may increase clinical pregnancy. Fertil Steril. 2005;83:710–4.
79. Kato O, Takatsuka R, Asch RH. Transvaginal-transmyometrial embryo transfer: the Towako method; experiences of 104 cases. Fertil Steril. 1993; 59:51–3.
80. Martinez F, Coroleu B, Parriego M, Carreras O, Belil I, Parera N, Hereter L, Buxaderas R, Barri PN. Ultrasound-guided embryo transfer: immediate withdrawal of the catheter versus a 30 second wait. Hum Reprod. 2001;16:871–4.
81. Visser DS, Fourie FL, Kruger HF. Multiple attempts at embryo transfer: effect on pregnancy outcome in an in vitro fertilization and embryo transfer program. J Assist Reprod Genet. 1993;10:37–43.
82. Nabi A, Awonuga A, Birch H, Barlow S, Stewart B. Multiple attempts at embryo transfer: does this affect in-vitro fertilization treatment outcome? Hum Reprod. 1997;12:1188–90.
83. Amarin ZO, Obeidat BR. Bed rest versus free mobilisation following embryo transfer: a prospective randomised study. BJOG. 2004;111:1273–6.
84. Purcell KJ, Schembri M, Telles TL, Fujimoto VY, Cedars MI. Bed rest after embryo transfer: a randomized controlled trial. Fertil Steril. 2007;87:1322–6.
85. Bar-Hava I, Kerner R, Yoeli R, Ashkenazi J, Shalev Y, Orvieto R. Immediate ambulation after embryo transfer: a prospective study. Fertil Steril. 2005; 83:594–7.
86. Tremellen KP, Valbuena D, Landeras J, Ballesteros A, Martinez J, Mendoza S, Norman RJ, Robertson SA, Simon C. The effect of intercourse on pregnancy rates during assisted human reproduction. Hum Reprod. 2000;15:2653–8.
87. Mastenbroek S, Twisk M, Van Echten-Arends J, Sikkema-Raddatz B, Korevaar JC, Verhoeve HR, Vogel NE, Arts EG, de Vries JW, Bossuyt PM, Buys CH, Heineman MJ, Repping S, van der Veen F. In vitro fertilization with preimplantation genetic screening. N Engl J Med. 2007;357:9–17.
88. Blake DA, Farquhar CM, Johnson N, Proctor M. Cleavage stage versus blastocyst stage embryo transfer in assisted conception. Cochrane Database Syst Rev. 2007:CD002118.
89. Grifo JA, Flisser E, Adler A, McCaffrey C, Krey LC, Licciardi F, Noyes N, Kump LM, Berkeley AS. Programmatic implementation of blastocyst transfer in a university-based in vitro fertilization clinic: maximizing pregnancy rates and minimizing triplet rates. Fertil Steril. 2007;88:294–300.
90. Schoolcraft WB, Treff NR, Stevens JM, Ferry K, Katz-Jaffe M, Scott Jr RT. Live birth outcome with trophectoderm biopsy, blastocyst vitrification, and single-nucleotide polymorphism microarray-based comprehensive chromosome screening in infertile patients. Fertil Steril. 2011;96:638–40.
91. Practice Committee of Society for Assisted Reproductive Technology, Practice Committee of American Society for Reproductive Medicine. Guidelines on number of embryos transferred. Fertil Steril. 2009;92:1518–9.
92. Magli MC, van den Abbeel E, Lundin K, Royere D, van der Elst J, Gianaroli L. Revised guidelines for good practice in IVF laboratories. Hum Reprod. 2008;23:1253–62.
93. Chang HJ, Suh CS. Ectopic pregnancy after assisted reproductive technology: what are the risk factors? Curr Opin Obstet Gynecol. 2010;22:202–7.
94. Strandell A, Thorburn J, Hamberger L. Risk factors for ectopic pregnancy in assisted reproduction. Fertil Steril. 1999;71:282–6.
95. Clayton HB, Schieve LA, Peterson HB, Jamieson DJ, Reynolds MA, Wright VC. Ectopic pregnancy risk with assisted reproductive technology procedures. Obstet Gynecol. 2006;107:595–604.
96. Society for Assisted Reproductive Technology, American Society for Reproductive Medicine. Assisted reproductive technology in the United States: 2001 results generated from the American Society for Reproductive Medicine/Society for Assisted Reproductive Technology registry. Fertil Steril. 2007;87:1253–66.
97. Mantzavinos T, Kanakas N, Zourlas PA. Heterotopic pregnancies in an in-vitro fertilization program. Clin Exp Obstet Gynecol. 1996;23:205–8.
98. Svare J, Norup P, Grove Thomsen S, Hornnes P, Maigaard S, Helm P, Petersen K, Nyboe Andersen A. Heterotopic pregnancies after in-vitro fertilization and embryo transfer—a Danish survey. Hum Reprod. 1993;8:116–8.
99. Reece EA, Petrie RH, Sirmans MF, Finster M, Todd WD. Combined intrauterine and extrauterine gestations: a review. Am J Obstet Gynecol. 1983;146: 323–30.
100. Clayton HB, Schieve LA, Peterson HB, Jamieson DJ, Reynolds MA, Wright VC. A comparison of heterotopic and intrauterine-only pregnancy outcomes after assisted reproductive technologies in the United States from 1999 to 2002. Fertil Steril. 2007;87: 303–9.
101. Barnhart KT, Sammel MD, Rinaudo PF, Zhou L, Hummel AC, Guo W. Symptomatic patients with an early viable intrauterine pregnancy: HCG curves redefined. Obstet Gynecol. 2004;104:50–5.
102. Doubilet PM, Benson CB. Outcome of first-trimester pregnancies with slow embryonic heart rate at 6–7 weeks gestation and normal heart rate by 8 weeks at US. Radiology. 2005;236:643–6.
103. Morse CB, Sammel MD, Shaunik A, Allen-Taylor L, Oberfoell NL, Takacs P, Chung K, Barnhart KT. Performance of human chorionic gonadotropin curves in women at risk for ectopic pregnancy: exceptions to the rules. Fertil Steril. 2012;97(101–6):e2.
104. Bachman EA, Barnhart K. Medical management of ectopic pregnancy: a comparison of regimens. Clin Obstet Gynecol. 2012;55:440–7.
105. Hajenius PJ, Mol F, Mol BW, Bossuyt PM, Ankum WM, van der Veen F. Interventions for tubal ectopic pregnancy. Cochrane Database Syst Rev. 2007: CD000324.
106. Sills ES, Perloe M, Kaplan CR, Sweitzer CL, Morton PC, Tucker MJ. Uncomplicated pregnancy and normal

singleton delivery after surgical excision of heterotopic (cornual) pregnancy following in vitro fertilization/embryo transfer. Arch Gynecol Obstet. 2002;266:181–4.
107. Wang CN, Chen CK, Wang HS, Chiueh HY, Soong YK. Successful management of heterotopic cesarean scar pregnancy combined with intrauterine pregnancy after in vitro fertilization-embryo transfer. Fertil Steril. 2007;88(706):e13–6.
108. Doubilet PM, Benson CB, Frates MC, Ginsburg E. Sonographically guided minimally invasive treatment of unusual ectopic pregnancies. J Ultrasound Med. 2004;23:359–70.

Moving Toward Single Embryo Transfer

5

Kevin S. Richter, Robert J. Stillman, and Eric A. Widra

Introduction

Since 1998, SET has been advocated as the only truly effective means by which to avoid multiple pregnancy in IVF cycles [1]. Since then, numerous publications have investigated and promoted the practice of elective single embryo transfer (eSET) [1–6] including a comprehensive Practice Committee Opinion from the Society for Reproductive Technology and the American Society of Reproductive Medicine Practice in 2012 [7]. However, throughout the three-decade history of IVF treatment, eSET has been the exception, rather than the norm. In order to compensate for low rates of implantation for individual embryos and achieve "acceptable" pregnancy rates, multiple embryos have been routinely transferred in the vast majority of patients undertaking IVF in the USA and most other countries. Consequently, IVF as generally practiced, carries a high risk of multiple pregnancy and its associated adverse effects on mother and child. There are numerous issues that must be addressed in order to maximize the efficacy of eSET and to improve its acceptability and utilization among clinicians and patients.

K.S. Richter, Ph.D. (✉) • R.J. Stillman, M.D.
Shady Grove Fertility Reproductive Science Center, 15001 Shady Grove Road, Suite 340, Rockville, MD 20850, USA
e-mail: Kevin.richter@integramed.com; Robert.stillman@integramed.com

E.A. Widra, M.D.
Shady Grove Fertility Reproductive Science Center, Washington, DC 20006, USA
e-mail: widra@georgetown.edu

Changing Policy and Practice

In the year 2000, more than two-thirds of all embryo transfers performed in the United Sates were of three or more embryos. Practice guidelines from the Society for Assisted Reproductive Technology (SART) and the American Society for Reproductive Medicine (ASRM) were published in 2004 and revised in 2009 [8]. In 2004, a maximum of two embryos was recommended for transfer in women 35 and younger, but in 2006 this was strengthened to a maximum of one embryo in women <35 year of favorable prognosis if blastocyst transfer (having a higher implantation rate) was performed, and additional recommendations now include patients with embryos to cryopreserve. From 1999 to 2008, the proportion of transfers with three or more embryos declined from 70 to 39%, with transfers of four or more embryos declining from 36 to 14%. However, the proportion of double embryo transfers increased from 23% in 1999 to 50% in 2008. The proportion of single embryo transfers also doubled from 6 to 12%. It must be noted, however, that prior to 2002 almost all single embryo transfers were nonelective (i.e., cycles in which only one embryo was available). Therefore the increase in single embryo transfers was

E.S. Ginsburg and C. Racowsky (eds.), *In Vitro Fertilization: A Comprehensive Guide*,
DOI 10.1007/978-1-4419-9848-4_5, © Springer Science+Business Media New York 2012

Table 5.1 ART outcomes 2003 through 2010

	2003	2004	2005	2006	2007	2008	2009	2010
Live birth rate/cycle (%)	37.5	36.6	37.1	38.8	39.9	41.3	41.4	41.7
Twin live birth rate (%)	33.5	32.7	33	32.3	32.9	33.3	32.9	32.4
Triplet live birth rate (%)	6.4	4.9	4.3	2	1.8	1.9	1.6	1.5
Average embryos transferred (*n*)	2.6	2.5	2.4	2.3	2.2	2.2	2.1	2
eSET (%)	0.7	1.2	2.1	3.3	4.5	5.2	7.9	9.6

Adapted from www.sart.org

mainly due to increases in elective SET. As shown in Table 5.1, the percentage of cycles with eSET rose from 0.7 in 2003 to 9.6 in 2010.

The USA has lagged behind much of the world with regard to eSET, only in part due to legislation restricting the number of embryos that may be cultured and transferred in other countries [9]. In 2007, 21% of cycles reported to ESHRE (the European Society of Human Reproduction and Embryology) had transfer of a single embryo [10].

Efficacy of Single Embryo Transfer

The largest single randomized trial comparing double to single embryo transfer was published by Thurin et al. in 2004 [3]. This was a blinded multi-center trial in 11 Swedish clinics which randomized 661 women to double or single embryo transfer. Subjects were ≤ 36 years old, on their first or second IVF attempt, and had at least two good quality embryos on day 2 or 3. Subjects randomized to the eSET group who did not have live birth from their fresh cycle underwent a subsequent transfer of a single thawed embryo. Therefore the maximum number of embryos transferred to each group was two. Birth rates were significantly lower following fresh transfer of one versus two embryos (28% vs. 43%, RR 0.64). However, when delivery from the frozen transfer was included, live birth rates in the 1 fresh +1 thawed group was 38%, which was not significantly different from that following double transfer of fresh embryos (43%, RR 0.90, $p=0.30$). Several other randomized controlled trials have compared birth rates between transfers of one versus two embryos and these have been reviewed in a Cochrane Review [11] and two meta-analyses [12, 13]. These showed similar results, with live birth rates of 26 and 42–43% with single and double embryo transfer respectively, with all but one included study employing cleavage-stage transfer. Gardner et al. [2] randomized patients to blastocyst transfer of one or two embryos on day 5, with ongoing pregnancy rates of 61% vs. 76% RR = 0.80; this result was likely not significant due to small sample size. The twin pregnancy rate in the double embryo transfer group was 47%. These results are similar to observational data reported from a large clinical practice performing blastocyst eSET in women <37 year over a 6-year period. The live birth rate with eSET was 56% vs. 54% for double embryo transfer, with a twinning rate of 44% in the double embryo transfer group [14]. Considering all studies, it is clear that the twining rate is over tenfold higher after transfer of two versus one embryo in good prognosis patients; the twining rate after single embryo transfer is very low, and due to monochorionic twinning.

In current clinical practice, eSET is reported by SART. Table 5.1 and Fig. 5.1 show data reflecting current practice and outcomes in the USA.

The Importance of Avoiding Multiple Pregnancy

The proportion of ART births that were multiple births in women <35 dropped somewhat from 39.9 to 33.9% over the last 8 years. Although

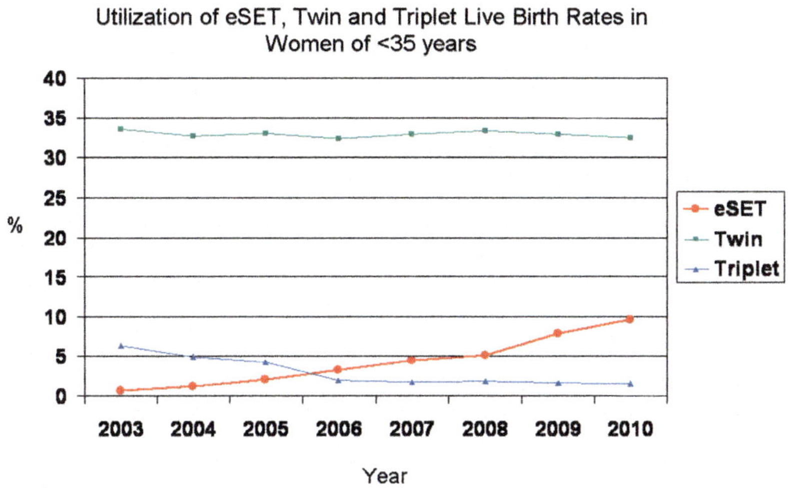

Fig. 5.1 Utilization of eSET, twin, and triplet live birth rates in women of <35 years. Adapted from www.sart.org

the rate of triplets decreased from 6.4 to 1.5%, the percentage of twin live births was essentially unchanged at 33.5 to 32.4% (Fig. 5.1) despite increases in eSET and an overall reduction in the average number of embryos transferred (Table 5.1). There is no debate about the fact that triplets are high-risk pregnancies and should be avoided, but there is more debate about the relative desirability of twin pregnancies. Natural twinning occurs in approximately 1% of all births, and the majority of twins born in the USA are therefore not from IVF treatment. However, IVF and other ovarian stimulation medications have notably increased the incidence of multiple births.

Maternal complications during pregnancy and delivery are higher with multiple pregnancy [15]. Mortality rates are two to three times higher with multiple compared to singleton pregnancies [16–18]. Serious complications include gestational diabetes [19], gestational hypertension [20, 21] preeclampsia [22] and eclampsia [23] which are two to three times higher with twins. Risks are almost doubled for post-partum hemorrhage, thromboembolism, pulmonary embolism, stroke, more than tripled risk of myocardial infarction, sevenfold increased in pulmonary edema, and 13-fold increase in heart failure [17, 24]. Rates of cesarian delivery [25, 26] and hysterectomy [27] are also three or more times higher, and overall the costs of multiple pregnancies are much higher [24].

Fetal and neonatal risk increase dramatically with twin pregnancies. The average gestational age of twins at birth is three and a half weeks less than singletons, and average birth weight is 30% lower [28]. The risk of low birth weight (<2500 g) is six times greater, very low birth weight (<1500 g) is five times greater, and preterm birth (<37 weeks) is more than four times greater for ART twins compared to ART singletons [29]. Two-thirds of all ART twins are born preterm, and the majority (57%) suffer from low birth weight, and 9% from very low birth weight [28]. Fetal mortality [30] is also higher than for singletons, and stillbirths [31] are more than twice as frequent. Neonatal mortality is six times higher for twins [32] and infant mortality [30] is five times higher. The risks of a wide range of congenital malformations including hydrocephaly, anencephaly, neural tube defects, cardiovascular, urogenital, gastrointestinal, and musculoskeletal malformations are increased in twins, with most relative risks being between 1.5 and 3 [33, 34]. In addition to these immediate risks, surviving infants are at increased risk of long-term medical and developmental problems. Compared to singletons, twins are 70% more likely to have a severe handicap, five times more likely to be diagnosed with cerebral palsy [29, 35, 36] and have impaired language [37] and cognitive development [38], and impaired academic [39, 40] and social behavior [41].

Other issues related to twin, and other multiple births are the increased stresses on the parents. Mothers of twins have more anxiety, depression, and fatigue, even after the infancy period is over and fathers have more depression, anxiety, social dysfunction, and sleeping difficulties [42].

There is also evidence that the transfer of multiple embryos may result in adverse outcomes even when a singleton live birth occurs. Singletons resulting from transfer of one embryo versus two are less likely to be premature and have low birth weight [43, 44]. It has been hypothesized that this is related to the effect of vanishing twins on the development of the surviving fetus. Rates of preterm birth and low birth weight among singletons were significantly higher when more than one heartbeat was observed on early ultrasound examination [43].

Indications for Single Embryo Transfer

Medical Indications

It is prudent to recommend single embryo transfer for patients with medical conditions which make them at particularly high risk if carrying a twin gestation, such as patients with comorbidities such as diabetes, hypertension, obesity, congenital uterine anomalies, history of premature delivery, or cervical incompetence.

Elective Indications

Elective SET is recommended by ASRM guidelines in patients <35 with favorable prognosis, i.e., first cycle, good quality embryos, excess embryos for cryopreservation and history of IVF success [8]. This may be a conservative recommendation. Jungheim et al. reported a 54% delivery rate for patients requested eSET despite only 15% of these cycles meeting ASRM guidelines for eSET [45]. A Belgian study found only a slight decrease in pregnancy rates per transfer (27.4% vs. 30.7%) after more than tripling their use of single embryo transfer to account for well over half of all cycles [46]. In another study the cumulative pregnancy rate per oocyte retrieval, including transfers of cryopreserved embryos, reportedly did not decline even after expanding the use of single embryo transfer to more than 90% of all ART cycles [47].

The primary indication for elective single embryo transfer is the availability of good to excellent quality embryos with high implantation potential. Single embryo transfer is most applicable to transfers of blastocyst-stage embryos on day 5 or 6 after oocyte retrieval, as blastocysts tend to have higher rates of implantation than cleavage-stage embryos [48, 49]. Morphologically top-quality blastocysts (those expanding by day 5 after oocyte retrieval with a high-quality inner cell mass and trophectoderm) may implant at rates of 70% or greater [50, 51]. Triplet pregnancy rates of 2% have been reported for double blastocyst transfers [14], indicating the risk of high order multiple pregnancy after monochorionic twinning. High-quality cleavage-stage embryos (7 or 8 cells with no multinucleation and minimal fragmentation) may implant at rates of 50% or more [52]. Clearly young patients, and women using donor oocytes, will be at highest risk of multiple gestation with transfer of two high-quality embryos. Indeed, there is clear age-related decline in twin rate when two embryos are transferred (Table 5.2).

Physician and Staff Education

One component necessary to expand the utilization of eSET is education of treating physicians and staff. Clinicians are often reluctant to encourage eSET out of concerns that pregnancy rates will suffer as a result [53]. All members of the team including physicians, embryologists and nurses must be aware that the literature

Table 5.2 Multiple pregnancy rates by maternal age

	<35	35–37	38–40	41–42	≥43
Average No. Embryos Transferred	2	2.2	2.6	3.0	3.1
Twin Live Birth Rate (%)	32.5	27.2	22.1	16.9	9.6
Triplet Live Birth Rate (%)	1.5	1.5	1.1	1.1	0.9

Data taken from the SART CORS reporting system: www.sart.org

demonstrates that high pregnancy rates can be maintained while increasing the health of the resulting children by performing eSET in good prognosis patients.

Patient Education

Patient education is vital for encouraging eSET, and presents a particular challenge. Not only are patients understandably concerned about potential reductions in pregnancy rates with only one embryo transferred, but numerous studies have found that the majority of patients prefer twin pregnancies over singleton pregnancies for a variety of reasons [54, 55]. Such attitudes may be largely due to misconceptions that underestimate the efficacy of eSET and the risks and health consequences associated with multiple pregnancy. Increased education has been shown to make eSET a more acceptable option to patients. When both male and female patients are educated regarding relative risks of pre-eclampsia, low birth weight, postpartum depression, the desire for twin pregnancy declined and eSET became the preferred option [56, 57]. Providing patients with educational material that contains a written description of the advantages of eSET has been shown to increase patient acceptance and triple use [58].

Reducing Financial Incentives

The prospect of limiting the number of high-cost IVF attempts may be an incentive to transfer more than one embryo and risk multiple pregnancy [55]. Educating patients about both the risks and costs of carrying a multiple pregnancy, and the increased risk of loss of work may assist in patient education. Long-term costs to society of multiple pregnancy, which includes both neonatal hospital care as well as care for long-term medical needs are clear. Insurance coverage for IVF treatment has been shown to reduce the number of embryos transferred [59]. Shared-risk programs, where good prognosis patients pay a fixed fee, with a guaranteed refund if treatment does not result in live birth, may increase patient acceptance of eSET [60].

Importance of the IVF Laboratory in eSET

It is critical that the IVF laboratory and embryologists are able to culture embryos successfully, and effectively grade and select the "best" embryo for transfer. In addition, an excellent cryopreservation program is essential in order to maximize the delivery rate per ovarian stimulation when eSET is employed. Embryo culture and grading are described in Chap. 7, and cryopreservation technology is discussed in Chap. 10.

Conclusions

Randomized controlled trials have demonstrated that birth rates are significantly higher with the transfer of two versus one embryo at the costs of much higher rates of multiple pregnancy. Twin pregnancies are associated with significantly increased risks of adverse outcomes and a large increase in financial costs. The only effective means of preventing multiple pregnancy in ART is to perform SET. eSET has been proven to be highly effective among appropriately selected patients; cumulative pregnancy rates per retrieval including transfers of cryopreserved embryos can be equivalent or higher for single compared to double embryo transfers. The primary indication for eSET is the availability of two or more high-quality embryos, particularly for blastocyst-stage transfer. Due to the high implantation potential of embryos derived from donor oocytes, single embryo transfer should be encouraged in donor oocyte cycles, unless embryo quality is poor. eSET should be the primary recommendation for younger women with good embryo quality and no history of repeated failed cycles despite good embryo quality. eSET should be offered to women as old as 40 years particularly if high-quality blastocyts are available and/or the couple has had a previous IVF or naturally conceived pregnancy.

References

1. Coetsier T, Dhont M. Avoiding multiple prengnancies in in-vitro fertilization; who's afraid of single embryo transfer? Hum Reprod. 1998;13:2663–4.
2. Gardner DK, Surrey E, Minjarez D, Leitz A, Stevens J, Schoolcraft WB. Single blastocyst transfer: a prospective randomized trial. Fertil Steril. 2004;81:551–5.
3. Thurin A, Hausken J, Hillensjo T, Jablonowska B, Pinborg A, Strandell A, et al. Elective single embryo transfer versus double embryo transfer in in-vitro fertilization. N Engl J Med. 2004;351:2392–402.
4. Lukassen HG, Braat DD, Wetzels AM, Zielhuis GA, Adang EM, Scheenjes E, et al. Two cycles with single embryo transfer versus one cycle with double embryo transfer: a randomized controlled trial. Hum Reprod. 2005;20:702–8.
5. Ryan GL, Sparks AE, Sipe CS, Syrop CH, Dokras A, Van Voorhis BJ. A mandatory single blastocyst transfer policy with educational campaign in a United States IVF program reduces multiple gestation rates without sacrificing pregnancy rates. Fertil Steril. 2007;88:354–60.
6. Devroey P, Pellicer A, Nyboe Andersen A, Arce JC. A randomized assessor-blind trial comparing highly purified hMG and recombinant FSH in a GnRH antagonist cycle with compulsory single-blastocyst transfer. Menopur in GnRH antagonist cycles with single embryo transfer trial group. Fertil Steril. 2012;97:561–71.
7. Practice Committee of the Society for Assisted Reproductive Technology and the American Society for Reproductive Medicine. Elective single embryo transfer. Fertil Steril. 2012;97:835–42.
8. Practice committee of the American Society for Reproductive Medicine and the Society for Assisted Reproductive Technology. Guidelines on number of embryos transferred. Fertil Steril. 2009;92:1518–9.
9. Maheshwari A, Griffiths S, Bhattacharya S. Global variations in the uptake of single embryo transfer. Hum Reprod Update. 2011;17:107–20.
10. de Mouzon J, Goossens V, Bhattacharya S, Castilla JA, Ferraretti AP, Korsak V, Kupka M, Nygren KG, Andersen AN, European IVF-Monitoring (EIM), Consortium for the European Society on Human Reproduction and Embryology (ESHRE). Assisted reproductive technology in Europe, 2007: results generated from European registers by ESHRE. Hum Reprod. 2012;27:954–66.
11. Pandian Z, Battacharya S, Ozturk O, Serour G, Templeton A. Number of embryos for transfer following in-vitro fertilization or intra-cytoplasmic sperm injection. Cochrane Database Syst Rev. 2009;CD003416
12. Gelbaya TA, Tsoumpou I, Nardo LG. The likelihood of live birth and multiple birth after single versus double embryo transfer at the cleavage stage: a systemic review and meta-analysis. Fertil Steril. 2010;94:936–45.
13. McLernon DJ, Harrild K, Bergh C, Davies MJ, de Neubourg D, Dumoulin JC, et al. Clinical effectiveness of elective single versus double embryo transfer: a metanalysis of individual patient data from randomised trials. BMJ. 2010;341:c6945.
14. Stillman RJ, Richter KS, Banks NK, Graham JR. Elective single embryo transfer: a 6 year progressive implementation of 784 single blastocyst transfers and the influence of payment method on patient choice. Fertil Steril. 2009;92:1895–906.
15. Practice Committee of the American Society for Reproductive Medicine. Multiple gestation associated with infertility therapy: an American Society for Reproductive Medicine Practice Committee opinion. Fertil Steril. 2012;97:825–34.
16. Senat MV, Ancel PY, Bouvier-Colle MH, Breart G. How does multiple pregnancy affect maternal mortality and morbidity? Clin Obstet Gynecol. 1998;41:78–83.
17. Conde-Agudelo A, Belizan JM, Lindmark G. Maternal morbidity and mortality associated with multiple gestations. Obstet Gynecol. 2000;95:899–904.
18. Walker MC, Murphy KE, Pan S, Yang Q, Wen SW. Adverse maternal outcomes in multifetal pregnancies. BJOG. 2004;111:1294–6.
19. Schwartz DB, Daoud Y, Zazula P, Goyert G, Bronsteen R, Wright D, et al. Gestational diabetes mellitus: metabolic and blood glucose parameters in singleton versus twin pregnancies. Am J Obstet Gynecol. 1999;181:912–4.
20. Day MC, Barton JR, O'Brien JM, Istwan NB, Sibai BM. The effect of fetal number on the development of hypertensive conditions of pregnancy. Obstet Gynecol. 2005;106:927–31.
21. Hernandez-Diaz S, Werler MM, Mitchell AA. Gestational hypertension in pregnancies supported by

infertility treatments: role of infertility, treatments, and multiple gestations. Fertil Steril. 2007;88:438–45.
22. Sibai GM, Hauth J, Caritis S, Lindheimer MD, MacPherson C, Klebanoff M, et al. Hypertensive disorders in twin versus singleton gestations. National Institute of Child Health and Human Development Network of Maternal-Fetal Medicine Units. Am J Obstet Gynecol. 2000;182:938–42.
23. Krotz S, Fajardo J, Ghandi S, Patel A, Keith LG. Hypertensive disease in twin pregnancies: a review. Twin Res. 2002;5:8–14.
24. Ros HS, Lichtenstein P, Bellocco R, Petersson G, Cnattingius S. Pulmonary embolism and stroke in relation to pregnancy: how can high-risk women be identified? Am J Obstet Gynecol. 2002;186: 198–203.
25. Collins J. Cost efficiency of reducing multiple births. Reprod Biomed Online. 2007;15 Suppl 3:35–9.
26. Pinborg A, Loft A, Nyboe Andersen A. Neonatal outcome in a Danish national cohort of 8602 children born after in vitro fertilization or intracytoplasmic sperm injection: the role of twin pregnancy. Acta Obstet Gynecol Scand. 2004;83:1071–8.
27. Francois K, Ortiz J, Harris C, Foley MR, Elliott JP. Is peripartum hysterectomy more common in multiple gestations? Obstet Gynecol. 2005;105:1369–72.
28. Martin JA, Hamilton BE, Sutton PD, Ventura SJ, Menacker F, Kirmeyer S, et al. Births: final data for 2006. Natl Vital Stat Rep. 2009;57:1–102.
29. Wright VC, Chang J, Jeng G, Macaluso M. Assisted reproductive technology surveillance—United States, 2005. MMWR Surveill Summ. 2008;57:1–23.
30. Scher AI, Petterson B, Blair E, Ellenberg JH, Grether JK, Haan E, et al. The risk of mortality or cerebral palsy in twins: a collaborative population-based study. Pediatr Res. 2002;52:671–81.
31. Doyle P. The outcome of multiple pregnancy. Hum Reprod. 1996;11 Suppl 4:110–7.
32. Alexander GR, Slay Wingate M, Salihu H, Kirby RS. Fetal and neonatal mortality risks of multiple births. Obstet Gynecol Clin North Am. 2005;32:1–16. vii.
33. Doyle PE, Beral V, Botting B, Wale CJ. Congenital malformation I twins in England and Wales. J Epidemiol Community Health. 1991;45:43–8.
34. Mastroiacovo P, Castilla EE, Arpino C, Botting B, Cocchi G, Goujard J, et al. Congenital malformations in twins: an internationals study. Am J Med Genet. 1999;83:117–24.
35. Petterson B, Nelson KB, Watson L, Stanley F. Twins, triplets, and cerebral palsy in births in Western Australia in the 1980s. BMJ. 1993;307:1239–43.
36. O'Callaghan ME, MacLennan AH, Gibson CS, McMichael GL, Haan EA, Broadbent JL, Goldwater PN, Dekker GA, Australian Collaborative Cerebral Palsy Research Group. Epidemiologic associations with cerebral palsy. Obstet Gynecol. 2011;118(3): 576–82.
37. Hay DA, Prior M, Collett S, Williams M. Speech and language development in preschool twins: implications for development. Twin Res. 2000;3:234–41.
38. Deary IJ, Pattie A, Wilson V, Whalley LJ. The cognitive cost of being a twin: two whole-population surveys. Twin Res Hum Genet. 2005;8:376–83.
39. Tsou MT, Tsou MW, Wu MP, Liu JT. Academic achievement of twins and singletons in early adulthood: Taiwanese cohort study. BMJ. 2008;337:a438.
40. Voracek M, Haubner T. Twin-singleton difference in intelligence: a meta-analysis. Psychol Rep. 2008;102: 951–62.
41. Di Lalla LF. Social development of twins. Twin Res Hum Genet. 2006;9:95–102.
42. Vilska S, Unkila-Kallio L, Punamäki RL, Poikkeus P, Repokari L, Sinkkonen J, Tiitinen A, Tulppala M. Mental health of mothers and fathers of twins conceived via assisted reproduction treatment: a 1-year prospective study. Hum Reprod. 2009;24(2):367–77.
43. Weng YA, Sullivan EA, Healy DL, Black DA. Perinatal outcomes after assisted reproductive technology treatment in Australia and New Zealand: single versus double embryo transfer. Med J Aust. 2009;190:234–7.
44. Luke B, Brown MB, Grainger DA, Stern JE, Klein N, Cedars MI. The effect of early fetal losses on singleton assisted-conception pregnancy outcomes. Fertil Steril. 2009;91:2578–85.
45. Jungheim ES, Ratts VS, Change AS, Moley KH, Lazendorf SE, Odem RR. Encouraging patient-driven single-embryo-transfer. Fertil Steril. 2008;90: 1266–8.
46. Van Landuyt L, Verheyen G, Tournaye H, Camus M, Devroey P, Van Steirtegham A. New Belgian embryo transfer policy leads to sharp decrease in multiple pregnancy rate. Reprod Biomed Online. 2006;13:765–71.
47. Sunde A. Significant reduction of twins with single embryo transfer in IVF. Reprod Biomed Online. 2007;15 Suppl 3:28–34.
48. Papanikolaou EG, Camus M, Kolibianakis EM, Van Landuyt L, Van Stierteghem A, Devroey P. In vitro fertilization with single blastocyst-stage versus single cleavage-stage embryos. N Engl J Med. 2006;354: 1139–46.
49. Blake DA, Farquahar CM, Johnson N, Proctor M. Cleavage stage versus blastocyst stage embryo transfer in assisted conception. Cochrane Database Syst Rev. 2007;CD002118
50. Criniti A, Thyer A, Chow G, Lin P, Klein N, Soules M. Elective single blastocyst transfer reduces twin rates without compromising pregnancy rates. Fertil Steril. 2005;84:1613–9.
51. Gardner DK, Lane M, Stevens J, Schlenker J, Schoolcraft WB. Blastocyst score affects implantation and pregnancy outcome; towards a single blastocyst transfer. Fertil Steril. 2000;73:1155–8.
52. Dennis SJ, Thomas MA, Williams DB, Robins JC. Embryo morphology score on day 3 is predictive of implantation and live birth rates. J Assist Reprod Genet. 2006;23:171–5.
53. Van Peperstraten AM, Nelen WL, Hermens RP, Jansen L, Scheenjes E, Braat DD, et al. Why don't we perform elective single embryo transfer? A qualitative

study among IVF patients and professionals. Hum Reprod. 2008;23:2036–42.
54. Grobman WA, Milad MP, Stout J, Klock SC. Patient perceptions of multiple gestations; an assessment of knowledge and risk aversion. Am J Obstet Gynecol. 2001;185:920–4.
55. Hojgaard A, Ottosen LD, Kesmodel U, Ingerslev HJ. Patient attitudes towards twin pregnancies and single embryo transfer- a questionnaire study. Hum Reprod. 2007;22:2673–8.
56. Ryan GL, Zhang SH, Dokras A, Syrop CH, Van Voorhis BJ. The desire of infertile patients for multiple births. Fertil Steril. 2004;81:500–4.
57. Newton CR, McBride J, Feyeles V, Tekpetey F, Power S. Factors affecting patients attitudes toward single- and multiple-embryo transfer. Fertil Steril. 2007;87:269–78.
58. Coetzee K, Stewart B, Peek J, Hutton JD. Acceptance of single-embryo transfer by patients. Fertil Steril. 2007;87:207–9.
59. Jain T, Harlow BL, Hornstein MD. Insurance coverage and outcomes of in vitro fertilization. N Engl J Med. 2002;347:661–6.
60. The Ethics Committee of the American Society for Reproductive Medicine. Shared-risk or refund programs in assisted reproduction. Fertil Steril. 2004;82 Suppl 1:S249–50.

Oocyte Insemination and Culture

6

Roberta Maggiulli, Filippo Ubaldi, and Laura F. Rienzi

Introduction

During the pre-ovulatory period, the follicular environment nurtures growth and development of the oocyte in the dominant follicle to produce a meiotically competent oocyte capable of resuming meiosis and progressing through meiosis to metaphase II. The cumulus-corona cells that surround the oocyte are critically important in sustaining oocyte nutrition and maturation, and providing essential metabolites, hormones, and growth factors [1–4]. After exposure to the pre-ovulatory surge of luteinizing hormone, considerable changes in the organization of these surrounding layers occur. Corona cell processes retract from the oolemma, gap junctions throughout the cumulus complex are disrupted, and glycosaminoglycans, predominantly hyaluronic acid, are secreted causing considerable expansion of the cumulus corona mass. At the time of follicular rupture, this mass will protect the oocyte from exposure to the transitional chemical and physical conditions that it will encounter during its journey along the fallopian tube.

The single most important goal of the IVF laboratory is to create an environment for the gametes and resulting embryos that is focused on maximizing their safety and developmental competence. Safety and maintenance of the oocytes from the moment of follicular aspiration, through insemination and embryo growth is paramount to IVF success. Due to the extreme sensitivity of these cells, even to slight changes in environmental conditions, all IVF handling and culture procedures should minimize oocyte exposure to biophysical and chemical fluctuations.

Oocyte Collection

The Procedure

In stimulated IVF cycles, oocyte retrieval is usually performed 36 h after hCG administration by ultrasound-guided transvaginal aspiration. Several factors including variables such as pump vacuum, velocity, needle lumen size and length, follicular pressure and size, and collection technique may affect oocyte competence and should be monitored and recorded before and during the retrieval procedure (reviewed by Horne et al. [5]). During collection, a maximum vacuum pressure of about 120 mmHg is recommended to dampen the risk of damage to the oocytes [6]. Moreover, to minimize changes in temperature, the collection tubes should be kept in a tube warmer maintained at 37°C before being connected to the collection system.

R. Maggiulli, B.Sc., Ph.D. • F. Ubaldi, M.D., M.Sc. • L.F. Rienzi, B.Sc., M.Sc. (✉)
GENERA Center for Reproductive Medicine, Clinica Valle Giulia, Via G. De Notaris 2B, Rome 00197, Italy
e-mail: maggiulli@generaroma.it; ubaldi.fm@tin.it; rienzi@generaroma.it

E.S. Ginsburg and C. Racowsky (eds.), *In Vitro Fertilization: A Comprehensive Guide*,
DOI 10.1007/978-1-4419-9848-4_6, © Springer Science+Business Media New York 2012

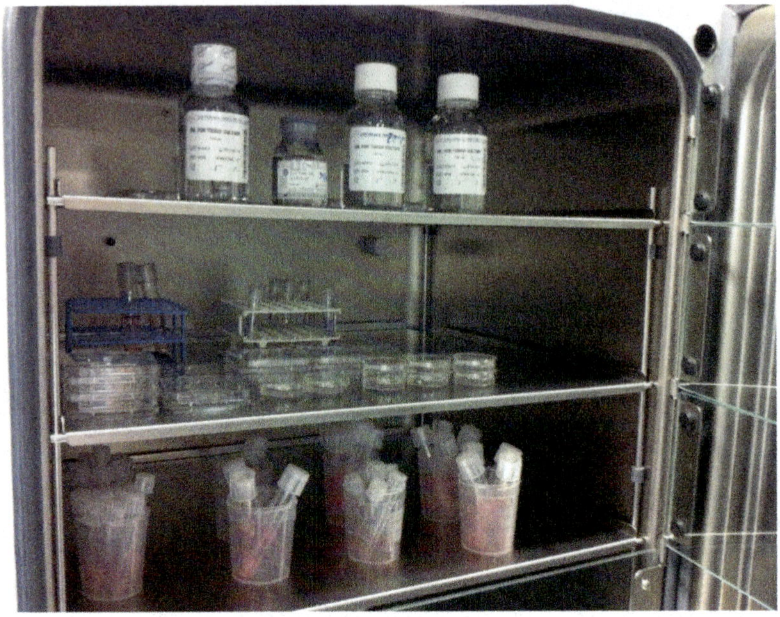

Fig. 6.1 Media and dish preincubation in daily IVF laboratory practice

The follicles are aspirated in a systematic manner with each tube containing aspirate passed off to the laboratory immediately after it is full. The adjoining laboratory examines the follicular fluid in sterile plastic dishes. Cumulus–corona–oocyte complexes (CCOC) are identified, rinsed in pre-equilibrated medium in order to remove any blood residue from follicular fluid, and the CCOCs are then transferred to dishes containing pre-equilibrated medium and incubated in a defined atmosphere (see Oxygen concentration during embryo culture below) at 37°C.

The cohort of oocytes collected after ovarian hyperstimulation represents a range of maturational stages that may have specific nutritional requirements. However, the standard IVF protocol is to use the same medium for all oocytes after collection unless some are specifically designated for in vitro maturation. The collection and holding media must contain glucose (in the range of 2.0–5.5 mmol/l) as the cumulus cells require this glycolytic substrate as an energy source. The electrolytic and the osmotic needs are met by most balanced salt solutions [7].

QA Considerations

Human oocytes are exquisitely sensitive to any environmental perturbations including both physical stresses, as well as chemical stresses such as temperature and pH fluctuations, and environmental air contamination. Temperature oscillations associated with handling oocytes outside the incubator may impair the oocyte microtubular system. Changes in spindle organization have been observed in mature human oocytes exposed to room temperature even for only few minutes [8–10]. Notwithstanding the ability of the meiotic spindle to reassemble when the temperature is reestablished, the risk of aneuploidy occurrence is potentially increased after a temperature-induced depolymerization [9].

Because of the extreme sensitivity of human oocytes, all the equipment in use (including Petri dishes and Pasteur pipettes) should be pre-warmed at 37°C (Fig. 6.1). In order to maintain a stable temperature in the dishes, the working areas (hood and microscope) and the thermo plates should be calibrated regularly. Daily, in the early morning, an external calibrated certified thermometer should be used to monitor the temperature of all the heating devices. The observed values should be reported and compared to the tolerance limits defined for each instrument. For a detailed discussion on quality management issues, see Chap. 15.

As mentioned by Mortimer et al. [11], a poorly recognized aspect of temperature maintenance is that most disposable plastic platforms are designed in a way that does not allow the medium to come into direct contact with the microscope stage. This air gap reduces the efficacy of heated stages, making it very difficult to stabilize the temperature when using standard IVF dishes.

One of the most important roles of the handling media is to prevent a pH shift. Although there is agreement regarding the need to monitor pH during IVF culture, there seems to be a less consensus regarding the actual correct value. In 1998, Dale et al. [12] demonstrated that the baseline intracellular pH (pHi) of the human oocyte is 7.4 ± 0.1 in HCO_3^-/CO_2-buffered medium. Recently, a lower pH (approximately 7.30) was found to be the optimum for culturing up to the pronuclear stage [13]. Unlike cleavage-embryos that have mechanisms for pH regulation, human oocytes lack the ability to regulate their internal pH; a problem that is even more marked in the cumulus-corona-free oocyte. Therefore, excursions in the extracellular pH can easily translate into deleterious intracellular perturbations that can compromise subsequent embryogenesis. Only 2–3 h after fertilization does the oocyte begin to recover the exchanger activity and the consequent ability to regulate its pH. The extracellular pH is generated by dynamic equilibrium between the CO_2 concentration in the incubator and the amount of bicarbonate in the media. For that reason, monitoring and stabilizing the extracellular pH is particularly challenging during the handling of oocytes and embryos outside the incubator.

Specific buffer systems are currently used in commercially available handling media for assisted reproduction treatment: 4-(2-hydroxyethyl)-1-piperazineethanesulphonic acid (HEPES) and 3-(*N*-morpholino)-propanesulphonic acid (MOPS). Since concerns have been raised regarding potential detrimental effects of these organic buffers on gamete competence [14, 15], media containing bicarbonate/CO_2 buffers are preferable, although they require controlled chambers to maintain a 5–7% CO_2 atmosphere. However, it is essential to note that many of the adverse effects of these buffer systems are largely dependent on interactions with other compounds in the media, and are not due to toxicity of the buffers themselves [16]. Regardless of the buffer chosen, it is crucial to maintain an appropriate and constant temperature, since temperature itself may alter the buffering ability of these compounds.

Cumulus–Corona–Oocyte Complex Grading

At the end of the retrieval process, the maturational stage of the oocyte may be evaluated. Several scoring systems of the cumulus corona oocyte complex have been introduced to predict the nuclear maturity of the enclosed oocytes and identify the proper timing for insemination [17–24], although it is generally acknowledged that these assessment systems are not perfect.

Early studies from Rattanachaiyanont et al. [17], performed on oocytes collected for IVF treatment, reported no correlation between oocyte–corona–cumulus complex morphology and nuclear maturity, fertilization rate, and embryo cleavage. On the contrary, other authors reported that CCOC scoring was related to fertilization and pregnancy rates [22] as well as to blastocyst quality and development [23]. Lin and colleagues [23], proposed a grading system for CCOCs based on the morphology of the oocyte cytoplasm, cumulus mass, corona cells, and membrane granulosa cells, to select oocytes prior to insemination by conventional IVF. Five grades (*Mature Group, Approximately Mature, Immature, Post-mature, and Atretic*) were described. The authors reported higher fertilization rates for the oocytes belonging to the Mature Group compared to those belonging to the other groups. Moreover, the Immature Group was characterized by a higher incidence of poor morphology day 3 embryos as compared to the Mature Group.

It has also been suggested that the presence of either CCOC anomalies such as amorphous

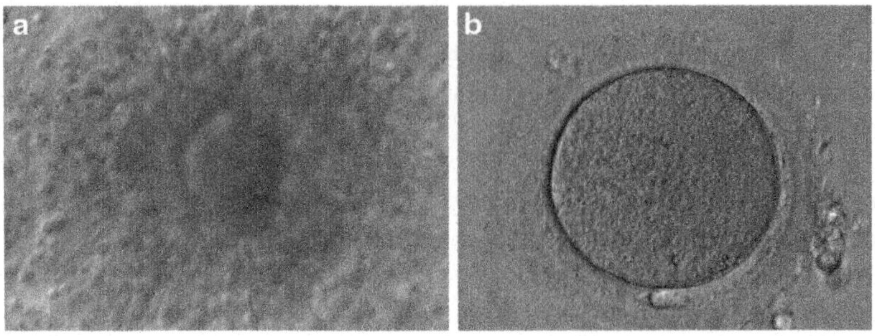

Fig. 6.2 A mature human oocyte (**a**) before cumulus removal; (**b**) after cumulus-corona removal

clumps, or blood clots, may be an index of a suboptimal follicular maturation [25, 26], and may impair the ability of the embryo to develop to the blastocyst stage. Oocytes from these CCOCs showed a significant alteration in the cytoplasmic texture probably related to the reduced fertilization rate obtained when those oocytes are used for insemination [26, 27]. Moreover, variations in temperature and pH as well as reactive oxygen species induced by the presence of blood clots have been suggested as responsible for the compromised competence of those oocytes [20].

Although cumulus-corona mass assessment is limited in terms of its ability to accurately predict oocyte maturity and competence, there is clearly some association between cumulus-corona disposition and meiotic status, with a fully expanded "sun burst" cumulus mass being associated with a mature oocyte (Fig. 6.2). Therefore, a careful assessment of CCOC morphology may be a useful tool to aid in oocyte selection when the oocytes are destined for standard insemination, rather than ICSI.

Insemination Procedures

Fertilization is achieved by conventional in vitro insemination procedure or ICSI according to the patients' history and sperm parameters. Although both these procedures are well established, there is no universal agreement regarding the elapsed number of hours to perform them after oocyte retrieval. We observed that a pre-incubation period of 3 h after oocyte retrieval may improve the fertilization rate and embryo quality after ICSI [28]. Other studies have been published regarding the time of injection post-retrieval, but without reaching consistent conclusions [29–35]. Oocyte nuclear maturity can be easily assessed before ICSI by visualization of the first polar body, which is a characteristic of the mature, MII oocyte. However, nuclear and cytoplasmic maturation are acquired independently during oocyte maturation and both of them are required for normal fertilization [36]. Therefore oocyte preincubation prior to IVF or ICSI may induce cytoplasmic maturation that could eventually increase fertilization and also pregnancy rates. Balakier and colleagues [37] reported that human oocytes progressively develop the ability for full activation and normal development during the MII arrest stage. An improvement in fertilization rates was obtained when ICSI was carried out 6–8 h after the polar body extrusion. Presumably, the different optimum time intervals identified in the various studies reflect differences in patient populations and stimulation regimens used and, possibly, variations in culture systems.

Conventional insemination can be carried out using various platforms including multi-well dishes, microdrops, or tubes. Our current approach is to perform insemination in Nunc four-well dishes containing 600 μl of fertilization medium with an oil overlay. Up to three oocytes/well are inseminated with about 120,000–150,000 spermatozoa/mL. After 16–18 h of incubation, oocytes are then denuded to assess fertilization. Some studies have hypothesized a detrimental effect of prolonged oocyte exposure to spermatozoa in vitro due to the production of free oxygen radicals, present especially in high concentrations of spermatozoa [38–41]. Therefore, reducing exposure of oocytes to spermatozoa has been proposed to improve embryo viability, possibly due to decreasing potential damage from sperm metabolic waste products [42].

Embryo Culture

Media and Platforms

Efforts to improve culture conditions have resulted in a substantial breakthrough in the past 10 years, with widespread application of new approaches including the use of atmospheric oxygen (so-called low oxygen tension), elimination of toxic components, and the introduction of sequential and single medium systems to culture embryos to the blastocyst stage. As a result, culture to the blastocyst stage has become an achievable goal which, in turn, has facilitated selection of the most viable embryos. This approach allows for single blastocyst transfer with acceptably high pregnancy and birth rates, at least in selected good prognosis patients.

Embryo Culture Media Composition

In the last decade, knowledge acquired from several studies regarding embryo physiology and biochemistry has led to significant improvements in media formulations used for embryo culture, resulting in a remarkable increase in efficiency of human assisted reproduction all over the world [43].

Media for human embryo culture should contain the following basic components: pure water, common salts, plus sodium bicarbonate as a buffer, sodium salt of EDTA or another chelator, pyruvate and lactate, amino acids, macromolecules, and antibiotics. However, commercially available human embryo culture media use different concentrations of each component, and many include other constituents as well. There are marked differences even in concentrations of the simplest elements, such as potassium chloride and magnesium sulphate [44]. Similarly, the optimal osmolality for development of human embryos in culture has not yet been determined. Moreover, almost all media require supplementation with chemically undefined or partially defined factors as albumin or synthetic serum substitutes.

The composition of the majority of IVF media is based on one of three physiological salines: Earle's balanced salt solution, Krebs-Ringer bicarbonate, and Tyrode's solution [45–47]. So far, two major approaches have been used to determine the media composition and concentration of each compound. The first approach is the "empirical optimization" of components by bioassays—also known as "let the embryos choose" principle—established by Biggers and colleagues [48]. The common principles of this approach are: (1) that only a single medium is used to support development from the zygote to blastocyst stage; and (2) the concentration of constituents is defined according to bioassays using a systematic approach to measure the response of embryos to several combinations and concentrations of test components. The concentration and type of component selected for the medium is usually that which gives a maximum response. One of the limitations of the "empirical optimization" approach is the theoretical requirement of astronomic numbers of experiments and some compromises in the interpretation of the mathematical models to determine the most suitable medium composition [48, 49]. Nevertheless, $KSOM^{AA}$, the optimum medium for mouse embryo culture, was developed using this approach (reviewed by [49]), and a slightly modified version of this formulation (Global medium) is a very effective medium for culturing human embryos to the blastocyst stage.

In contrast to the "let the embryos choose" approach, the "back to nature" approach uses the concentration of a substance that approximates the concentration to which the embryo is naturally exposed [50]. This approach was introduced by Leese [51]. The major problem with this principle is the extremely low amounts of the fluids in the oviduct and uterus available for assay, and the technical and ethical problems related to its collection and measurement. So far, investigations have been performed in vivo (by micropuncture, chronic, or acute in situ cannulation) or in vitro (by vascular and luminar perfusion). However, the composition of oviduct and uterine fluids likely differ from the in vivo microenvironment around the embryo [52].

Numerous studies supporting the efficacy of both sequential and single media have been published [48, 49, 53–62], and the overall weight of the evidence indicates that probably neither system is superior to the other for growth of human embryos to the blastocyst stage. Indeed, both systems are used worldwide, with each having potential advantages and disadvantages (reviewed by Vajta et al. [63]). As a side note, since most of the data used for development of commercially available human media are derived from experiments performed on animal embryos, it is likely that a more intensive dialogue between human and domestic animal embryologists may eventually improve the composition of human media [64].

Oxygen Concentration During Embryo Culture

Until recently, human embryos have been cultured under atmospheric oxygen (20%), a procedure adapted from earlier somatic tissue culture protocols [65]. However, in the early 1990s three different research groups observed the beneficial effect of reduced oxygen concentration (5%) on embryo development in a protein-free medium without somatic cell support [66–68].

Supporting evidence of using reduced oxygen concentrations for human embryo culture is the low oxygen concentration measured within the oviduct and uterus of different mammalian species (2–8%) [69–71]. Moreover, by continuous assessment of embryo development, using time-lapse microscopy, the temporal effect of atmospheric oxygen on embryo development has been studied and the embryos response to either static or changing concentration of oxygen has been evaluated [72]. Authors have showed detrimental effects of atmospheric oxygen on mouse embryos during in vitro culture, as reflected by slower cleaving embryos and decreased cell numbers in cleavage-stage embryos, and poorer blastocyst development [72]. Compared with embryos cultured in 5% oxygen, embryos cultured in 20% oxygen were delayed at the first cleavage by 0.45 h ($P<0.05$), at the second cleavage by 0.84 h ($P<0.01$) and at the third cleavage by 3.19 h ($P<0.001$). Importantly, these detrimental effects of atmospheric oxygen were irreversible, as switching the embryo to reduced oxygen concentration for the second 48 h of development (post-compaction) did not alleviate the developmental perturbations induced during the initial 48 h. A prospective, randomized study conducted by Waldenstrom et al. [73] on human embryos showed that blastocyst culture with low-oxygen (5%) versus high-oxygen (19%) concentration yielded a higher conversion rate to blastocyst and a marked improvement in birth rate. Recently, a meta-analysis has been accomplished to clarify whether or not the low O_2 concentration significantly improves clinical outcomes compared to atmospheric O_2 concentration [74]. When embryos were transferred on days 5 and 6, the meta-analysis showed a statistically significantly higher implantation rate in the group of embryos cultured at low oxygen tension as compared with those cultured in 20% oxygen ($P=0.006$) [74].

The above published data suggest that, unless a future strong contra-indication is documented, low oxygen concentration should be a principle for culture of human embryos in all ART laboratories. This is one of the few questions where a definite answer is available and a worldwide consensus is currently being formed. However, a further decrease in oxygen concentration below 5% may have negative consequences. In fact, setting the oxygen concentration at 2%, although leading to increased blastocyst rates, may cause developmental abnormalities in ruminants [75]. On the other hand, there is no evidence that embryos need a continuous gas supply. A gas mixture volume of 50 ml in a closed system generously covers the requirements of 200 bovine embryos for 1 week, from the zygote to the blastocyst stage [76].

Embryo Culture Platforms

In sharp contrast to the widespread research regarding the design and utilization of optimum culture media, very little attention has been paid to devices used for embryo culture.

In routine IVF, gametes and embryos are cultured on inert surfaces such as glass or plastic polymers of varying configuration considered as "static" platforms, since they do not employ active means to agitate or stimulate embryo or media movement [77]. Usually, the media preparation consists of placing media in disposable polystyrene multiwell or Petri dishes, in 10–80 μl drops covered with oil with a subsequent overnight equilibration in the proper gas mixture at 37°C to stabilize the pH, temperature and achieve proper saturation with gasses. In most systems, the medium is changed on Day 3 (Day 0 being the day of oocyte retrieval), whether to a fresh drop of the same medium (the one-step system) or to a drop of a second growth medium (the sequential system). As discussed above, there is no consensus as to whether one of these systems affords an advantage over the other. As previously described [78], what is perhaps of greater importance is the fact that fundamental differences exist between these conventional culture systems and the oviduct. During the progression through the female tract, embryos are exposed to changing components of oviductal fluid. In addition, embryos in vivo develop in a dynamic environment and are subjected to changing gravitational positions. In contrast, in the in vitro environment, embryos are submerged in modified salt solutions, where autocrine factors are often diluted, and some of them diffuse into the oil layer; any change in composition of media occurs only once during the culture period, and not necessarily according to the proper metabolic needs of the embryo; no dynamic movements are ensured. Moreover, most dishes are not developed for embryological purposes, and the standard embryo culture system is based on monolayer culture methods developed more than 50 years ago for primary cultures of somatic cells and cell lines.

Fortunately, serious efforts are currently being focused on exploring the physical requirements of the embryo in the hope of optimizing embryo development in vitro. New culture platforms have been developed utilizing lower volumes of media with a limited surface area since it has been found in many animal models that co-culture of embryos in reduced volumes improves development, potentially through secretion of autocrine/paracrine factors [79–81]. However, this approach requires careful attention in media handling since shifts in pH and osmolality are more frequent.

In order to exploit the potential beneficial effects of increased embryo density, other platforms that combine the communal effect while allowing individual identification of embryos have been established. The Well of the Well or WOW system consists of small microwells produced on the bottom of a culture dish aiming to create a small microenvironment for individual embryos, while allowing them to share a larger common culture media reservoir above [80–82]. Improvement in the percentage of embryos developing into blastocysts can be achieved in WOWs compared to traditional cultures (56% vs. 37%, respectively), and promising pregnancy and birth rates have also been reported [82].

As an alternative to microwells, use of microchannels has been proposed for culturing embryos. The Glass Oviduct or GO system proposed by Thouas [81] is based on an open-ended 2 μl sterile capillary with 200 μm inner diameter. The GO system is an extremely simplified and static version of the microchannel system that allows embryos to be cultured vertically promoting increased cell contact.

Recently some special specialized surface-coated dishes have been proposed as intriguing means of potentially improving current in vitro embryo culture systems (reviewed by Swain and Smith [77]), however their application remains modest. Special surface treatments of dishes do not seem to have obvious benefits; therefore, further studies are required before drawing any conclusion regarding their true potential.

In order to implement a radically new embryo culture system, the possibility to employ dynamic culture platforms has been investigated, including those specifically engineered to stimulate controlled media flow/movement. Macroscopically, the usual microfluidic device consists of the following parts: a glass microscopic slide base; a plastic (for example polydimethylsiloxane) layer with the channels and valves; and connections to mechanical or pneumatic pumps. Sporadic and isolated attempts in the past decade to improve culture systems have demonstrated that microfluids are suitable to perform almost all steps of human IVF varying from selection of motile spermatozoa, oocyte cumulus removal, in vitro fertilization by insemination and embryo culture [83–85]. Initial steps to assemble the isolated steps into a production line have also been successfully performed. Accordingly, there is a chance to make complex procedures completely automated including the whole human IVF laboratory process [83]. The only unproven step that would need to be adopted into the microfluidic system is ICSI; however, this procedure may ultimately be replaced with alternative solutions, or performed in a semi-automated way [86].

Embryo Grading and Selection

Static Morphology Evaluation

Embryo morphological grading remains the standard method for evaluation and selection because of its simplicity and cost-effectiveness, and due to the failure of recent "-omics" technologies (metabolomics, transcriptomics, and proteomics) to improve selection (reviewed by [87]). Different morphological criteria for cleavage embryo assessment have been described through the years and a variety of characteristics have been proposed as indicative of embryo viability: early cleavage [88–108], cleavage rate [95–98], blastomere size [96, 97, 99], presence of multinucleation [99–104], extent of fragmentation [96, 97, 105–109] and distribution of fragments [107, 108].

One of the most critical factors in the evaluation of cleavage-stage embryos is the strict timing for the assessment. For standardization, a European consensus was reached to perform the 2-day and 3-day evaluation respectively at 44 ± 1 and 68 ± 1 h post insemination [110]. Early cleavage in two daughter cells has been associated with higher development and pregnancy and implantation rates [88, 90–93], indicating its use as a valuable additional embryo selection criterion.

A great number of embryo morphology scoring systems have been proposed [111–115]. However, at present the lack of standardization (in the nomenclature used as well as the number of characteristics considered and the calculated threshold values) is an obstacle for an easy and unequivocal interpretation of the different results. Therefore, two consensus groups have proposed standardized systems for staging the embryos, one group from the Society for Assisted Reproductive Technology/American Society for Reproductive Medicine (SART/ASRM) [116], the other from Alpha [110]. In addition, both groups proposed the simple categories of "good," "fair," and "poor" as related to embryo quality [110, 116], and the Alpha group further defined these categories with regards to blastomere number, degree of fragmentation, extent of blastomere asymmetry, and presence of multinucleation (Fig. 6.3) [110].

It has been also suggested that the capacity of the embryo to reach the blastocyst stage could have additional prognostic value in identifying the best embryo(s). Indeed, increases in pregnancy and implantation rates have been reported after both fresh and cryopreserved blastocyst transfers [117–121]. However data are still controversial, since some authors found comparable results after cleavage embryo transfers [113, 122, 123]. Moreover, a large number of embryos fail to develop to the blastocyst stage in extended culture and it is not possible to know which of these embryos would have implanted if they had been replaced earlier [113, 124].

Since blastocyst development is dynamic, grading should be evaluated 112–114 h post insemination when a defined inner cell mass, a blastocoel cavity, and a ring of evenly spaced and sized trophectoderm cells should be observed [110].

Different scoring systems for blastocysts have been described [125–127] however, the most commonly used is that described by Gardner et al. [125]. The authors defined an alphanumeric scoring system on the basis of degree of blastocyst expansion and hatching status, the development of the inner cell mass and the development of the trophectoderm (Figs. 6.4 and 6.5).

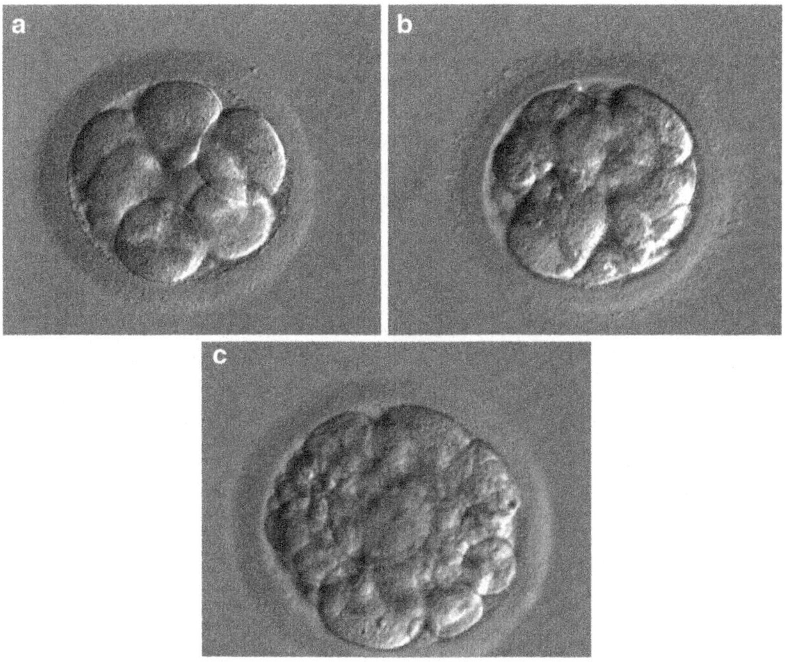

Fig. 6.3 Day 3 embryos of varying quality: (**a**) Good quality, characterized by mild fragmentation (<10%), stage-specific cell size and absence of multinucleation; (**b**) Fair quality, characterized by the presence of moderate fragmentation (10–25%), stage-specific cell size for the majority of blastomeres and no evidence of multinucleation; (**c**) Poor quality, characterized by severe fragmentation (>25%), cell size not stage-specific and evidence of multinucleation

Time-Lapse Imaging

One major limitation to classic morphology grading is the static evaluation of the embryos at one, or at the most, a few discrete time points. Continual monitoring by means of time-lapse cinematography allows noninvasive, dynamic imaging of embryo morphological changes and permits correlations to be made among morphokinetics, further development and clinical fate. Indeed, timing of different embryonic developmental events post-insemination has been proposed as an additional criterion in embryo selection [128–130]. A recent study revealed that an optimal time range (time window) exists for every early cell division, supporting the hypothesis that viable embryos undergo tightly regulated cellular events [130].

Various combinations of different morphological criteria, from the oocyte, to the cleavage-stage embryo, to the blastocyst have been evaluated, and many have proven to have predictive power for selecting developmentally competent embryos (reviewed by [87]). Indeed, morphological grading remains the first-line method for evaluation and selection of embryos in clinical IVF.

Noninvasive Media Profiling

Improving knowledge about gamete and embryo physiology should allow the identification of novel markers of embryo quality that may be useful as additional selection criteria. In this regard, targeted approaches that measure specific components in the culture medium (such as amino acids [131]), as well as the application of recent "-omics" technologies [132, 133] hold promise. Among these new methods, the employment of a noninvasive screening technology using near infrared spectroscopy to analyze the metabolomic

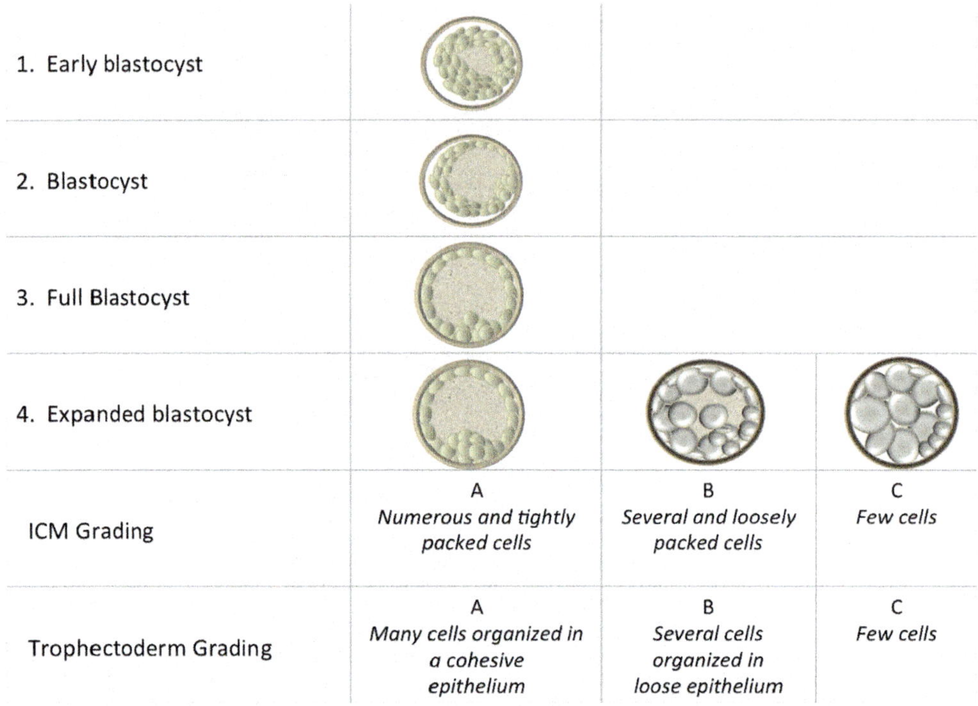

Fig. 6.4 Blastocyst grading according to Gardner and Schoolcraft. Blastocysts are classified by a numerical score from 1 to 6 on the basis of their degree of expansion and hatching status: (1) an early blastocyst with a blastocoel that is less than half of the volume of the embryo; (2) a blastocyst with a blastocoel that is half of or greater than half of the volume of the embryo; (3) a full blastocyst with a blastocoel completely filling the embryo; (4) an expanded blastocyst with a blastocoel volume larger than that of the early embryo, with a thinning zona. For fully developed blastocysts, the development of the inner cell mass is assessed: (A) tightly packed, many cells; (B) loosely grouped, several cells; (C) very few cells. The trophectoderm is assessed according to the number and appearance of trophectoderm cells: (A) many cells forming a cohesive epithelium; (B) few cells forming a loose epithelium; (C) very few large cells. Adapted from Sakkas and Gardner, *Textbook of Assisted Reproductive Techniques: Laboratory and Clinical Perspectives, Second Ed.*

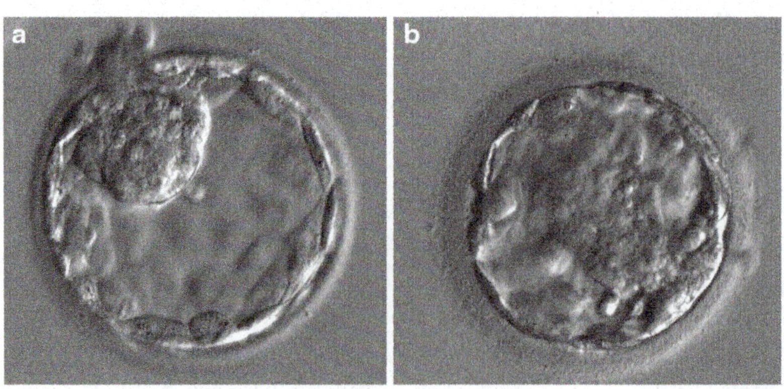

Fig. 6.5 Examples of blastocysts of contrasting stage and quality: (**a**) Blastocyst with grade 4AA; (**b**) Blastocyst with grade of 3CC

profiling of embryo culture medium has been proposed as one of the most promising selection methods. However, besides the initial benefits reported in retrospective studies [132, 134–139], recent prospective randomized studies have shown that the evaluation of metabolomic profiles by near infrared spectroscopy does not improve implantation rates [140, 141].

Concluding Remarks

Applications of new culture approaches including use of atmospheric oxygen level and the introduction of single-step and sequential media have resulted in several significant breakthroughs in the clinical IVF laboratory. The ability to improve preservation of embryonic developmental potential has increased the likelihood of obtaining a consistent number of embryos reaching the blastocyst stage. With these improvements, application of single blastocyst transfer should continue to increase, at least in good prognosis patients. This, in turn, will continue to decrease the incidence of multiple pregnancies while preserving the overall efficiency of the treatment.

Notwithstanding the demonstrated benefits of innovative and sophisticated platforms, the widespread use of these technologies is currently limited due to the costs of these devices and design pitfalls that can make them more labor intensive to utilize. In a futuristic view, a complex, automated system may be established to perform all steps that lead to embryo production [77]. The system could also be enhanced with a time lapse imaging system to allow noninvasive detailed analysis of embryo development and with various sensors to measure, for instance, embryo-derived biomarkers (metabolomics) or gene expression profiles (transcriptomics). The enormous amount of information derived from morphological (including phase-contrast) images and time-lapse videos together with biochemical parameters may prove invaluable for determining the optimal time for embryo transfer, for selecting the best embryo(s) for transfer, and for comparison of various versions of culture methods and parameters.

Although improvements in the IVF culture system have resulted in significantly improved clinical outcomes, one of the major limitations in IVF laboratory technology still relates to identification of the most viable embryo(s) to transfer. Currently, selection of the best embryo(s) is based on static assessment of morphological features, but most of the embryos transferred fail to implant. In the future, implementation of current culture systems with time lapse cinematography and "-omics" technology may improve the identification of novel markers of embryo quality to provide additional selection criteria. Furthermore, preimplantation genetic screening may help in the determination of embryonic "health" through screening the genetic constitution of the embryo (see Chap. 8). However, this technology is still far from being routinely used in IVF clinics and further investigations are needed to ensure the reliability and sensitivities of these methods.

References

1. Biggers JD, Whittingham DG, Donahue RP. The pattern of energy metabolism in the mouse oöcyte and zygote. Proc Natl Acad Sci USA. 1967;58(2): 560–7.
2. Donahue RP, Stern S. Follicular cell support of oocyte maturation: production of pyruvate in vitro. J Reprod Fertil. 1968;17(2):395–8.
3. Brower PT, Schultz RM. Intercellular communication between granulosa cells and mouse oocytes: existence and possible nutritional role during oocyte growth. Dev Biol. 1982;90(1):144–53.
4. Haghighat N, Van Winkle LJ. Developmental change in follicular cell-enhanced amino acid uptake into mouse oocytes that depends on intact gap junctions and transport system Gly. J Exp Zool. 1990;253(1): 71–82.
5. Horne R, Bishop CJ, Reeves G, et al. Aspiration of oocytes for in-vitro fertilization. Hum Reprod Update. 1996;2:77–85.
6. Edwards RG, Steptoe PC, Fowler RE, Baillie J. Observations on preovulatory human ovarian follicles and their aspirates. Br J Obstet Gynaecol. 1980;87(9):69–79.
7. Pool TB, Ord VA. Oocyte treatment: from retrieval to insemination. In: Gardner DK, Weissman A, Howles CM, Shoham Z, editors. Textbook of assisted reproductive techniques. 2nd ed. Philadelphia, PA: Taylor & Francis; 2004. p. 107–14.

8. Sathananthan AH, Trounson A, Freemann L, Brady T. The effects of cooling human oocytes. Hum Reprod. 1988;3:968–77.
9. Pickering SJ, Braude PR, Johnson MH, Cant A, Currie J. Transient cooling to room temperature can cause irreversible disruption of the meiotic spindle in the human oocyte. Fertil Steril. 1990;54:102–8.
10. Almeida PA, Bolton VN. The effect of temperature fluctuations on the cytoskeletal organisation and chromosomal constitution of the human oocyte. Zygote. 1995;3:357–65.
11. Mortimer D, Mortimer ST. Quality and risk management in the IVF laboratory. Cambridge: Cambridge University Press; 2005.
12. Dale B, Menezo Y, Cohen J, DiMatteo L, Wilding M. Intracellular pH regulation in the human oocyte. Hum Reprod. 1998;13(4):964–70.
13. Hentemann M, Mousavi K, Bertheussen K. Differential pH in embryo culture. Fertil Steril. 2011;95:1291–4.
14. Iwasaki T, Kimura E, Totsukawa K. Studies on a chemically defined medium for in vitro culture of in vitro matured and fertilized porcine oocytes. Theriogenology. 1999;51:709–20.
15. Morgia F, Torti M, Montigiani M, Piscitelli C, Giallonardo A, Schimberni M, Giannini P. Sbracia Use of a medium buffered with N-hydroxyethylpiperazine-N-ethanesulfonate (HEPES) in intracytoplasmic sperm injection procedures is detrimental to the outcome of in vitro fertilization. Fertil Steril. 2006;85(5):1415–9.
16. Swain JE. Optimizing the culture environment in the IVF laboratory: impact of pH and buffer capacity on gamete and embryo quality. Reprod Biomed Online. 2010;21(1):6–16.
17. Rattanachaiyanont M, Leader A, Léveillé MC. Lack of correlation between oocyte-corona-cumulus complex morphology and nuclear maturity of oocytes collected in stimulated cycles for intracytoplasmic sperm injection. Fertil Steril. 1999;71(5):937–40.
18. Veeck LL. The morphologic estimation of mature oocytes and their preparation for insemination. In: Jones Jr HW, Jones GS, et al., editors. In-vitro fertilization—Norfolk. Baltimore, MD: Williams and Wilkins; 1986. p. 81.
19. Wolf DP. Oocyte quality and fertilization. In: Wolf DP, editor. In-vitro fertilization and embryo transfer. New York: Plenum; 1988. p. 129–38.
20. Daya S, Kohut J, Gunby J, et al. Influence of blood clots in the cumulus complex on oocyte fertilization and cleavage. Hum Reprod. 1990;5:744–6.
21. Veeck LL. The morphological assessment of human oocytes and early conception. In: Keel BA, Webster BW, editors. Handbook of the laboratory diagnosis and treatment of infertility. Boca Raton, FL: CRC; 1990. p. 353–69.
22. Ng ST, Chang TH, Wu TC. Prediction of the rates of fertilization, cleavage, and pregnancy success by cumulus-coronal morphology in an in vitro fertilization program. Fertil Steril. 1999;72:412–7.
23. Lin YC, Chang SY, Lan KC, et al. Human oocyte maturity in vivo determines the outcome of blastocyst development in vitro. J Assist Reprod Genet. 2003;20:506–12.
24. Balaban B. Urman B Effect of oocyte morphology on embryo development and implantation. Reprod Biomed Online. 2006;12:608–15.
25. Motta PM, Nottola SA, Pereda J, et al. Ultrastructure of human cumulus oophorus: a transmission electron microscopic study on oviductal oocytes and fertilized eggs. Hum Reprod. 1995;10:2361–7.
26. Ebner T, Moser M, Shebl O, Sommergruber M, Yaman C, Tews G. Blood clots in the cumulus-oocyte complex predict poor oocyte quality and post-fertilization development. Reprod Biomed Online. 2008;16(6):801–7.
27. Kahraman S, Yakin K, Donmez E, et al. Relationship between granular cytoplasm of oocytes and pregnancy outcome following intracytoplasmic sperm injection. Hum Reprod. 2000;15:2390–3.
28. Rienzi L, Ubaldi F, Anniballo R, et al. Preincubation of human oocytes may improve fertilization and embryo quality after intracytoplasmic sperm injection. Hum Reprod. 1998;13:1014–9.
29. Yanagida K, Yazawa H, Katayose H, et al. Influence of oocyte preincubation time on fertilization after intracytoplasmic sperm injection. Hum Reprod. 1998;13:2223–6.
30. Van de Velde H, de Vos A, Joris H, et al. Effect of timing of oocyte denudation and micro-injection on survival, fertilization and embryo quality after intracytoplasmic sperm injection. Hum Reprod. 1998;13: 3160–4.
31. Jacobs M, Stolwijk AM, Wetzels AM. The effect of insemination/injection time on the results of IVF and ICSI. Hum Reprod. 2001;16:1708–13.
32. Ho JY, Chen MJ, Yi YC, et al. The effect of preincubation period of oocytes on nuclear maturity, fertilization rate, embryo quality, and pregnancy outcome in IVF and ICSI. J Assist Reprod Genet. 2003;9: 358–64.
33. Isiklar A, Mercan R, Balaban B, et al. Impact of oocyte pre-incubation time on fertilization, embryo quality and pregnancy rate after intracytoplasmic sperm injection. Reprod Biomed Online. 2004;6: 682–6.
34. Dozortsev D, Nagy P, Abdelmassih S, et al. The optimal time for intracytoplasmic sperm injection in the human is from 37 to 41 hours after administration of human chorionic gonadotropin. Fertil Steril. 2004;6: 1492–6.
35. Falcone P, Gambera L, Pisoni M, et al. Correlation between oocyte preincubation time and pregnancy rate after intracytoplasmic sperm injection, Gynecol Endocrinol. 2008;6:295–9.
36. Eppig JJ, Schultz RM, O'Brien M, Chesnel F. Relationship between the developmental programs controlling nuclear and cytoplasmic maturation of mouse oocytes. Dev Biol. 1994;164:1–9.

37. Balakier H, Sojecki A, Motamedi G, Librach C. Time dependent capability of human oocytes for activation and pronuclear formation during metaphase II arrest. Hum Reprod. 2004;19:982–7.
38. Aitken JR, Clarkson JS. Cellular basis of defective sperm function and its association with the genesis of reactive oxygen species by human spermatozoa. J Reprod Fertil. 1987;81:459–69.
39. Dumoulin JCM, Bras M, Land JA, Pieters M, Enginsu ME, et al. Effect of the number of inseminated spermatozoa on subsequent human and mouse embryonic development in vitro. Hum Reprod. 1992;7:1010–3.
40. Parinaud J, Labal B, Mieusset R, Rkhoilley G, Vieitez G. Influence of sperm parameters on embryo quality. Fertil Steril. 1993;60:888–92.
41. Aitken JR. A free radical theory of male infertility. Reprod Fertil Dev. 1994;6:19–24.
42. Gianaroli L, Fiorentino A, Magli MC, et al. Prolonged sperm–oocyte exposure and high sperm concentration affect human embryo viability and pregnancy rate. Hum Reprod. 1996;11:2507–11.
43. Quinn P. The development and impact of culture media for assisted reproductive technologies. Fertil Steril. 2004;81:27–9.
44. Gardner DK, Lane M. Culture of the mammalian preimplantation embryo. In: Gardner DK, Lane M, Watson AJ, editors. A laboratory guide to the mammalian embryo. Oxford, NY: Oxford University Press; 2004. p. 41–61.
45. Earle WR. Production of malignancy in vitro. IV. The mouse fibroblast cultures and changes in living cells. J Natl Cancer Inst. 1943;4:165–212.
46. Krebs HA, Henseleit K. Untersuchungen uÈ ber die Harnstoffbildung im Tierkorper. Z Physiol Chem. 1932;210:33–66.
47. Tyrode MV. The mode of action of some purgative salts. Arch Int Pharmacodyn. 1910;20:205–23.
48. Biggers JD, McGinnis LK. Evidence that glucose is not always an inhibitor of mouse preimplantation development in vitro. Hum Reprod. 2001;16:153–63.
49. Summers MC, Biggers JD. Chemically defined media and the culture of mammalian preimplantation embryos: historical perspective and current issues. Hum Reprod Update. 2003;9(6):557–82.
50. Gardner DK, Lane M. Development of viable mammalian embryos in vitro: evolution of sequential media. In: Cibelli J, Lanza RP, Campbell KHS, West MD, editors. Principles of cloning. NY: Academic; 2002. p. 187–213.
51. Leese HJ. Human embryo culture: back to nature. J Assist Reprod Genet. 1998;15:466–8.
52. Leese HJ, Tay JI, Reischl J, et al. Formation of fallopian tubal fluid: role of a neglected epithelium. Reproduction. 2001;121:339–46.
53. Gardner DK, Lane M. Culture and selection of viable blastocysts: a feasible proposition for human IVF? Hum Reprod Update. 1997;3:367–82.
54. Gardner DK, Lane M. Blastocyst transfer. Clin Obstet Gynaecol. 2003;46:231–8.
55. Gardner DK. Dissection of culture media for embryos: the most important and less important components and characteristics. Reprod Fertil Dev. 2008;20:9–18.
56. Gardner DK, Lane M. Embryo culture systems. In: Gardner DK, editor. In vitro fertilization: a practical approach. New York: Informa Healthcare; 2007. p. 221–82.
57. Lane M, Gardner DK. Embryo culture medium: which is the best? Best Pract Res Clin Obstet Gynaecol. 2007;21:83–100.
58. Pool TB. An update on embryo culture for human assisted reproductive technology: media, performance, and safety seminars. Semin Reprod Med. 2002;23:309–18.
59. Pool TB. Recent advances in the production of viable human embryos in vitro. Reprod Biomed Online. 2005;4:294–302.
60. Biggers JD, McGinnis LK, Lawitts JA. One-step versus two-step culture of mouse preimplantation embryos: is there a difference? Hum Reprod. 2005;20:3376–84.
61. Biggers JD, Summers MC. Choosing a culture medium: making informed choices. Fertil Steril. 2008;90:473–83.
62. Sepu´lveda S, Garcia J, Arriaga E, et al. In vitro development and pregnancy outcomes for human embryos cultured in either a single medium or in a sequential media system. Fertil Steril. 2008;91:1765–70.
63. Vajta G, Rienzi L, Cobo A, Yovich J. Embryo culture: can we perform better than nature? Reprod Biomed Online. 2010;20:453–69. Review.
64. Bavister BD. How animal embryo research led to the first documented human IVF. Reprod Biomed Online. 2002;4 Suppl 1:24–9.
65. Edwards RG. Test-tube babies. Nature. 1981;293: 253–6.
66. Nagao Y, Saeki K, Hoshi M, et al. Effects of oxygen concentration and oviductal epithelial tissue on the development of in vitro matured and fertilized bovine oocytes cultured in protein-free medium. Theriogenology. 1994;41:681–7.
67. Trounson A, Pushett D, Maclellan LJ, et al. Current status of IVM/IVF and embryo culture in humans and farm animals. Theriogenology. 1994;41:57–66.
68. Voelkel SA, Hu YX. Effect of gas atmosphere on the development of one-cell bovine embryos in two culture systems. Theriogenology. 1992;37:1117–31.
69. Fischer B, Bavister BD. Oxygen tension in the oviduct and uterus of rhesus monkeys, hamsters and rabbits. J Reprod Fertil. 1993;99:673–9.
70. Maas DH, Storey BT, Mastroianni Jr L. Oxygen tension in the oviduct of the rhesus monkey (Macaca mulatta). Fertil Steril. 1976;27:1312–7.
71. Mastroianni Jr L, Jones R. Oxygen Tension within the Rabbit Fallopian Tube. J Reprod Fertil. 1965;9: 99–102.
72. Wale PL, Gardner DK. Time-lapse analysis of mouse embryo development. Reprod Biomed Online. 2010;21(3):402–10.

73. Waldenstrom U, Engstrom AB, Hellberg D, Nilsson S. Low-oxygen compared with high-oxygen atmosphere in blastocyst culture, a prospective randomized study. Fertil Steril. 2009;91(6):2461–5.
74. Gomes Sobrinho DB, Oliveira JB, Petersen GC, et al. IVF/ICSI outcomes after culture of human embryos at low oxygen tension: a meta-analysis. Reprod Biol Endocrinol. 2011;9:143.
75. Thompson JG, Peterson AJ. Bovine embryo culture in vitro: new developments and post-transfer consequences. Hum Reprod. 2000;15 Suppl 5:59–67.
76. Vajta G, Holm P, Greve T, et al. The submarine incubation system, a new tool for in vitro embryo culture. A technique report. Theriogenology. 1997;48:1379–85.
77. Swain JE, Smith GD. Advances in embryo culture platforms: novel approaches to improve preimplantation embryo development through modifications of the microenvironment. Hum Reprod Update. 2011;17(4):541–57.
78. Rienzi L, Vajta G, Ubaldi F. New culture devices in ART. Placenta. 2011;32 Suppl 3:S248–51.
79. Lane M, Gardner DK. Effect of incubation volume and embryo density on the development and viability of mouse embryos in vitro. Hum Reprod. 1992;7: 558–62.
80. Vajta G, Peura TT, Holm P, et al. New method for culture of zona-included and zone-free embryos: the Well of the Well (WOW) system. Mol Reprod Dev. 2000;55:256–64.
81. Thouas GA, Jones GM, Trounson AO. The 'GO' system–a novel method of microculture for in vitro development of mouse zygotes to the blastocyst stage. Reproduction. 2003;126:161–9.
82. Vajta G, Korösi T, Du Y, et al. The Well-of-the-Well system: an efficient approach to improve embryo development. Reprod Biomed Online. 2008;17:73–81.
83. Beebe DJ, Wheeler M, Zeringue H, et al. Microfluidic technology for assisted reproduction. Theriogenology. 2002;57:125–35.
84. Smith GD, Takayama S. Gamete and embryo isolation and culture with microfluidics. Theriogenology. 2007;68S:S190–5.
85. Thompson JG. Culture without the Petri dish. Theriogenology. 2007;67:16–20.
86. Wang W, Liu X, Gelinas D, Ciruna B, Sun Y. A fully automated robotic system for microinjection of zebrafish embryos. PLoS One. 2007;2(9):e862.
87. Machtinger R, Racowsky C. The bioinformatics of embryo development and assessment. RBMOnline (In Press).
88. Shoukir Y, Campana A, Farley T, et al. Early cleavage of in-vitro fertilized human embryos to the 2-cell stage: a novel indicator of embryo quality and viability. Hum Reprod. 1997;12:1531–6.
89. Sakkas D, Shoukir Y, Chardonnens D, et al. Early cleavage of human embryos to the two-cell stage after intacytoplasmic sperm injection as an indicator of embryo viability. Hum Reprod. 1998;13:182–7.
90. Sakkas D, Percival G, D'Arcy Y, et al. Assessment of early cleaving in vitro fertilized human embryos at the 2-cell stage before transfer improves embryo selection. Fertil Steril. 2001;76:1150–6.
91. Salumets A, Hyden-Granskog C, Makinen S, et al. Early cleavage predicts the viability of human embryos in elective single embryo transfer procedures. Hum Reprod. 2003;18:821–5.
92. Neuber E, Rinaudo P, Trimarchi JR, et al. Sequential assessment of individually cultured human embryos as an indicator of subsequent good quality blastocyst development. Hum Reprod. 2003;18:1307–12.
93. Van Montfoort AP, Dumoulin JC, Kester AD, et al. Early cleavage is a valuable addition to existing embryo selection parameters: a study using single embryo transfers. Hum Reprod. 2004;19:2103–8.
94. Guerif E, Le Gouge A, Giraudeau B, et al. Limited value of morphological assessment at day 1 and 2 to predict blastocyst development potential: a prospective study based on 4042 embryos. Hum Reprod. 2007;22:1973–81.
95. Lewin A, Schenker JG, Safran A, et al. Embryo growth rate in vitro as an indicator of embryo quality in IVF cycles. J Assist Reprod Genet. 1994;11:500–3.
96. Giorgetti C, Terriou P, Auquier P, et al. Embryo score to predict implantation after in-vitro fertilization: based on 957 single embryo transfers. Hum Reprod. 1995;10:2427–31.
97. Ziebe S, Petersen K, Lindberg S, et al. Embryo morphology or cleavage stage: how to select the best embryos for transfer after in-vitro fertilization. Hum Reprod. 1997;12:1545–9.
98. Desai NN, Goldstein J, Rowland DY, et al. Morphological evaluation of human embryos and derivation of an embryo qyality scoring system specific for day 3 embryos: a preliminary study. Hum Reprod. 2000;15:2190–6.
99. Handarson T, Hanson C, Sjögren A, et al. Human embryos with unevenly sized blastomeres have lower pregnancy and implantation rates: indications for aneuploidy and multinucleation. Hum Reprod. 2001;16:313–8.
100. Kligman I, Benavida C, Alikani M, et al. The presence of multinucleated blastomeres in human embryos is correlated with chromosomal abnormalities. Hum Reprod. 1996;11:1492–8.
101. Jackson KV, Ginsburg ES, Hornstein MD, et al. Multinucleation in normally fertilized embryos is associated with an accelerated ovulation induction response and lower implantation and pregnancy rates in in vitro fertilization-embryo transfer cycles. Fertil Steril. 1998;70:60–6.
102. Palmstierna M, Murkes D, Csemiczky G, et al. Zona pellucida thickness variation and occurrence of visible mononucleated blastomers in preembryos are associated with a high pregnancy rate in IVF treatment. J Assist Reprod Genet. 1998;15:70–5.
103. Pelinck MJ, De Vos M, Dekens M, et al. Embryos cultured in vitro with multinucleated blastomeres

have poor implantation potential in human in-vitro fertilization and intracytoplasmic sperm injection. Hum Reprod. 1998;13:960–3.

104. Van Royen E, Mangelschots K, Vercruyssen M, et al. Multinucleation in cleavage stage embryos. Hum Reprod. 2003;18:1062–9.
105. Staessen C, Camus M, Bollen N, et al. The relationship between embryo quality and the occurrence of multiple pregnancies. Fertil Steril. 1992;57: 626–30.
106. Roseboom TJ, Vermeiden JP, Schoute E, et al. The probability of pregnancy after embryo transfer is affected by the age of the patient, cause of infertility, number of embryos transferred and the average morphology score, as revealed by multiple logistic regression analysis. Hum Reprod. 1995;10: 3035–41.
107. Alikani M, Cohen J, Tomkin G, et al. Human embryo fragmentation in vitro and its implications for pregnancy and implantation. Fertil Steril. 1999;71: 836–42.
108. Antczak M, Van Blerkom J. Temporal and spatial aspects of fragmentation in early human embryos: possible effects on developmental competence and association with the differential elimination of regulatory proteins from polarized domains. Hum Reprod. 1999;14:429–47.
109. Van Royen E, Mangelschots K, De Neuborg D, et al. Characterization of a top quality embryo, a step towards single-embryo transfer. Hum Reprod. 1999;14:2345–9.
110. Alpha Scientists in Reproductive Medicine and ESHRE Special Interest Group of Embryology. The Istanbul consensus workshop on embryo assessment: proceedings of an expert meeting. Hum Reprod. 2011;26:1270–83.
111. Veeck LL. Preembryo grading and degree of cytoplasmic fragmentation. In: Veeck LL, editor. An Atlas of Human Gametes and Conceptuses. New York: Parthenon Publishing Group; 1999. p. 46–50.
112. Fisch JD, Rodriguez H, Ross R, et al. The Graduated Embryo Score (GES) predicts blastocyst formation and pregnancy rate from cleavage-stage embryos. Hum Reprod. 2001;16:1970–5.
113. Rienzi L, Ubaldi F, Iacobelli M, et al. Significance of morphological attributes of the early embryo. Reprod Biomed Online. 2005;10:669–81.
114. Cutting R, Morrol D, Roberts SA, et al. Elective single embryo transfer: guidelines for practice British Fertility Society and Association of Clinical Embryologists. Hum Fertil. 2008;11:131–46.
115. Stensen MH, Tanbo T, Storeng R, et al. Routine morphological scoring systems in assisted reproduction treatment fail to reflect age-related impairment of oocyte and embryo quality. Reprod Biomed Online. 2010;21:118–25.
116. Racowsky C, Vernon M, Mayer J, et al. Standardization of grading embryo morphology. Fertil Steril. 2010;94(3):1152–3.
117. Gardner DK, Lane M, Stevens J, et al. Blastocyst score affects implantation and pregnancy outcome: towards a single blastocyst transfer. Fertil Steril. 2000;73:1155–8.
118. Schoolcraft WB, Gardner DK. Blastocyst culture and transfer increases the efficiency of oocyte donation. Fertil Steril. 2000;74:482–6.
119. Langley MT, Marek DM, Gardner DK, et al. Extended embryo culture in human assisted reproduction treatments. Hum Reprod. 2001;16:902–8.
120. Schwarzler P, Zech H, Auer M, et al. Pregnancy outcome after blastocyst transfer as compared to early cleavage stage embryo transfer. Hum Reprod. 2004;19:2097–102.
121. Blake DA, Farquhar CM, Johnson N, et al. Cleavage stage versus blastocyst stage embryo transfer in assisted conception. Cochrane Database Syst Rev. 2007; CD002118
122. Coskun S, Hollanders J, Al-Hassan S, et al. Day 5 versus day 3 embryo transfer: a controlled randomized trial. Hum Reprod. 2000;15:1947–52.
123. Huisman GJ, Fauser BC, Eijkemans MJ, et al. Implantation rates after in vitro fertilization and transfer of a maximum of two embryos that have undergone three to five days of culture. Fertil Steril. 2000;73:117–22.
124. Alper M, Brinsden P, Fischer R, et al. To blastocyst or not to blastocyst? That is the question. Hum Reprod. 2001;16:617–9.
125. Gardner DK, Schoolcraft WB. *In vitro* culture of human blastocysts. In: Jansen R, Mortimer D, editors. Towards reproductive certainty: fertility and genetics beyond. London: Parthenon Publishing; 1999. p. 378–88.
126. Veeck LL, Zaninovic N. Grading criteria for human blastocysts. An atlas of human blastocysts. New York: Parthenon Publishing; 2003. p. 118.
127. Stephenson EL, Braude PR, Mason C. International community consensus standard for reporting derivation of human embryonic stem cell lines. Regen Med. 2007;2:349–62.
128. Lemmen JG, Agerholm I, Ziebe S. Kinetic markers of human embryo quality using time-lapse recordings of IVF/ICSI-fertilized oocytes. Reprod Biomed Online. 2008;17:385–91.
129. Wong CC, Loewke KE, Bossert NL, et al. Non-invasive imaging of human embryos before embryonic genome activation predicts development to the blastocyst stage. Nat Biotechnol. 2010;28:1115–21.
130. Meseguer M, Herrero J, Tejera A, et al. The use of morphokinetics as a predictor of embryo implantation. Hum Reprod. 2011;26:2658–71.
131. Brison DR, Houghton FD, Falconer D, Roberts SA, Hawkhead J, Humpherson PG, Lieberman BA, Leese HJ. Identification of viable embryos in IVF by non-invasive measurement of amino acid turnover. Hum Reprod. 2004;19:2319–24.
132. Seli E, Sakkas D, Scott R, Kwok SC, Rosendahl SM, Burns DH. Noninvasive metabolomic profiling of

embryo culture media using Raman and near-infrared spectroscopy correlates with reproductive potential of embryos in women undergoing in vitro fertilization. Fertil Steril. 2007;88:1350–7.

133. Katz-Jaffe MG, McReynolds S, Gardner DK, Schoolcraft WB. The role of proteomics in defining the human embryonic secretome. Mol Hum Reprod. 2009;15:271–7.
134. Seli E, Vergouw CG, Morita H, Botros LL, Roos P, Lambalk CB, Yamashita N, Kato O, Sakkas D. Noninvasive metabolomic profiling as an adjunct to morphology for noninvasive embryo assessment in women undergoing single embryo transfer. Fertil Steril. 2010;94:535–42.
135. Seli E, Bruce C, Botros LL, Henson M, Roos P, Judge K, Hardarson T, Ahlström A, Harrison P, Henman M, et al. Receiver operating characteristic (ROC) analysis of day 5 morphology grading and metabolomics viability Score on predicting implantation outcome. J Assist Reprod Genet. 2011;28:137–44.
136. Nagy ZP, Sakkas D, Behr B. Non-invasive assessment of embryo viability by metabolomic profiling of culture media ('metabolomics'). Reprod Biomed Online. 2008;17:502–7.
137. Nagy ZP, Jones-Colon S, Roos P, Botros L, Greco E, Dasig J, Behr B. Metabolomic assessment of oocyte viability. Reprod Biomed Online. 2009;18: 219–25.
138. Vergouw CG, Botros LL, Roos P, Lens JW, Schats R, Hompes PGA, Burns DH, Lambalk CB. Metabolomic profiling by near infrared spectroscopy as a tool to assess embryo viability: a novel, non-invasive method for embryo selection. Hum Reprod. 2008;23:1499–504.
139. Ahlström A, Wikland M, Rogberg L, Barnett JS, Tucker M, Hardarson T. Cross-validation and predictive value of near-infrared spectroscopy algorithms for day-5 blastocyst transfer. Reprod Biomed Online. 2011. doi:10.1016/j.rbmo.2011.01.009.
140. Hardarson T, Ahlstrom A, Rogberg L, et al. Non-invasive metabolomic profiling of Day 2 and 5 embryo culture medium: a prospective randomized trial. Hum Reprod. 2012;27(1):89–96.
141. Vergouw CG, Kieslinger DC, Kostelijik EH, et al. Day 3 embryo selection by metabolomic profiling of culture medium with near-infrared spectroscopy as an adjunct to morphology: a randomized controlled trial. Hum Reprod. 2012;27:2304–11.

Micromanipulation: Intracytoplasmic Sperm Injection and Assisted Hatching

7

Gianpiero D. Palermo, Queenie V. Neri, Devin Monahan, and Zev Rosenwaks

Background

Since the first human birth following in vitro fertilization (IVF) in 1978, this procedure has been used extensively for alleviation of infertility. However, because spermatozoa cannot fertilize in many cases of male factor infertility, a number of supplementary techniques have been developed to overcome this inability; these techniques are generally referred to as assisted fertilization, microsurgical fertilization, or simply micromanipulation. The application of micromanipulation to human gametes has not only allowed fertilization in cases of severe oligo-zoospermia and even defective spermatozoa, it has also provided a powerful tool for a more comprehensive understanding of the basic elements of oocyte maturation, fertilization, and early development. Micromanipulation techniques also now permit the diagnosis and sometimes even the correction of genetic anomalies, as well as optimization of implantation rates in certain cases.

When sperm density, motility, or morphology is inadequate, various techniques have been proposed to bypass the zona pellucida. The practical use of micromanipulation started in the mid-1980s with zona drilling (ZD) and partial zona dissection (PZD). Since then, this field has undergone such a rapid evolution that these early approaches have largely been abandoned in favor of intracytoplasmic sperm injection (ICSI), with the use of PZD confined to the 4–8 cell embryo stage (i.e., assisted hatching) in an effort to promote implantation. Zona drilling (ZD) first reported by Gordon and Talansky [1] involved the creation of a circumscribed opening in the zona by acid Tyrode's solution applied through a fine glass micropipette. After insemination, more than one spermatozoon frequently entered such drilled zonae. Moreover, the use of acidic medium had a deleterious effect on the oocyte—an effect not seen to the same extent in cleavage stage embryos using the "hatching" procedure, discussed later. At the same time as ZD was being tested, mechanical cutting of a hole in the zona was introduced as another technique for nuclear manipulation of fertilized oocytes [2]. Alternative but similar procedures were zona cracking, in which the zona was breached mechanically with two fine glass hooks controlled by a micromanipulator [3] and zona softening performed by a brief exposure to trypsin [4] or pronase. PZD [5], used extensively for a period in cases of fertilization failure, involved cutting the zona with

G.D. Palermo, M.D., Ph.D. (✉)
Ronald O. Perelman and Claudia Cohen Center for Reproductive Medicine, New York, NY 10021, USA
e-mail: gdpalerm@med.cornell.edu

Q.V. Neri, M.Sc., B.Sc. • D. Monahan, B.Sc.
Z. Rosenwaks, M.D.
Ronald O. Perelman and Claudia Cohen Center for Reproductive Medicine, Weill Cornell Medical College, New York, NY 10021, USA
e-mail: qneri@med.cornell.edu; dem2020@med.cornell.edu; zrosenw@med.cornell.edu

E.S. Ginsburg and C. Racowsky (eds.), *In Vitro Fertilization: A Comprehensive Guide*,
DOI 10.1007/978-1-4419-9848-4_7, © Springer Science+Business Media New York 2012

glass pipettes shortly before exposure of the treated oocytes to spermatozoa.

For all the above techniques, spermatozoa had to be progressively motile and to have undergone, or to have the potential to undergo, an acrosome reaction. The techniques also carried a distinct risk of injury to the oocytes and the need to produce an opening in the zona of optimal size. Localized laser photoablation of the zona also has been used to produce a gap of precise dimensions in the zona, and this has resulted in a few healthy offspring [6, 7]. However, not only did all these early procedures produce only a moderate fertilization rate, with PZD being the most useful in that regard, they were associated with a significant incidence of polyspermy. Mechanical insertion of spermatozoa directly into the perivitelline space—subzonal sperm injection (SUZI) [8] was introduced as another way of overcoming inadequacies of sperm concentration and motility, and this proved to be more effective than ZD or PZD, particularly following prior induction of the acrosome reaction [9–11]. However, SUZI also remained limited by an inability to overcome acrosomal abnormalities or dysfunction of the sperm-oolemma fusion process, and, ultimately, by unacceptably low rates of normal fertilization with formation of two pronuclei.

Intracytoplasmic Sperm Injection (ICSI) involves insertion of a single selected spermatozoon directly into the oocyte, bypassing all the preliminary steps of fertilization. The technique was pioneered in animals, initially by Hiramoto [12] in the sea urchin, then by Lin [13] in mammalian (mouse) oocytes. Later, Uehara and Yanagimachi [14] observed relatively high rates of sperm nucleus decondensation after microinjection of human or golden hamster spermatozoa into hamster eggs, and subsequently ICSI was used to study the determinants of male pronucleus formation [15, 16]. This approach also caused oocyte injury and lysis [17], and in early studies only about 30% of injected mouse eggs survived the procedure, even when fine micropipettes were used under ideal conditions [18].

Because the membrane fusion step of fertilization is bypassed in ICSI, male pronucleus development generally requires oocyte activation in most species tested. This can be provoked by energetic suction of some cytoplasm immediately before or during sperm nucleus insertion [19].

The first live offspring using ICSI were obtained in the rabbit following the transfer of sperm-injected eggs into the oviduct of a pseudopregnant female [20], and soon after that the first ICSI live birth was reported in the bovine [21]. Although applied to human gametes some years earlier [22, 23], the first human pregnancies with ICSI occurred only in 1992 [10, 11].

In this chapter, we review the different techniques of sperm and oocyte manipulation that are employed for ICSI currently and consider the techniques that hold promise in the treatment of oocyte/embryo abnormalities.

Indications for ICSI

Despite agreement in some areas, no universal standards for patient selection for ICSI have been defined. However, there is a general consensus that ICSI be adopted when an extremely poor sperm sample is noted, or following fertilization failure or unacceptably low fertilization using in vitro insemination techniques.

Although oocytes that failed to fertilize with standard IVF techniques can be reinseminated, this introduces a risk of fertilizing aged eggs [24]. In our own limited experience, 6 of 8 pregnancies established by micromanipulation of such oocytes miscarried, and cytogenetic studies performed on the aborted fetuses provided evidence of chromosomal abnormalities. Thus, notwithstanding a few reports of normal pregnancies [25, 26] the reinsemination of unfertilized oocytes is currently not advised for routine clinical application.

When the initial sperm concentration in the ejaculate is $<5\times10^6$/ml, the likelihood of fertilization with standard IVF is significantly reduced [27], and therefore such couples should be considered unsuitable for this procedure, particularly where <1% normal forms are observed. However, fertilization of mature oocytes may still fail to occur in the presence of normal sperm [28] because of a hardening of the zona pellucida [29], or when oocytes contain ooplasmic inclusions [30, 31], or in cases of unknown etiology [32]. Abnormalities of the zona pellucida prevent sperm fusion with the oolemma [33] thus justifying sperm injection. In most instances, however, failure of fertilization is due to coexisting sperm abnormalities, presenting ICSI as the only treatment option [34, 35].

Early experience showed that isolated nuclei of testicular and epididymal hamster spermatozoa decondensed soon after injection into mature hamster oocytes, and formed pronuclei in activated eggs [36]. Although in vitro fertilization of human oocytes was accomplished in men with epididymal spermatozoa recovered in cases of obstructive azoospermia [37, 38], only with the advent of ICSI was it possible to obtain consistent fertilization with them [39–42]. Testicular biopsy was employed to obtain sperm cells from men who had a scarred epididymis and, therefore, no chance of retrieval through that route [43, 44]. However, the therapeutic possibilities of ICSI go even further since immotile testicular spermatozoa and even spermatids have been successfully used [45].

Some men produce only round-headed spermatozoa which have no acrosome and can neither bind to nor penetrate zona-free hamster oocytes [22, 23, 46]. However, ICSI has enabled even such acrosomeless spermatozoa to establish pregnancies [47–51].

The dependability of ICSI has broadened its initial use from a technique capable of overriding the dysfunctionality of spermatozoa to one that may often, although not always, compensate for problems with the oocyte [32]. ICSI has allowed successful fertilization when only a few and/or abnormal oocytes were available [52]. Stripping cumulus cells from oocytes allows a direct assessment of maturation, thus potentially offering a woman with a limited number of oocytes a much greater chance of successful fertilization. In fact, the availability of ICSI has been instrumental in some European countries, including Italy and Germany, in circumventing restrictive legislation that limits the number of oocytes inseminated or embryos to be replaced [53–55].

ICSI has also made possible more consistent fertilization of cryopreserved oocytes [56]—overcoming the problem that freezing can lead to a premature exocytosis of cortical granules, resulting in zona hardening and inhibition of natural sperm penetration [57–60]. ICSI is also the preferred fertilization method during the application of preimplantation genetic diagnosis (PGD) because it avoids DNA contamination from additional sperm adhering to the zona, and it enhances the number of fertilizable oocytes and ultimately embryos available for screening [61].

ICSI also has an impact in the arena of HIV infection. Three-quarters of individuals infected by HIV or HCV are in their reproductive years. Male-to-female transmission of HIV is estimated to be only 1 per 1,000 acts of unprotected intercourse [62] and even fewer in HCV infected patients [63]. Moreover, because of antiretroviral therapies, the course of HIV-1 infection has shifted from a lethal acquired immunodeficiency syndrome to a chronic manageable disease. Many patients infected with HIV-1 are interested in beginning a family, but serodiscordant couples are concerned, with the possibility of both horizontal and vertical transmission of the virus. In such cases, intrauterine insemination (IUI) with spermatozoa processed by double gradient centrifugation followed by swim up has been the suggested method of treating serodiscordant couples with an HIV-1-infected male partner [64]. However, the use of ICSI has been proposed by several groups because of its negligible oocyte exposure to semen, thereby reducing the risk of viral transmission [65, 66]. Advantages of ICSI over IUI also include the considerably higher success rate [65], requiring fewer attempts to achieve pregnancy while reducing viral exposure [67]. Fortunately, so far, no seroconversions have been reported following ICSI treatments or IUIs [68, 69].

Finally, because only a single spermatozoon is needed for each oocyte, ICSI has allowed treatment of men who are virtually azoospermic (also defined as cryptozoospermic) [70]. Such cases of spermatogenic arrest have necessarily involved the injection of immature spermatozoa or even spermatogonia [44, 45, 71, 72]. Nonetheless, where fertilization occurs in such cases, the embryo implantation rate occurs at a similar incidence, at least in our experience, to that seen in IVF.

Techniques for Sperm Isolation

Semen samples are collected by masturbation after at least 3 days of abstinence; they are then allowed to liquefy for about 20 min at 37°C prior to analysis. Other methods of semen collection such as electroejaculation and retrograde ejaculation have been described elsewhere [39, 40].

The sample is washed by centrifugation at 500 × *g* for 5 min in HTF medium supplemented with 0.4% plasma protein (Plasmanate®, BDI Pharma). The resuspended pellet is layered on a discontinuous density gradient (Isolate®, Irvine Scientific) on two (90 and 45%) or single (90%) layers, and then centrifuged at 300 × *g* for 20 min when samples have a sperm density of $<5 \times 10^6$/ml spermatozoa and <20% motile spermatozoa. The sperm-rich fraction is rinsed by adding 4 ml of culture medium and centrifuged at 500–1,800 × *g* for 5 min to remove silica gel particles. For spermatozoa with poor kinetic characteristics, the sperm suspension is exposed to a 3 μM solution of pentoxifylline at time of the ICSI procedure. The concentration of the assessed sperm suspension is adjusted to $1–1.5 \times 10^6$/ml, when necessary, by the addition of HTF medium, and subsequently incubated at 37°C in 5% CO_2 in air.

Azoospermia can be indicative of epididymal vas obstruction or absence (obstructive azoospermia) or a failure of spermatogenesis (nonobstructive azoospermia). Obstructive azoospermia is characterized by normal sperm production and is often caused by congenital malformation or absence of the vas deferens, often associated with a cystic fibrosis gene mutation(s). The treatment for these men is microsurgical epididymal sperm aspiration (MESA), or when the epididymal access is lacking, direct testicular sampling is undertaken. On the other hand, nonobstructive azoospermia is characterized by a varying degree of spermatogenetic failure and may be associated with certain chromosomal or genetic abnormalities [73, 74] (see Chap. 3). The only method to retrieve spermatozoa in this setting is by a direct extraction of sperm or germ cells from a testis.

The infertility of men due to irreparable obstructive azoospermia has been treated successfully by MESA [75, 76] or percutaneous testicular retrieval of spermatozoa [77]. In the MESA procedure, 1–5 μl of fluid is aspirated from the lumen of an individual epididymal tubule in the mid-portion of the obstructed epididymis with a 300–350 μm glass pipette. The epididymal fluid is diluted with 300 μl of culture medium. Additional proximal punctures of the epididymis are performed until enough spermatozoa are obtained. Because sperm concentration in the epididymal fluid often reaches over 1×10^6/μl, only microliter quantities generally suffice. Epididymal fluid is diluted in 500 μl culture medium and processed like ejaculated spermatozoa. After removal of the density gradient medium, a 1 μl aliquot of the final suspension at approximately 1×10^6/ml is placed in the injection dish [39, 40, 78].

The procedure for direct microscopic identification of functioning seminiferous tubules is referred to as microdissection TESE [79, 80]. As with the standard multi-biopsy approach, optical magnification (6–8 power) is used to visualize blood vessels under the surface of the tunica vaginalis, allowing testis biopsy incisions to be made in avascular regions. Each biopsy specimen is first rinsed in culture medium to remove red blood cells, separated into individual tubules on sterile glass slides, and minced using fine scissors. The resulting suspension of seminiferous tubules is then sequentially passed through a 24 gauge angiocatheter to further disrupt the tubules. Individual testicular samples are distributed in 5.0 ml centrifuge tubes (Falcon, Becton Dickinson and Company, Lincoln Park, NJ, USA) containing an excess of culture medium. To assess for the presence of spermatozoa, a small amount (~5 μl) of suspension medium is carefully studied under a phase contrast microscope at 200–400×. In preparation for ICSI, the shredded testicular tissue is removed and the suspension medium subsequently centrifuged at 500–1,800 × *g* for 5 min, with the pellet being subjected to a single-layer density gradient centrifugation.

When no spermatozoa are identified, testicular tissue is placed in 1 ml of prewarmed medium supplemented with 5% HSA, 1.6 mM $CaCl_2$ (Sigma Chemical Co., St Louis, MO), 25 μg/ml DNase (Sigma Chemical Co.), and 1,000 IU/ml collagenase type IV (Sigma Chemical Co) [81]. DNase is added to the incubation medium to prevent clotting of the resulting cell suspension due to the release of free DNA from apoptotic cells [82, 83]. Testicular tissue is exposed to collagenase and incubated at 37°C for 1 h. The suspension is pipetted every 10–15 min to enhance enzymatic digestion. Large portions of tubular walls are removed with fine tweezers. The digested suspension is then centrifuged twice at 500 × *g* for 5 min. The supernatant is removed and the pellet resuspended in 100–500 μl of sperm cell medium.

Preparation of Oocytes for ICSI

Superovulation is performed by administration of gonadotropins in association with agonist or antagonist protocols in the standard fashion [84] (see Chap. 4). Immediately after the oocyte retrieval, under the inverted microscope at 100×, the cumulus corona cell complexes are scored as mature, slightly immature, completely immature, or slightly overmature [34, 35, 85]. Thereafter, the oocytes are incubated for more than 4 h. Immediately prior to micromanipulation, the cumulus corona cells are removed by exposure to HTF-HEPES-buffered medium containing 40 IU/ml of ICSI Cumulase®. For final removal of the residual corona cells, the oocytes are repeatedly aspirated in and out of a hand-drawn Pasteur pipette with an inner diameter of ~200 μm. Each oocyte is then examined under the microscope to assess the maturation stage and its integrity, metaphase II (MII) being assessed according to the absence of the germinal vesicle and the presence of an extruded polar body. ICSI is performed only in oocytes that have reached this level of maturity.

The ICSI Procedure

The holding and injection pipettes are inserted into the respective micromanipulation tool holders mounted on an inverted microscope. The controllers are pneumatic for the holding pipette and oil-filled for the injection pipette. Using the coarse motorized controllers, the pipettes are positioned in the center of the microscopic field at 20×, then the magnification is gradually increased while maintaining the tools in focus by adjusting the hydraulic controllers. Under the highest magnification (400×), correct pipette positioning is achieved only by the use of the hydraulic joysticks, and both pipettes should be able to course through the entire optical field. With regards to tool tip angles, the distal bent portions of both microtools should be slightly above parallel to avoid the elbows touching the bottom of the dish and interfering with control. This also allows prompt immobilization and visual control of the spermatozoon inside the injection pipette. Once properly aligned, the pipettes are raised by means of the coarse motorized controllers to allow placement of the ICSI dish on the microscope stage.

Nine drops containing 8 μl of injection medium (G-MOPS™ + 6% G-MM™; Vitrolife) are placed in a petri dish, with one in the center radially surrounded by the other eight. The drops should then be gently overlaid with culture oil to prevent evaporation. Using a red non-embryo toxic wax pencil, the 12 o'clock position is marked, a circle drawn around the central drop, and the drops are sequentially numbered starting from the 12 o'clock position, moving counter clockwise. This allows easy navigation between droplets during ICSI. ICSI dishes are stored at 37°C until use ([86] in press; [87] in press).

Immediately prior to the injection, under a stereomicroscope, the central drop is removed and replaced with 1 μl of sperm suspension diluted in 4 μl of 7% PVP. Using a hand-pulled Pasteur pipette, MII oocytes are aspirated from the culture dish and a single oocyte is placed in each drop.

The spermatozoon is positioned at 90° with respect to the tip of the injection pipette, and the principal piece of the tail is compressed by gently lowering the cylindrical tip and by rolling the posterior flagellum over the bottom of the Petri dish. If initially unsuccessful, the procedure is repeated until the tail is clearly kinked, looped, or convoluted. It is important to note, however, that a misshapen tail may adhere to the dish or to the inner surface of the pipette. The spermatozoon is aspirated tail first.

The oocyte is held in place by suction through the holding pipette and, using both tools, the oocyte is rotated slowly to locate the polar body and the area of cortical rarefaction (or polar granularity). When the equatorial plane of the oocyte is located, the depth of the holding pipette is adjusted to have its internal opening in the same plane to allow for greater support of the oocyte in a position opposite to the penetration point. The injection pipette is lowered and focused with the outer right border of the oolemma on the equatorial plane at 3 o'clock. When the spermatozoon is close to the beveled opening of the injection pipette, the injection pipette is pressed against the zona to begin penetration, and then thrust forward to the inner surface of the oolemma at 9 o'clock. At this point, a break in the membrane should occur at the approximate center of the egg. Such a break is indicated by a sudden quivering of the convexities of the oolemma (at the site of invagination) above and below the penetration point, as well as by the proximal flow of cytoplasmic organelles and the spermatozoon back into the pipette. The spermatozoon is then ejected with the cytoplasmic component.

To optimize its interaction with the cytoplasm, the spermatozoon should be ejected past the tip of the pipette to ensure a close intermingling with the ooplasmic lattices, which helps maintain the sperm in place while withdrawing the pipette. To facilitate oocyte activation, additional ooplasm is aspirated back and forth with the injection pipette. It is paramount to remove residual medium following spermatozoon insertion by applying a mild suction to the injection tool while withdrawing it, so that the cytoplasmic structures can envelop the sperm, thereby reducing the size of the breach. Once the pipette is extracted, the edges of the entry point should maintain a funnel shape with the tip towards the center of the egg. If the border of the oolemma becomes everted, the cytoplasmic organelles can leak out and the oocyte may lyse. The average time required to accomplish a single oocyte injection is about 30–40 s.

Assisted Hatching

Assisted hatching (AH) is based on the hypothesis that weakening of the zona pellucida, by drilling a hole through it, by thinning it, or by altering its stability, will promote hatching of embryos which are otherwise unable to escape from their zonae during blastocyst expansion [88, 89]. This approach was suggested by the observation that cleaved embryos with a good prognosis for implantation had a reduced zona thickness, and presumably therefore an increased potential for escape from it [90]; and particularly that microsurgically fertilized embryos with artificial gaps in their zonae appeared to have higher rates of implantation [91].

Ideally, the embryo is positioned to present the zona above the larger perivitelline space not occupied with blastomeres or containing enucleated fragments. The hatching procedure may be performed by use of a laser (reviewed by [92]) or by delivery of a small volume of Acid Tyrode's to the localized region of the zona. In our program, we use Acid Tyrode's. The microneedle is front-loaded in an adjacent droplet contained in the same dish, then acidic medium is expelled gently at 3 o'clock over a small area of zona of approximately 30 μm, while the needle presses slightly against it and at the same time is moved up and down in a limited pendular movement to avoid excess acid over any one point in the equatorial plane. Expulsion of the acidic Tyrode's medium should cease immediately when the innermost layer of the zona appears eroded. If embryo fragments are present these are removed, but this is best accomplished after moving the embryo to a fresh area of the droplet where the concentration of acid Tyrode solution is minimal. The micromanipulated embryos should be quickly rinsed then placed in fresh culture medium until they are transferred into the uterine cavity.

Clinical Outcomes with ICSI

According to the 2010 SART data, ICSI was performed in 66% of all cycles in reporting programs, and in 87% of cycles performed for male factor infertility (www.sart.org- national summary report). There are a multitude of papers on ICSI and ICSI outcomes. As in IVF, the main predictor of implantation, clinical pregnancy, and live birth rates is maternal age. Although, sperm source does play a role. Fertilization rates are similar with fresh or frozen epididymal specimens, however, epididymal samples resulted in higher fertilization and pregnancy rates than testicular spermatozoa obtained from men with non-obstructive azoospermia [93].

A SART database study of 465,046 ART cycles performed from 2004 to 2008 identified 77,432 performed for male factor of which 93.6% underwent ICSI. However, of all cycles, 272,526 (58.6%) employed ICSI, of which 50.1% were performed for female factor infertility. Live birth rates were similar for male factor infertility that did or did not employ ICSI, despite the fact that more severely defective spermatozoa were likely injected. Birth weights were also equivalent for male factor cycles using ICSI versus conventional IVF. In addition, when ICSI was performed in tubal ligation patients with no male factor indications, outcomes were equivalent to when ICSI was performed for male factor. Furthermore, whether the sperm used were ejaculated, from biopsy, retrograde ejaculation, or electroejaculation, live birth rates were the same [94].

A disadvantage of national registry studies is that detailed patient information is not available. In order to provide up to date clinical data on ICSI outcomes, an analysis of experience over the last 18 years at Cornell, has been undertaken for this chapter. We have performed a total of 33,170 ART cycles with an average maternal age for IVF of 37.6 ± 4 years and for ICSI of 35.8 ± 5 years, and mean paternal ages of 39.6 ± 6 years and 40.8 ± 8 years, respectively. Of those cycles, 32.2% (10,667) included the standard in vitro insemination of 11,490 oocytes from 6,036 couples with a fertilization rate of 60.4% and a clinical pregnancy rate of 40.5%. In vitro insemination was generally performed in patients with ideal semen parameters, while ICSI has been used to treat couples with suboptimal spermatozoa, a history of poor fertilization, and/or limited numbers of oocytes.

Of 12,763 couples treated by ICSI, the average number of oocytes retrieved was 10.6 per cycle (n = 237,498), of which 188,217 (79.2%) were at metaphase II and, therefore, subjected to ICSI. Of the oocytes injected, 94.7% (178,241/188,217) survived and 138,911 (73.8%) developed two pronuclei (PN). Of the oocytes that were abnormally fertilized, 4,951 (2.6%) displayed 1PN and 6,137 (3.3%) 3PN. The types of mature spermatozoa included 18,201 ejaculated samples, 2,023 cryopreserved, 83 obtained by electroejaculation, and 37 by bladder catheterization. Among the collection/cryopreservation methods, fertilization rates ranged from 67.3 to 83.5%. The clinical pregnancy rate was comparable in all groups ranging from 35.1 to 50.8%.

When more immature forms of spermatozoa were utilized, for example those surgically retrieved, the fertilization rate of 62.5% was satisfactory but lower than that with ejaculated spermatozoa (P = 0.0001) (Table 7.1). While the clinical pregnancy rate was lower in the ejaculated group in comparison to the surgically retrieved spermatozoa, this difference may be attributed to the maternal age. The etiology of the vas deferens or efferens obstruction, congenital (n = 513) or acquired (n = 429), had no effect on fertilization after ICSI giving an overall rate of 71.6% and a clinical pregnancy rate of 51.2%. However, after cryopreservation of epididymal spermatozoa, the clinical pregnancy was clearly impaired compared with fresh epididymal specimens (from 61.0 to 45.8%; P = 0.0001; Table 7.2).

In testicular extraction cases (n = 1,217), the spermatozoa recovered generated a fertilization rate of 55.0% and a clinical pregnancy rate of

Table 7.1 Fertilization and pregnancy rates according to semen origin

No. of	Spermatozoa Ejaculated	Surgically retrieved
Maternal age (M ± SD years)	36.9 ± 5[a]	34.7 ± 5[a]
Cycles	20,344	2,159
Fertilization (%)	126,401/168,191 (75.2)[b]	12,510/20,025 (62.5)[b]
Clinical pregnancies (%)	8,101 (39.8)[c]	965 (44.7)[c]

[a]Student's *t*-test, two independent samples, $P < 0.001$
[b, c]χ^2, 2×2, 1 *df*, Effect of spermatozoal source on fertilization and clinical pregnancy rates, $P = 0.0001$

Table 7.2 Spermatozoal parameters and ICSI outcome according to specimen source and storage

	Spermatozoa			
	Epididymal		Testicular	
	Fresh	Frozen/thawed	Fresh	Frozen/thawed
Cycles	333	609	892	325
Density (10^6/ml SD)	36.9 ± 44	23.4 ± 27	0.4 ± 3	0.2 ± 0.6
Motility (% ± SD)	18.8 ± 16[a]	3.4 ± 8[a]	3.5 ± 8	1.1 ± 4
Morphology (% ± SD)	1.7 ± 2	1.2 ± 2	0	0
Fertilization (%)	2,471/3,404 (72.6)	3,908/5,622 (70.9)	4,717/8,222 (57.4)[c]	1,334/2,777 (48.0)[c]
Clinical pregnancies (%)	203 (61.0)[b]	279 (45.8)[b]	368 (41.3)[d]	49 (35.4)[d]

[a]Student's *t*-test, two independent samples; Effect of cryopreservation on sperm motility, $P < 0.0001$
[b]χ^2, 2×2, 1 *df*, Effect of cryopreservation of epididymal spermatozoa on clinical pregnancy, $P = 0.0001$
[c, d]χ^2, 2×2, 1 *df*, Effect of cryopreservation of testicular spermatozoa on fertilization and clinical pregnancy rates, $P = 0.0001$

Table 7.3 Pregnancy characteristics of 22,503 ICSI cycles

No. of		No. of positive outcomes	
ICSI cycles	22,503		
Embryo replacements	20,995		
Positive hCGs	11,791	Pregnancy	52.4% (11,791/22,503)
Biochemical pregnancies	1,887		
Blighted ova	726		
Ectopic pregnancies	112		
Positive fetal heartbeats	9,066	Clinical pregnancy	40.3% (9,066/22,503)
Miscarriages/therapeutic abortions	860		
Deliveries and ongoing pregnancies	8,206		

39.7%. When comparing fresh versus cryopreserved spermatozoa in testicular cycles, the clinical pregnancy rate was lower in those that were cryopreserved (41.3 vs. 35.4%; $P = 0.0001$; Table 7.2).

Of the 22,503 ICSI cycles analyzed, 11,791 resulted in a positive ßhCG (52.4%) and in 40.3% of all cycles the presence of at least one fetal heartbeat was observed (Table 7.3). Among the positive ßhCG, 1,887 (16.0%) were biochemical pregnancies, 726 (6.2%) were anembryonic, and 112 (0.9%) were ectopic. Among the 9,066 cycles with a fetal heart, 799 spontaneously miscarried. This left an ongoing pregnancy rate of 36.5% per retrieval (8,206/22,503) and 39.1% per embryo replacement procedure (8,206/20,995).

When pregnancy rate from 21,028 ICSI cycles (after exclusion of the donor egg cycles) was plotted as a function of increasing maternal age, there was a progressive decrease in pregnancy ($P = 0.0001$) (Fig. 7.1) and consequently delivery rates ($P = 0.0001$). As predicted, there was a higher

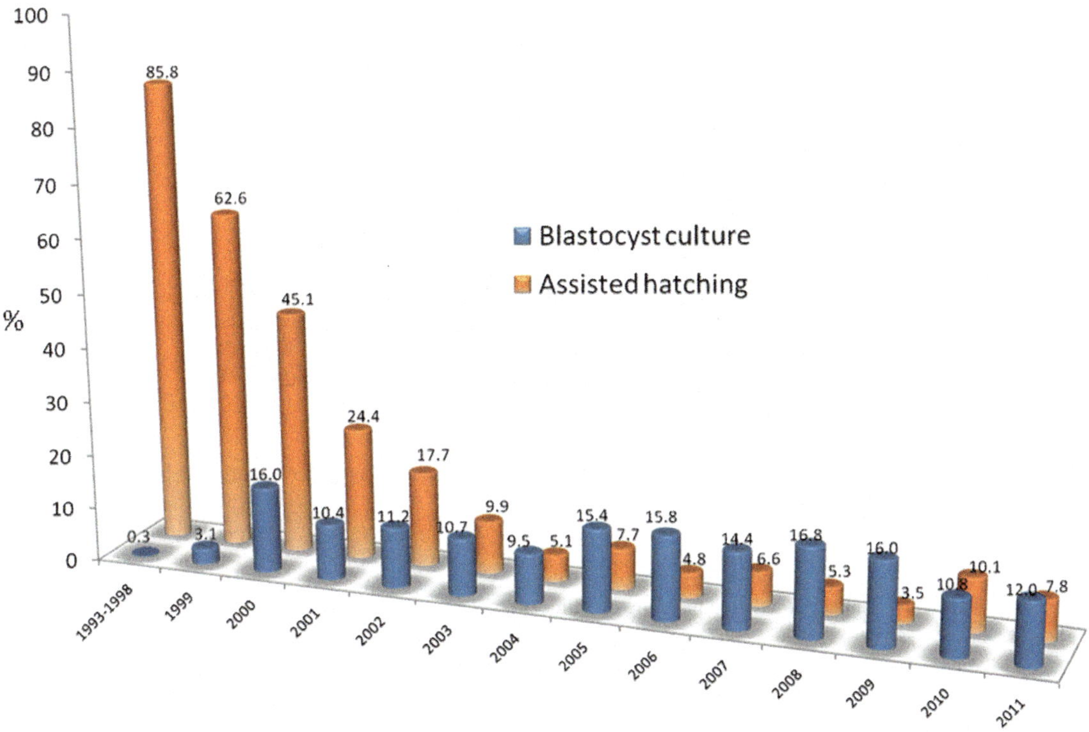

Fig. 7.1 Yearly variation of the proportion of ICSI cycles with at least one artificially hatched conceptus (*orange*). Correspondent implementation of blastocyst culture (*blue*)

incidence of miscarriages, therapeutic abortions, and overall pregnancy losses as a function of age of the female partner ($P=0.0001$), pregnancy wastage being 2.6 times greater in women ≥ 40 years compared to those of <35 years.

A total of 7,422 ICSI patients delivered 9,150 babies comprising 4,606 males and 4,521 females (with 23 unknown genders). A total of 3.6% (330) exhibited congenital abnormalities at birth, of which 174 were major and 156 were minor. IVF children ($n=5{,}183$) had a comparable overall malformation rate (104 major and 83 minor). Major malformations ranged from cardiac defects to multiorgan diseases including central nervous system anomalies, chromosomal abnormalities (gonosomal trisomies such as 47, XXX; 47, XXY and autosomal trisomies such as chromosomes 7, 18, 21), and urogenital disorders requiring surgery such as severe hypospadias and undescended testes. Examples of minor malformations were café-au-lait spots, urethral defects, and very mild forms of clubfoot.

Clinical Outcomes with Assisted Hatching

A Cochrane analysis of 28 randomized clinical trials (RCTs) found higher implantation rates when assisted hatching was performed; however, the higher-order gestation rate was significantly higher in the hatched versus unhatched group (OR 1.67, 95% CI 1.24–2.26) [95]. The issue as to whether assisted hatching enhances implantation rates is still open for discussion and a more recent interpretation of the key studies [92] emphasizes that selection of patients for assisted hatching is important and that the laser technique may be superior to the earlier methods.

We have analyzed our own program data for this chapter in order to provide an overview of the clinical experience at our center. Assisted hatching was established at our center in the early 1990s and, at that time, was being performed on at least one embryo in over 89% of all the cases (Fig. 7.2). Use of assisted

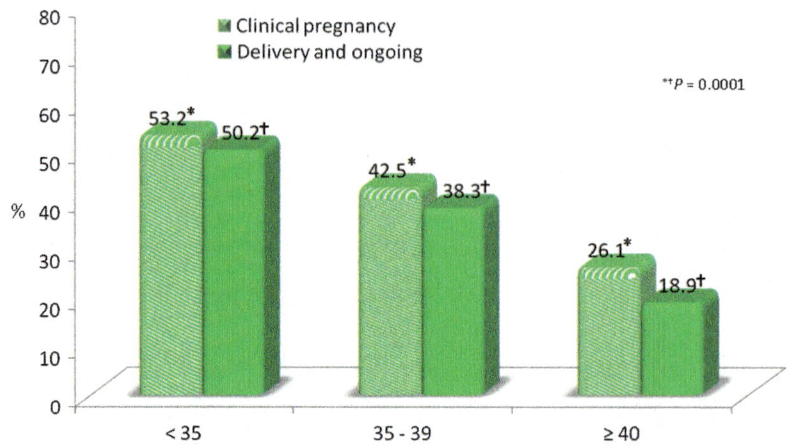

Fig. 7.2 Clinical outcome per oocyte retrieval grouped according to maternal age. Clinical pregnancy is considered as the presence of at least one fetal heartbeat

Table 7.4 Impact of assisted hatching on clinical outcome

	Assisted hatching performed	
No. of (%)	All embryos	None
Cycles	2,625	16,890
Maternal age (mean ± SD)	37.9 ± 4	37.3 ± 5
Implantation rate (%)	1,421/8,239 (17.2)[a]	10,102/45,979 (22.0)[a]
Clinical pregnancy (+FHB) (%)	820 (31.2)[b]	6,401(37.9)[b]
Delivery (%)	678 (25.8)[c]	5,725 (33.9)[c]

[a, b, c] χ^2, 2×2, 1 *df*, Effect of assisted hatching on clinical outcome, $P = 0.0001$

hatching in our center dropped to 63% in 1999 when we began blastocyst culture and has subsequently declined further to 12% as more extended culture has been performed. To determine if assisted hatching did in fact increase implantation rates, we reviewed ICSI cases utilizing fresh ejaculated samples that had either all the embryos with assisted hatching ($n = 2{,}625$) or not ($n = 16{,}890$) (Table 7.4). No difference in maternal age was observed, however, implantation rate was significantly higher in the cohort where embryos were left intact ($P = 0.0001$) and the same findings were reflected in clinical pregnancy and delivery rates ($P = 0.0001$). No difference in pregnancy losses was observed between the two groups (13.1 vs. 12.1%, respectively). To remove a potential female confounding factor, we assessed only those cycles that were ≤35 years old. In cases that had all their embryos hatched, the implantation rate was 26.3% (513/1,950) which was lower than their nonmanipulated counterparts (33.5%, 3,619/10,807; $P = 0.0001$). The clinical pregnancies and deliveries were also higher in the cases where assisted hatching was not performed ($P = 0.0001$).

The above findings from our program experience may appear to be in contradiction to the Cochrane analysis previously cited. We would point out that in IVF laboratories, and in our program, patients are not randomly assigned to undergo assisted hatching; the technique is performed based on patient and embryo characteristics. Finally, patients must be apprised that assisted hatching appears to increase the risk of monochorionic twinning in cycles utilizing standard insemination (OR 2.23, 95% CI 1.06–4.67) [95, 96].

Safety and Conclusions

Notwithstanding the large number of babies born following ICSI worldwide, concerns still exist as to whether either the procedure itself or the use of suboptimal spermatozoa can result in genomic or phenotypic abnormalities in the progeny [97]. In one of the earlier studies on the outcome of pregnancies after ICSI, it was observed that the rate of malformation was 2.6% after ICSI [34, 35]. An extension of the Cornell series which included a total of 14,333 ART children examined found that the incidence of overall malformation was comparable between the IVF and ICSI, consistent with prior published results [98–100].

These qualms are not only limited to the inheritance of specific traits that bear on fertility but, most importantly, they relate to the postnatal well-being of the offspring as reflected in growth [101] and cognitive development [102]. A complete child development evaluation is labor intensive and costly, and therefore one study employed a standardized parent-administered questionnaire(Ages and Stages Questionnaire®, ASQ), as an alternative method to evaluate children for developmental delays that are considered serious in their first 5 years of life [103, 104]. In screening a large number of children using the ASQ the great majority of the 3-year-old children analyzed in the ICSI and IVF groups had normal cognitive abilities, socio-emotional development, and motor skill scores [100]. Of the children that had developmental delays, the large majority originated from high-order gestation ($P<0.01$). This further solidifies the theory that single embryo transfer is essential in ensuring a healthy baby. Interestingly, children whose fathers' gametes were harvested surgically appeared to score better than those conceived with ejaculated spermatozoa by both IVF and ICSI [105]. Thus far, studies of children ranging from 5 to 12 years of age [99, 106–109] have been reassuring in terms of perinatal outcome, IQ, and physical development [98].

The specific concerns with regards to ICSI, whether real or theoretical [110–113], include the insemination method, the use of spermatozoa with genetic or structural defects, and the possible introduction of foreign genes. Several epidemiological studies of assisted reproduction children report a twofold increase in infant malformations [114], a recurrent reduction in birth weight [115], certain rare syndromes related to imprinting errors [116–120] and even a higher frequency of some cancers [121]. However, such observations do not prove that there is an increased risk of imprinting disorders and even less so childhood cancers in ICSI children [113]. A recent Australian study of 308, 974 total births, of which 6,163 were a result of assisted reproductive technology, found 513 defects (8.3%) in ART deliveries as compared with pregnancies not involving assisted conception (17,546 defects, 5.8%) with multivariate-adjusted odds ratio of 1.28 (95% CI, 1.16–1.41). The corresponding odds ratios with standard iVF (165 birth defects, 7.2%) was 1.07 (95% CI, 0.90–1.26), and the odds ratios with ICSI (139 defects, 9.9%) of 1.57 (95% CI, 1.30–1.90). A history of infertility, either with or without assisted conception, was also significantly associated with birth defects. The authors concluded that the findings could also be attributable to residual confounders not adjusted for in the model [122]. Thus assessment of the health of ART offspring is still ongoing and new information continues to become available. Although the abnormalities may be linked to the genetics or infertile status of the parents rather than the conception method employed, it is important to alert patients of a possible causal relationship with the technology *per se* [123].

Thus far, Beckwith-Wiedemann Syndrome (BWS) is the only epigenetic disorder that has been clearly associated with ART procedures [124] and the incidence has been found to be equally distributed among the in vitro conception methods. Epigenetic imbalances have been similarly linked to the exposure of the embryos to long term culture [98, 125]. At present, there is no evidence that the ICSI insemination itself is responsible for any increase in epigenetic disorders, findings that have been confirmed in animal studies [126].

In summary, the most important factor that may lead to adverse outcomes in offspring conceived by IVF or ICSI is high-order pregnancies.

However, the introduction of single embryo transfer has reduced this considerably. Although perinatal outcomes such as prematurity, low birth weight, perinatal mortality, and increased incidence of malformations have been linked to the techniques of IVF and ICSI, there is still the contribution of infertility itself. Overall, no significant long-term neurodevelopmental differences have been found in connection with the ARTs, though the risks associated with childhood cancer and future fertility still require further investigation.

Since the early establishment of in vitro insemination it became clear that a large portion of couples would not be capable of achieving fertilization. Now ICSI is generously applied worldwide for a variety of indications, and not exclusively for male factor infertility. ICSI has been shown to be the procedure of choice when spermatozoa, such as in azoospermic men, are directly retrieved from the epididymis and the testis. In fact in these men, as long as a viable spermatozoon is isolated, there is a chance of generating a viable pregnancy. The fertilization rates achieved with surgically retrieved specimens match those seen with optimal male gametes and similarly, embryo development is uncompromised. Concerns raised by ICSI have proved to be mainly unfounded as the health and developmental potential of offspring born from ICSI are comparable to those born after standard in vitro insemination. However, infertile men do have a higher incidence of chromosomal defects and particularly in azoospermic men, Yq microdeletion(s) may be present (see Chap. 3). Likewise, azoospermia is associated with a higher incidence of aneuploidy in the germ cells and with a possible increase in gonosomal disomies which can impact their offspring.

A meta-analysis of 28 RCTs confirmed that the application of assisted hatching yielded a higher clinical pregnancy than untreated embryos [95]. Other reports (Hellebaut et al. 1996; SART 2008) suggest that the execution of hatching on embryos of all ART couples is unwarranted. Current opinion is that targeted infertile couples may benefit from enhanced hatching even though the technique to be applied is still a matter of debate [92].

Once ART reins in the incidence of multiple gestations, available data indicate that the overall health of ART offspring will likely be highly comparable to those of children spontaneously conceived, even considering the older age of the female partners. In addition the frequencies of small for gestational age and prematurity in the ART population also will likely be similar to those occurring in spontaneous conceptions.

References

1. Gordon JW, Talansky BE. Assisted fertilization by zona drilling: a mouse model for correction of oligospermia. J Exp Zool. 1986;239:347–54.
2. Tsunoda Y, Yasui T, Nakamura K, Uchida T, Sugie T. Effect of Cutting the Zona-Pellucida on the Pronuclear Transplantation in the Mouse. J Exp Zool. 1986;240:119–25.
3. Odawara Y, Lopata A. A zona opening procedure for improving in vitro fertilization at low sperm concentrations: a mouse model. Fertil Steril. 1989;51:699–704.
4. Gordon JW, Grunfeld L, Garrisi GJ, Talansky BE, Richards C, Laufer N. Fertilization of Human Oocytes by Sperm from Infertile Males after Zona Pellucida Drilling. Fertil Steril. 1988;50:68–73.
5. Cohen J, Malter H, Fehilly C, Wright G, Elsner C, Kort H, Massey J. Implantation of Embryos after Partial Opening of Oocyte Zona Pellucida to Facilitate Sperm Penetration. Lancet. 1988;2:162–2.
6. Antinori S, Versaci C, Fuhrberg P, Panci C, Caffa B, Gholami GH. Seventeen live births after the use of an erbium-yytrium aluminum garnet laser in the treatment of male factor infertility. Hum Reprod. 1994;9:1891–6.
7. Feichtinger W, Strohmer H, Fuhrberg P, Radivojevic K, Antinori S, Pepe G, Versaci C. Photoablation of oocyte zona pellucida by erbium-YAG laser for in-vitro fertilisation in severe male infertility. Lancet. 1992;339:811.
8. Laws-King A, Trounson A, Sathananthan H, Kola I. Fertilization of human oocytes by microinjection of a single spermatozoon under the zona pellucida. Fertil Steril. 1987;48:637–42.
9. Palermo G, Van Steirteghem A. Enhancement of acrosome reaction and subzonal insemination of a single spermatozoon in mouse eggs. Mol Reprod Dev. 1991;30:339–45.
10. Palermo G, Joris H, Devroey P, Van Steirteghem AC. Pregnancies after intracytoplasmic injection of single spermatozoon into an oocyte. Lancet. 1992;340:17–8.
11. Palermo G, Joris H, Devroey P, Van Steirteghem AC. Induction of acrosome reaction in human spermatozoa used for subzonal insemination. Hum Reprod. 1992;7:248–54.

12. Hiramoto Y. Microinjection of the live spermatozoa into sea urchin eggs. Exp Cell Res. 1962;27:416–26.
13. Lin TP. Microinjection of mouse eggs. Science. 1966;151:333–7.
14. Uehara T, Yanagimachi R. Microsurgical injection of spermatozoa into hamster eggs with subsequent transformation of sperm nuclei into male pronuclei. Biol Reprod. 1976;15:467–70.
15. Naish SJ, Perreault SD, Foehner AL, Zirkin BR. DNA synthesis in the fertilizing hamster sperm nucleus: sperm template availability and egg cytoplasmic control. Biol Reprod. 1987;36:245–53.
16. Perreault SD, Wolff RA, Zirkin BR. The role of disulfide bond reduction during mammalian sperm nuclear decondensation in vivo. Dev Biol. 1984; 101:160–7.
17. Laufer N, Pratt BM, DeCherney AH, Naftolin F, Merino M, Markert CL. The in vivo and in vitro effects of clomiphene citrate on ovulation, fertilization, and development of cultured mouse oocytes. Am J Obstet Gynecol. 1983;147:633–9.
18. Thadani VM. Injection of sperm heads into immature rat oocytes. J Exp Zool. 1979;210:161–8.
19. Perreault SD, Zirkin BR. Sperm nuclear decondensation in mammals: role of sperm-associated proteinase in vivo. J Exp Zool. 1982;224:253–7.
20. Iritani A, Utsumi K, Miyake M, Hosoi Y, Saeki K. In vitro fertilization by a routine method and by micromanipulation. Ann N Y Acad Sci. 1988;541: 583–90.
21. Goto K, Kinoshita A, Takuma Y, Ogawa K. Fertilization of Bovine Oocytes by the Injection of Immobilized, Killed Spermatozoa. Vet Rec. 1990;127:517–20.
22. Lanzendorf S, Maloney M, Ackerman S, Acosta A, Hodgen G. Fertilizing potential of acrosome-defective sperm following microsurgical injection into eggs. Gamete Res. 1988;19:329–37.
23. Lanzendorf SE, Maloney MK, Veeck LL, Slusser J, Hodgen GD, Rosenwaks Z. A preclinical evaluation of pronuclear formation by microinjection of human spermatozoa into human oocytes. Fertil Steril. 1988;49:835–42.
24. Nagy ZP, Staessen C, Liu J, Joris H, Devroey P, Van Steirteghem AC. Prospective, auto-controlled study on reinsemination of failed-fertilized oocytes by intracytoplasmic sperm injection. Fertil Steril. 1995;64:1130–5.
25. Morton PC, Yoder CS, Tucker MJ, Wright G, Brockman WD, Kort HI. Reinsemination by intracytoplasmic sperm injection of 1-day-old oocytes after complete conventional fertilization failure. Fertil Steril. 1997;68:488–91.
26. Zhu L, Xi Q, Nie R, Chen W, Zhang H, Li Y. Rescue intracytoplasmic sperm injection: a prospective randomized study. J Reprod Med. 2011;56:410–4.
27. Yovich JL, Stanger JD. The limitations of in vitro fertilization from males with severe oligospermia and abnormal sperm morphology. J In Vitro Fert Embryo Transf. 1984;1:172–9.
28. Chia CM, Sathananthan H, Ng SC, Law HY, Edirisinghe WR. Ultrastructural investigation of failed in vitro fertilisation in idiopathic subfertility. Academy of Medicine: Singapore; 1984.
29. Defelici M, Siracusa G. Spontaneous Hardening of the Zona Pellucida of Mouse Oocytes during Invitro Culture. Gamete Res. 1982;6:107–13.
30. Bedford JM, Kim HH. Sperm/egg binding patterns and oocyte cytology in retrospective analysis of fertilization failure in vitro. Hum Reprod. 1993;8: 453–63.
31. Vanblerkom J, Henry G. Oocyte Dysmorphism and Aneuploidy in Meiotically Mature Human Oocytes after Ovarian Stimulation. Hum Reprod. 1992;7: 379–90.
32. Combelles CM, Morozumi K, Yanagimachi R, Zhu L, Fox JH, Racowsky C. Diagnosing cellular defects in an unexplained case of total fertilization failure. Hum Reprod. 2010;25:1666–71.
33. Lalonde L, Langlais J, Antaki P, Chapdelaine A, Roberts KD, Bleau G. Male infertility associated with round-headed acrosomeless spermatozoa. Fertil Steril. 1988;49:316–21.
34. Palermo GD, Cohen J, Rosenwaks Z. Intracytoplasmic sperm injection: a powerful tool to overcome fertilization failure. Fertil Steril. 1996;65:899–908.
35. Palermo GD, Colombero LT, Schattman GL, Davis OK, Rosenwaks Z. Evolution of pregnancies and initial follow-up of newborns delivered after intracytoplasmic sperm injection. JAMA. 1996;276:1893–7.
36. Uehara T, Yanagimachi R. Behavior of nuclei of testicular, caput and cauda epididymal spermatozoa injected into hamster eggs. Biol Reprod. 1977;16: 315–21.
37. Silber S, Ord T, Borrero C, Balmaceda J, Asch R. New treatment for infertility due to congenital absence of vas deferens. Lancet. 1987;2:850–1.
38. Temple-Smith PD, Southwick GJ, Yates CA, Trounson AO, de Kretser DM. Human pregnancy by in vitro fertilization (IVF) using sperm aspirated from the epididymis. J In Vitro Fert Embryo Transf. 1985;2:119–22.
39. Palermo GD, Cohen J, Alikani M, Adler A, Rosenwaks Z. Development and implementation of intracytoplasmic sperm injection (ICSI). Reprod Fertil Dev. 1995;7:211–7. discussion 217–218.
40. Palermo GD, Cohen J, Alikani M, Adler A, Rosenwaks Z. Intracytoplasmic sperm injection: a novel treatment for all forms of male factor infertility. Fertil Steril. 1995;63:1231–40.
41. Silber SJ, Nagy ZP, Liu J, Godoy H, Devroey P, Van Steirteghem AC. Conventional in-vitro fertilization versus intracytoplasmic sperm injection for patients requiring microsurgical sperm aspiration. Hum Reprod. 1994;9:1705–9.
42. Tournaye H, Devroey P, Liu JE, Nagy Z, Lissens W, Vansteirteghem A. Microsurgical Epididymal Sperm Aspiration and Intracytoplasmic Sperm Injection—a New Effective Approach to Infertility as a Result of

Congenital Bilateral Absence of the Vas-Deferens. Fertil Steril. 1994;61:1045–51.
43. Craft I, Bennett V, Nicholson N. Fertilising ability of testicular spermatozoa. Lancet. 1993;342:864.
44. Fishel S, Green S, Bishop M, Thornton S, Hunter A, Fleming S, al-Hassan S. Pregnancy after intracytoplasmic injection of spermatid. Lancet. 1995;345:1641–2.
45. Tesarik J, Mendoza C, Testart J. Viable embryos from injection of round spermatids into oocytes. N Engl J Med. 1995;333:525.
46. Lundin K, Sjogren A, Nilsson L, Hamberger L. Fertilization and pregnancy after intracytoplasmic microinjection of acrosomeless spermatozoa. Fertil Steril. 1994;62:1266–7.
47. Egashira A, Murakami M, Haigo K, Horiuchi T, Kuramoto T. A successful pregnancy and live birth after intracytoplasmic sperm injection with globozoospermic sperm and electrical oocyte activation. Fertil Steril. 2009;92(2037):e2035–9.
48. Heindryckx B, Van der Elst J, De Sutter P, Dhont M. Treatment option for sperm- or oocyte-related fertilization failure: assisted oocyte activation following diagnostic heterologous ICSI. Hum Reprod. 2005;20: 2237–41.
49. Liu J, Nagy Z, Joris H, Tournaye H, Devroey P, Van Steirteghem A. Successful fertilization and establishment of pregnancies after intracytoplasmic sperm injection in patients with globozoospermia. Hum Reprod. 1995;10:626–9.
50. Taylor SL, Yoon SY, Morshedi MS, Lacey DR, Jellerette T, Fissore RA, Oehninger S. Complete globozoospermia associated with PLCzeta deficiency treated with calcium ionophore and ICSI results in pregnancy. Reprod Biomed Online. 2010;20:559–64.
51. Tejera A, Molla M, Muriel L, Remohi J, Pellicer A, De Pablo JL. Successful pregnancy and childbirth after intracytoplasmic sperm injection with calcium ionophore oocyte activation in a globozoospermic patient. Fertil Steril. 2008;90(1202):e1201–5.
52. Ludwig M, al-Hasani S, Kupker W, Bauer O, Diedrich K. A new indication for an intracytoplasmic sperm injection procedure outside the cases of severe male factor infertility. Eur J Obstet Gynecol Reprod Biol. 1997;75:207–10.
53. Benagiano G, Gianaroli L. The new Italian IVF legislation. Reprod Biomed Online. 2004;9:117–25.
54. Ludwig M, Strik D, Al-Hasani S, Diedrich K. No transfer in a planned ICSI cycle: we cannot overcome some basic rules of human reproduction. Eur J Obstet Gynecol Reprod Biol. 1999;87:3–11.
55. Ludwig M, Schopper B, Al-Hasani S, Diedrich K. Clinical use of a pronuclear stage score following intracytoplasmic sperm injection: impact on pregnancy rates under the conditions of the German embryo protection law. Hum Reprod. 2000;15: 325–9.
56. Porcu E, Fabbri R, Seracchioli R, Ciotti PM, Magrini O, Flamigni C. Birth of a healthy female after intracytoplasmic sperm injection of cryopreserved human oocytes. Fertil Steril. 1997;68:724–6.
57. Johnson MH. The effect on fertilization of exposure of mouse oocytes to dimethyl sulfoxide: an optimal protocol. J In Vitro Fert Embryo Transf. 1989;6:168–75.
58. Schalkoff ME, Oskowitz SP, Powers RD. Ultrastructural observations of human and mouse oocytes treated with cryopreservatives. Biol Reprod. 1989;40:379–93.
59. Van Blerkom J, Davis PW. Cytogenetic, cellular, and developmental consequences of cryopreservation of immature and mature mouse and human oocytes. Microsc Res Tech. 1994;27:165–93.
60. Vincent C, Pickering SJ, Johnson MH. The hardening effect of dimethylsulphoxide on the mouse zona pellucida requires the presence of an oocyte and is associated with a reduction in the number of cortical granules present. J Reprod Fertil. 1990;89:253–9.
61. Harton GL, De Rycke M, Fiorentino F, Moutou C, SenGupta S, Traeger-Synodinos J, Harper JC. ESHRE PGD consortium best practice guidelines for amplification-based PGD. Hum Reprod. 2011;26: 33–40.
62. de Vincenzi I. A longitudinal study of human immunodeficiency virus transmission by heterosexual partners. European Study Group on Heterosexual Transmission of HIV. N Engl J Med. 1994;331: 341–6.
63. Garrido N, Meseguer M, Simon C, Pellicer A, Remohi J. Assisted reproduction in HIV and HCV infected men of serodiscordant couples. Arch Androl. 2004;50:105–11.
64. Bujan L, Daudin M, Pasquier C. Choice of ART programme for serodiscordant couples with an HIV infected male partner. Hum Reprod. 2006;21:1332–3. author reply 1333–1334.
65. Mencaglia L, Falcone P, Lentini GM, Consigli S, Pisoni M, Lofiego V, Guidetti R, Piomboni P, De Leo V. ICSI for treatment of human immunodeficiency virus and hepatitis C virus-serodiscordant couples with infected male partner. Hum Reprod. 2005;20: 2242–6.
66. Sauer MV, Chang PL. Establishing a clinical program for human immunodeficiency virus 1-seropositive men to father seronegative children by means of in vitro fertilization with intracytoplasmic sperm injection. Am J Obstet Gynecol. 2002;186:627–33.
67. Pena JE, Klein J, Thornton 2nd M, Chang PL, Sauer MV. Successive pregnancies with delivery of two healthy infants in a couple who was discordant for human immunodeficiency virus infection. Fertil Steril. 2002;78:421–3.
68. van Leeuwen E, Repping S, Prins JM, Reiss P, van der Veen F. Assisted reproductive technologies to establish pregnancies in couples with an HIV-1-infected man. Neth J Med. 2009;67:322–7.
69. Vitorino RL, Grinsztejn BG, de Andrade CA, Hokerberg YH, de Souza CT, Friedman RK, Passos SR. Systematic review of the effectiveness and safety of assisted reproduction techniques in couples serodiscordant for human immunodeficiency virus where the man is positive. Fertil Steril. 2011;95:1684–90.

70. Bendikson KA, Neri QV, Takeuchi T, Toschi M, Schlegel PN, Rosenwaks Z, Palermo GD. The outcome of intracytoplasmic sperm injection using occasional spermatozoa in the ejaculate of men with spermatogenic failure. J Urol. 2008;180:1060–4.
71. Edwards RG, Tarin JJ, Dean N, Hirsch A, Tan SL. Are spermatid injections into human oocytes now mandatory? Hum Reprod. 1994;9:2217–9.
72. Tsai MC, Takeuchi T, Bedford JM, Reis MM, Rosenwaks Z, Palermo GD. Alternative sources of gametes: reality or science fiction? Hum Reprod. 2000;15:988–98.
73. Girardi SK, Mielnik A, Schlegel PN. Submicroscopic deletions in the Y chromosome of infertile men. Hum Reprod. 1997;12:1635–41.
74. Reijo R, Seligman J, Dinulos MB, Jaffe T, Brown LG, Disteche CM, Page DC. Mouse autosomal homolog of DAZ, a candidate male sterility gene in humans, is expressed in male germ cells before and after puberty. Genomics. 1996;35:346–52.
75. Schlegel PN, Palermo GD, Alikani M, Adler A, Reing AM, Cohen J, Rosenwaks Z. Micropuncture retrieval of epididymal sperm with in vitro fertilization: importance of in vitro micromanipulation techniques. Urology. 1995;46:238–41.
76. Schlegel PN, Berkeley AS, Goldstein M, Cohen J, Alikani M, Adler A, Gilbert BR, Rosenwaks Z. Epididymal micropuncture with in vitro fertilization and oocyte micromanipulation for the treatment of unreconstructable obstructive azoospermia. Fertil Steril. 1994;61:895–901.
77. Pavlovich CP, Schlegel PN. Fertility options after vasectomy: a cost-effectiveness analysis. Fertil Steril. 1997;67:133–41.
78. Palermo G, Joris H, Derde MP, Camus M, Devroey P, Van Steirteghem A. Sperm characteristics and outcome of human assisted fertilization by subzonal insemination and intracytoplasmic sperm injection. Fertil Steril. 1993;59:826–35.
79. Ramasamy R, Reifsnyder JE, Bryson C, Zaninovic N, Liotta D, Cook CA, Hariprashad J, Weiss D, Neri Q, Palermo GD, et al. Role of tissue digestion and extensive sperm search after microdissection testicular sperm extraction. Fertil Steril. 2011;96: 299–302.
80. Schlegel PN. Nonobstructive azoospermia: a revolutionary surgical approach and results. Semin Reprod Med. 2009;27:165–70.
81. Reis MM, Tsai MC, Schlegel PN, Feliciano M, Raffaelli R, Rosenwaks Z, Palermo GD. Xenogeneic transplantation of human spermatogonia. Zygote. 2000;8:97–105.
82. Crabbe E, Verheyen G, Tournaye H, Van Steirteghem A. The use of enzymatic procedures to recover testicular germ cells. Hum Reprod. 1997;12:1682–7.
83. Crabbe E, Verheyen G, Silber S, Tournaye H, Van de Velde H, Goossens A, Van Steirteghem A. Enzymatic digestion of testicular tissue may rescue the intracytoplasmic sperm injection cycle in some patients with non-obstructive azoospermia. Hum Reprod. 1998;13:2791–6.
84. Dragisic KG, Davis OK, Fasouliotis SJ, Rosenwaks Z. Use of a luteal estradiol patch and a gonadotropin-releasing hormone antagonist suppression protocol before gonadotropin stimulation for in vitro fertilization in poor responders. Fertil Steril. 2005;84: 1023–6.
85. Veeck LL. The morphological assessment of human oocytes and early concepti. Boca Raton, Florida: CRC Press; 1990.
86. Neri QV, Monahan D, Palermo GD, Rosenwaks Z. IntraCytoplasmic Sperm Injection: Technical Aspects. United Kingdom: Informa UK Ltd; 2012.
87. Palermo GD, Neri QV, Monahan D, Takeuchi T, Schlegel PN, Rosenwaks Z. Intracytoplasmic Sperm Injection. New York: Springer; 2012.
88. Cohen J. Assisted Hatching of Human Embryos. J In Vitro Fertil Em. 1991;8:179–90.
89. Khalifa EAM, Tucker MJ, Hunt P. Cruciate Thinning of the Zona-Pellucida for More Successful Enhancement of Blastocyst Hatching in the Mouse. Hum Reprod. 1992;7:532–6.
90. Cohen J, Malter H, Wright G, Kort H, Massey J, Mitchell D. Partial Zona Dissection of Human Oocytes When Failure of Zona Pellucida Penetration Is Anticipated. Hum Reprod. 1989;4:435–42.
91. Cohen J, Alikani M, Trowbridge J, Rosenwaks Z. Implantation Enhancement by Selective Assisted Hatching Using Zona Drilling of Human Embryos with Poor Prognosis. Hum Reprod. 1992;7: 685–91.
92. Hammadeh ME, Fischer-Hammadeh C, Ali KR. Assisted hatching in assisted reproduction: a state of the art. J Assist Reprod Genet. 2011;28:119–28.
93. Palermo GD, Schlegel PN, Hariprashad JJ, Ergun B, Mielnik A, Zaninovic N, Veeck LL, Rosenwaks Z. Fertilization and pregnancy outcome with intracytoplasmic sperm injection for azoospermic men. Hum Reprod. 1999;14:741–8.
94. Nangia AK, Luke B, Smith JF, Mak W, Stern JE. National study of factors influencing assisted reproductive technology outcomes with male factor infertility. Fertil Steril. 2011;96:609–14.
95. Das S, Blake D, Farquhar C, Seif MM. Assisted hatching on assisted conception (IVF and ICSI). Cochrane Database Syst Rev 2009; CD001894.
96. Skiadas CC, Missmer SA, Benson CB, Gee RE, Racowsky C. Risk factors associated with pregnancies containing a monochorionic pair following assisted reproductive technologies. Hum Reprod. 2008;23:1366–71.
97. Ludwig M, Katalinic A. Malformation rate in fetuses and children conceived after ICSI: results of a prospective cohort study. Reprod Biomed Online. 2002;5:171–8.
98. Basatemur E, Sutcliffe A. Follow-up of children born after ART. Placenta. 2008;29(Suppl B): 135–40.
99. Basatemur E, Shevlin M, Sutcliffe A. Growth of children conceived by IVF and ICSI up to 12years of age. Reprod Biomed Online. 2010;20:144–9.
100. Palermo GD, Neri QV, Takeuchi T, Squires J, Moy F, Rosenwaks Z. Genetic and epigenetic characteristics of ICSI children. Reprod Biomed Online. 2008;17: 820–33.

101. Schieve LA, Rasmussen SA, Buck GM, Schendel DE, Reynolds MA, Wright VC. Are children born after assisted reproductive technology at increased risk for adverse health outcomes? Obstet Gynecol. 2004;103:1154–63.
102. Bowen JR, Gibson FL, Leslie GI, Saunders DM. Medical and developmental outcome at 1 year for children conceived by intracytoplasmic sperm injection. Lancet. 1998;351:1529–34.
103. Neri QV, Tanaka N, Wang A, Katagiri Y, Takeuchi T, Rosenwaks Z, Palermo GD. Intracytoplasmic sperm injection. Accomplishments and qualms. Minerva Ginecol. 2004;56:189–96.
104. Squires J, Carter A, Kaplan P. Developmental monitoring of children conceived by intracytoplasmic sperm injection and in vitro fertilization. Fertil Steril. 2003;79:453–4.
105. Neri QV, Williams-Pitman M, Rosenwaks Z, Palermo GD. Cognitive and behavioral profiles of ICSI children conceived from surgically retrieved spermatozoa. Fertil Steril. 2007;88:S39.
106. Belva F, Henriet S, Liebaers I, Van Steirteghem A, Celestin-Westreich S, Bonduelle M. Medical outcome of 8-year-old singleton ICSI children (born>or=32 weeks' gestation) and a spontaneously conceived comparison group. Hum Reprod. 2007;22:506–15.
107. Goldbeck L, Gagsteiger F, Mindermann I, Strobele S, Izat Y. Cognitive development of singletons conceived by intracytoplasmic sperm injection or in vitro fertilization at age 5 and 10 years. J Pediatr Psychol. 2009;34:774–81.
108. Knoester M, Helmerhorst FM, Vandenbroucke JP, van der Westerlaken LA, Walther FJ, Veen S, Leiden Artificial Reproductive Techniques Follow-up, P. Perinatal outcome, health, growth, and medical care utilization of 5- to 8-year-old intracytoplasmic sperm injection singletons. Fertil Steril. 2008;89: 1133–46.
109. Leunens L, Celestin-Westreich S, Bonduelle M, Liebaers I, Ponjaert-Kristoffersen I. Follow-up of cognitive and motor development of 10-year-old singleton children born after ICSI compared with spontaneously conceived children. Hum Reprod. 2008;23:105–11.
110. Cummins JM, Jequier AM. Treating male infertility needs more clinical andrology, not less. Hum Reprod. 1994;9:1214–9.
111. de Kretser DM. The potential of intracytoplasmic sperm injection (ICSI) to transmit genetic defects causing male infertility. Reprod Fertil Dev. 1995;7:137–41. discussion 141–132.
112. De Rycke M, Liebaers I, Van Steirteghem A. Epigenetic risks related to assisted reproductive technologies: risk analysis and epigenetic inheritance. Hum Reprod. 2002;17:2487–94.
113. Edwards RG, Ludwig M. Are major defects in children conceived in vitro due to innate problems in patients or to induced genetic damage? Reprod Biomed Online. 2003;7:131–8.
114. Hansen M, Kurinczuk JJ, Bower C, Webb S. The risk of major birth defects after intracytoplasmic sperm injection and in vitro fertilization. N Engl J Med. 2002;346:725–30.
115. Schieve LA, Meikle SF, Ferre C, Peterson HB, Jeng G, Wilcox LS. Low and very low birth weight in infants conceived with use of assisted reproductive technology. N Engl J Med. 2002;346:731–7.
116. DeBaun MR, Niemitz EL, Feinberg AP. Association of in vitro fertilization with Beckwith-Wiedemann syndrome and epigenetic alterations of LIT1 and H19. Am J Hum Genet. 2003;72:156–60.
117. Gicquel C, Gaston V, Mandelbaum J, Siffroi JP, Flahault A, Le Bouc Y. In vitro fertilization may increase the risk of Beckwith-Wiedemann syndrome related to the abnormal imprinting of the KCN1OT gene. Am J Hum Genet. 2003;72:1338–41.
118. Halliday J, Oke K, Breheny S, Algar E, J Amor D. Beckwith-Wiedemann syndrome and IVF: a case-control study. Am J Hum Genet. 2004;75:526–8.
119. Maher ER, Brueton LA, Bowdin SC, Luharia A, Cooper W, Cole TR, Macdonald F, Sampson JR, Barratt CL, Reik W, et al. Beckwith-Wiedemann syndrome and assisted reproduction technology (ART). J Med Genet. 2003;40:62–4.
120. Orstavik KH. Intracytoplasmic sperm injection and congenital syndromes because of imprinting defects. Tidsskr Nor Laegeforen. 2003;123:177.
121. Moll AC, Imhof SM, Schouten-van Meeteren AY, van Leeuwen FE. In-vitro fertilisation and retinoblastoma. Lancet. 2003;361:1392.
122. Davies MJ, Moore VM, Willson KJ, Van Essen P, Priest K, Scott H, Haan EA, Chan A. Reproductive technologies and the risk of birth defects. N Engl J Med. 2012;366:1803–13.
123. Wen J, Jiang J, Ding C, Dai J, Liu Y, Xia Y, Liu J, Hu Z. Birth defects in children conceived by in vitro fertilization and intracytoplasmic sperm injection: a meta-analysis. Fertil Steril. 2012;97(1331–1337): e1334.
124. Sutcliffe AG, Peters CJ, Bowdin S, Temple K, Reardon W, Wilson L, Clayton-Smith J, Brueton LA, Bannister W, Maher ER. Assisted reproductive therapies and imprinting disorders–a preliminary British survey. Hum Reprod. 2006;21:1009–11.
125. Rivera RM, Stein P, Weaver JR, Mager J, Schultz RM, Bartolomei MS. Manipulations of mouse embryos prior to implantation result in aberrant expression of imprinted genes on day 9.5 of development. Hum Mol Genet. 2008;17:1–14.
126. Wilson TJ, Lacham-Kaplan O, Gould J, Holloway A, Bertoncello I, Hertzog PJ, Trounson A. Comparison of mice born after intracytoplasmic sperm injection with in vitro fertilization and natural mating. Mol Reprod Dev. 2007;74:512–9.

Preimplantation Genetic Testing: Available and Emerging Technologies

8

Paul R. Brezina, Rony T. Elias, Glenn Schattman, and William G. Kearns

Introduction

Genetic defects in embryos, both aneuploidies and specific genetic disorders, are major barriers to achieving a healthy live born infant. Preimplantation genetic testing techniques have been developed to prevent the transfer of genetically abnormal embryos during in vitro fertilization (IVF) cycles [1–3]. These procedures determine the genetic status of embryos by analyzing one or more biopsied cell(s) from the developing embryo and then extrapolate the results of this analysis to the entire embryo (4-[4], [5], [6, 7]). Embryos believed to be free of abnormalities are then transferred into the woman's uterus.

P.R. Brezina, M.D., MBA
Division of Reproductive Endocrinology and Infertility, Department of Gynecology and Obstetrics, Johns Hopkins Medical Institutions, Phipps 264, 600N, Wolfe Street, Baltimore, MD 21287, USA

R.T. Elias, M.D.
The Center for Reproductive Medicine, Weill Cornell Medical College, 1305 York Avenue, 7th floor, New York, NY 10021, USA
e-mail: rta9002@med.cornell.edu

G. Schattman, M.D.
Department of OB/GYN, The Center for Reproductive and Infertility, Cornell Weill Medical Center, New York Presbyterian Hospital, Weill Medical College, Cornell University, 1305 York Avenue, New York, NY 10021, USA

W.G. Kearns, Ph.D (✉)
Department of Gynecology and Obstetrics, Johns Hopkins Medical Institutions, Phipps 264, 600N, Wolfe Street, Baltimore, MD 21287, USA

The Center for Preimplantation Genetics, LabCorp., Rockville, MD 20850, USA
e-mail: wkearns1@jhmi.edu; kearnsw@labcorp.com

When first introduced in 1990, preimplantation genetic testing was used exclusively to determine if embryos harbored specific genetic mutations that were known to exist from previous parental DNA analysis [1, 6, 8]. The practice of evaluating embryos for a known parental genetic defect was known as preimplantation genetic diagnosis (PGD), as a specific diagnosis is being investigated. As aneuploidy is the most significant reason for pregnancy failure, the technology of evaluating biopsied cells from embryos was then used to screen the ploidy status of embryos prior to embryo transfer [9, 10]. This evaluation of embryonic cells for aneuploidy, rather than for a known monogenetic defect from healthy parents, has therefore been termed PGS. Together, PGD and PGS are referred to as preimplantation genetic testing. PGD is useful to couples who wish to avoid passing a known inherited genetic condition on to their children. PGS has been proposed for couples who have a risk factor for aneuploidy, (i.e., advanced maternal age), recurrent pregnancy loss (RPL), or unsuccessful IVF cycles.

PGD or PGS is performed as part of an IVF cycle in which multiple oocytes are produced and retrieved from the woman's ovaries. Once retrieved, the oocytes are fertilized and embryo biopsy is performed [8, 11–13]. The biopsy

E.S. Ginsburg and C. Racowsky (eds.), *In Vitro Fertilization: A Comprehensive Guide*,
DOI 10.1007/978-1-4419-9848-4_8, © Springer Science+Business Media New York 2012

involves creating a defect in the zona pellucida layer surrounding the developing embryo in order to remove one or more cells from each embryo. This can be done mechanically, chemically (with acid Tyrode's solution), or with a laser and can be performed on polar bodies (extra chromosomal material that is the byproduct of oocyte maturation) fertilization blastomeres (cells taken from day 3 embryos, or trophectoderm, cells taken from embryos 5–6 days after fertilization, called blastocysts, [13, 14]). The biopsied cells are then sent to the testing laboratory where they are analyzed for the presence of genetic disorders. Through the use of advanced genetic testing technologyies, the samples free of abnormalities are identified. Results are usually available within 4–35 h, depending upon the technology employed [15].

Indications for Preimplantation Genetic Testing

Preimplantation Genetic Diagnosis

Single Gene Disorders

The genotype of a person is a set of alleles that make up his or her genetic constitution, either collectively at all loci, or more typically at a single locus. In contrast, the phenotype is the observable expression of the genotype as a morphological, clinical, cellular, or biochemical characteristic. The phenotype is usually thought of as the presence or absence of a disease, but a phenotype can refer to any manifestation, including characteristics that can be detected only by blood or tissue testing. In a more limited sense, the phenotype is the abnormality resulting from a particular mutant gene.

For the purpose of the present discussion, single gene disorders are DNA sequence variations in a gene that cause a specific type of genetic phenotype (i.e., delta F508 and cystic fibrosis). Single gene disorders are characterized by their patterns of transmission in families. To establish the pattern of transmission, the first step is to obtain information about the family history of the patient and to summarize the details in the form of a pedigree. A pedigree is a graphical representation of the family tree. The extended family depicted in such pedigrees is called a kindred. The member through whom the family with a genetic disorder is first brought to the attention of a geneticist is the proband. This is the person who is affected with the genetic disease segregating in the extended family (Fig. 8.1).

The pattern shown by single gene disorders and pedigrees depends chiefly on the following three factors:

1. Whether the phenotype is dominant. This means the phenotype is expressed when only one chromosome of a pair carries the mutant allele (i.e., Huntington disease) and the other chromosome has the wild type allele at the homologous chromosome locus
2. Whether the phenotype is recessive and is expressed only when both chromosomes of a homologous pair carry a mutation allele (i.e., cystic fibrosis)
3. The chromosome on which the gene locus is present. These loci may be on autosomal chromosomes (i.e., 1–22) or the sex chromosomes (X and Y). Single gene inheritance patterns include autosomal dominant (AD) inheritance, autosomal recessive (AR) inheritance, X-linked dominant inheritance, or X-linked recessive inheritance

In cases of single gene disorders, PGD is used to diagnose specific genetic mutations that are documented in the parents and that segregate within their extended family. This may be done by FISH (florescent in situ hybridization) but is now mostly accomplished using polymerase chain reaction (PCR) to amplify the DNA of the chromosome where the gene of interest resides and DNA sequencing [4, 16]. DNA sequencing identifies the specific altered DNA sequence and linkage analysis identifies surrounding markers used to determine recombination and whether the DNA of the sperm and oocyte amplified [17, 18].

Autosomal Dominant Disorders

More than half of all Mendelian disorders are inherited as an AD trait. The incidence of some autosomal disorders is high and this varies from

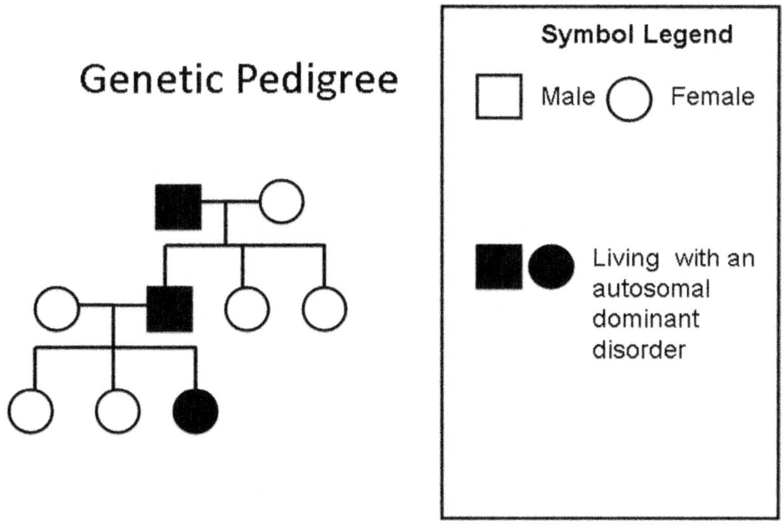

Fig. 8.1 Three-generation pedigree for an autosomal dominant disorder

region to region. An AD disorder is one in which one gene contains the mutant allele. The risk and severity of a dominantly inherited disease in the offspring depend on whether one or more parents are affected and whether the trait is strictly dominant or incompletely dominant.Affected carriers of an AD disorder have a 50% risk of having a child with that genetic disorder.

Autosomal Recessive Disorders

AR disease occurs in homozygotes who have the same abnormal allele at a particular locus location on a chromosome. Compound heterozygotes are individuals with two different mutant alleles at the same locus and no normal allele. In AR diseases, a heterozygote individual, with one normal gene copy, is able to compensate for the mutant allele and prevent the disease from occurring. If the husband and wife are both carriers of an autosomal recessive disorder, they have a 25% chance of having an affected child.

Sex Chromosome Linked Disorders

The X and Y chromosomes are responsible for sex determination and are distributed unequally in males and females. For this reason, phenotypes determined by genes on the X chromosome have a characteristic sex distribution and a pattern of inheritance that is usually easy to identify. Because females have two copies of the X chromosome, a female with a mutant allele on one X chromosome is termed heterozygous, or homozygous, if present on both X chrosomosomes. In contrast, a male, with only one X chromosome, is termed to be hemizygous for any given allele on the X chromosome. X-linked dominant and recessive patterns of inheritance are distinguished on the basis of the phenotype of heterozygous females. If this phenotype is consistently expressed in carriers (in female heterozygotes), it is considered an X-linked dominant disorder (i.e., in Rett syndrome).

Since females have two X chromosomes, one X chromosome undergoes X inactivation. If there is a disorder on one of the two X chromosomes, such as a CGG permutation repeat sequence as seen in fragile X syndrome, the X chromosome with the disorder is more likely to be inactivated. Therefore, approximately 99% of carrier females are unaffected carriers of an X-linked disorder. However, some women may be diagnosed with diseases caused by an X-linked recessive mutation (i.e., Hemophilia A) through skewed X chromosome inactivation in which the normal X chromosome undergoes X inactivation. X-linked disorders are expressed in males that only possess one X chromosome. Carrier females have a 50% chance of transmitting their mutant X chromosome to their daughters and a 50% chance of transmitting their mutant X chromosome to all their sons. Therefore, the chance of a female carrier having an affected embryo is 25% (one half of all affected male embryos).

Explanation of the phenotypic expression of single gene mutations depends upon the penetrance and expressivity of the mutated gene and is complicated. Patients who are affected by or carriers of genetic diseases should have consultation with genetic counselors, particularly prior to IVF for PGD as discussed later.

Testing for Single Gene Disorders

The most common method for testing single gene disorders is by genotyping or direct sequencing. Since only one or a few cells are biopsied for single gene testing, a DNA amplification step must be included in the analysis. For single gene testing the most common amplification step is by polymerase chain reaction (PCR) [19, 20]. Some laboratories, including ours, have employed a round of multiple displacement chain reaction followed by PCR for the gene being genotyped when doing single gene PGD and 23-chromosome PGS [21].

In order to confirm that the DNA from both the sperm and the egg has amplified within the reaction, one should also employ a modified linkage analysis assay which identifies polymorphic markers in the male and female samples for the chromosome where the gene mutation resides [21]. There is a risk of misdiagnosis with PGD that is introduced by failure to amplify genetic material (allele drop out, ADO), achieving only incomplete amplification (partial amplification), or contamination [22–24]. By incorporating a modified linkage analysis assay in the single gene mutation analysis, one greatly reduces the risk of ADO which is the leading cause of a single gene misdiagnosis [17, 18, 25, 26]. Some gene expansion mutations, such as fragile X, require the use of traditional linkage analysis incorporating multiple family generations to identify the mutant X-chromosome which contains the fragile X gene mutation.

PGD for HLA Typing

Another application for PGD is Human Leukocyte Antigen (HLA) typing [27, 28]. The major histocompatibility complex (MHC) is composed of a large cluster of genes located on the short arm of chromosome 6. These genes are categorized into three classes based upon structural and functional differences. The class I and class II genes correspond to the HLA genes. These genes encode cell surface proteins that play a critical role in the initiation of an immune response. The HLA alleles are codominant; each parent has two haplotypes and expresses both. These loci are located in close proximity and can be transmitted to gametes as a single block. As a result, the parent and child share only one haplotype and there is a 25% chance that two siblings will inherit the same haplotype from their parents. The testing for HLA is generally employed by parents who have a child affected by a particular disorder that could benefit from some sort of human tissue transplant. Due to the 25% chance that siblings will have an identical haplotype, genetic counseling is required to ensure that the couple has proper expectations, for example, when a child with leukemia requires a bone marrow transplant. In these cases, PGD has been employed as a modality to ensure that the next child that the couple conceives will be HLA compatible with their existing child with the given illness. This practice is relatively uncommon but has generated considerable debate regarding the ethics of HLA typing PGD [29].

Structural Chromosome Aberrations

PGD to detect structural chromosome imbalances in embryos are due to balanced parental chromosome rearrangements [30]. Parental chromosome rearrangements include reciprocal translocations, Robertsonian translocations, pericentric inversions, or paracentric inversions. Chromosomal rearrangements do not usually have a phenotypic effect if they are balanced because all of the chromosomal material is present even though it is packaged differently. Even when structural rearrangements in parents are truly balanced, they can pose a threat to their subsequent generation because carriers are likely to produce a high frequency of unbalanced gametes and therefore have an increased risk of having a miscarriage or an abnormal offspring with a genetic syndrome related to the unbalanced karyotype [31, 32]. The degree and severity of the phenotype observed in the offspring with the unbalanced karyotype depends upon the chromosomes (genes) involved in the structural chromosome imbalance [33].

Translocations

A translocation involves the exchange of chromosome segments between two usually nonhomologous chromosomes. There are two main types of translocations; reciprocal and Robertsonian.

Reciprocal Translocations

Reciprocal translocations result from the breakage of nonhomologous chromosomes, with reciprocal exchange of the broken segments [30]. Usually only two chromosomes are involved, and because the exchange is reciprocal, the total chromosome number is unchanged and the person harbors a balanced reciprocal rearrangement. Balanced rearrangements are usually harmless. Like other balanced structural rearrangements (i.e., inversions), balanced reciprocal translocations can result in unbalanced chromosomes in gametes leading to miscarriage or genetic syndromes. There are three main types of 2:2 chromosome segregation from carriers of reciprocal translocations [34]. 2:2 chromosome segregation is the normal distribution of entire nonhomologous or homologous chromosomes to daughter cells during cell division. Alternate segregation, the usual type of meiotic segregation, produces gametes that have either a normal chromosome complement or the two reciprocal chromosomes; both types of gametes are balanced. The other two types of segregation are called adjacent-1 or adjacent- 2, and these yield all unbalanced gametes. 3:1 chromosome segregation (the transmission to daughter cells of extra or too few nonhomologous or homologous chromosomes during cell division) can also occur; leading to gametes with either 22 or 24 chromosomes.

Robertsonian Translocations

Robertsonian translocations involve two acrocentric chromosomes, chromosome in which the centromere is located quite near one end, (i.e., chromosomes 13, 14, 15, 21, and 22) that fuse near the centromere with the loss of the short arms [35]. The short arms of acrocentric chromosomes contain ribosomal genes so there is no clinical significance. While Robertsonian translocations involving all acrocentric chromosomes have been reported, Robertsonian translocations involving chromosomes 13q and 14q or chromosomes 14q and 21q are the most common.

Inversions

An inversion occurs when a single chromosome undergoes two breaks and is reconstituted with the segment between the brakes inverted [31]. There are two types of inversions: pericentric inversions, which span the centromere; and paracentric inversions, which only occur on one arm of the chromosome (Figs. 8.2 and 8.3). An inversion does not usually cause an abnormal phenotype in carriers because it is a balanced rearrangement. The medical significance from either of these conditions pertains to the offspring of a parent with a balanced chromosomal aberration. A carrier of either type of inversion is at risk of producing abnormal gametes that may lead to genetically unbalanced offspring and reproductive failure, or to the birth of a child with a genetic syndrome.

Risk to Offspring

Parental carriers of translocations or inversions have an approximate 50% chance of producing unbalanced gametes. In couples with a possible recurrent pregnancy loss (RPL) and a documented balanced reciprocal or Robertsonian translocation or chromosomal inversion (paracentric or pericentric) in one or both parents, preimplantation genetic diagnosis (PGD) coupled with IVF has been shown to have some benefit in improving pregnancy and live birth rates [36–39].

Testing for Chromosome Imbalances

Traditionally, FISH has been used to identify the presence of translocation or inversion imbalances.

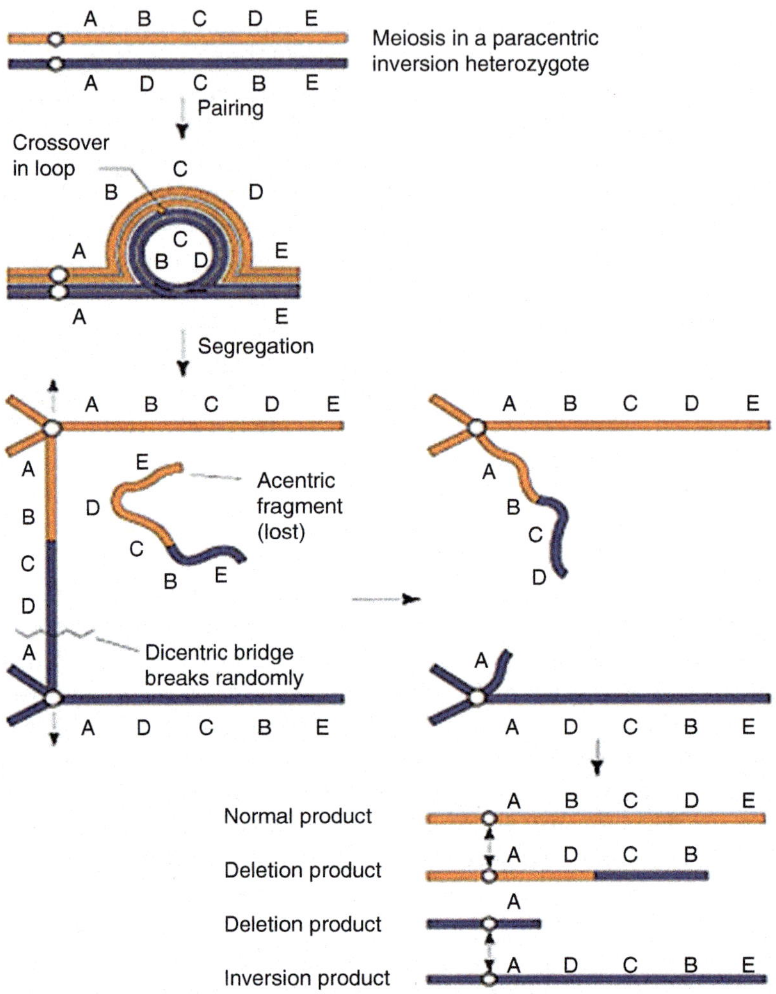

Fig. 8.2 Gamete formation for a paracentric inversion carrier; modified from http:www.fmv.uld.ac.be/genmol/MODGEN/Fig8_20.html. The image depicts the possible gamete formation following one crossing-over event during meiosis. Note the four possible gamete combinations (i.e., 25% dicentric chromosome, 25% acentric fragment, 25% normal chromosome, 25% inverted chromosome)

FISH is primarily able to differentiate between balanced and unbalanced chromosomal states. That is, it can tell if there is an extra piece or missing piece of chromosomal material in the cell (s) tested, but not if a cell has the balanced translocation of one of the parents. It is possible to employ specific chromosome breakpoint probes for reciprocal translocation or inversion carriers with FISH, to identify single cells with only the normal (nontranslocation or inversion chromosome). However, in recent years, microarrays are being increasingly utilized. Microarrays are able to evaluate all 23 pairs of chromosomes and thus evaluate the chromosomes involved in the structural aberration as well other chromosomes for aneuploidy or other imbalances [37, 39]. To a more limited extent, real-time PCR (discussed in a later section) [30] can be used Fig. 8.4 shows the application of FISH using telomere-specific probes for chromosomes involved in the structural chromosome imbalance along with centromeric markers of the appropriate chromosomes.

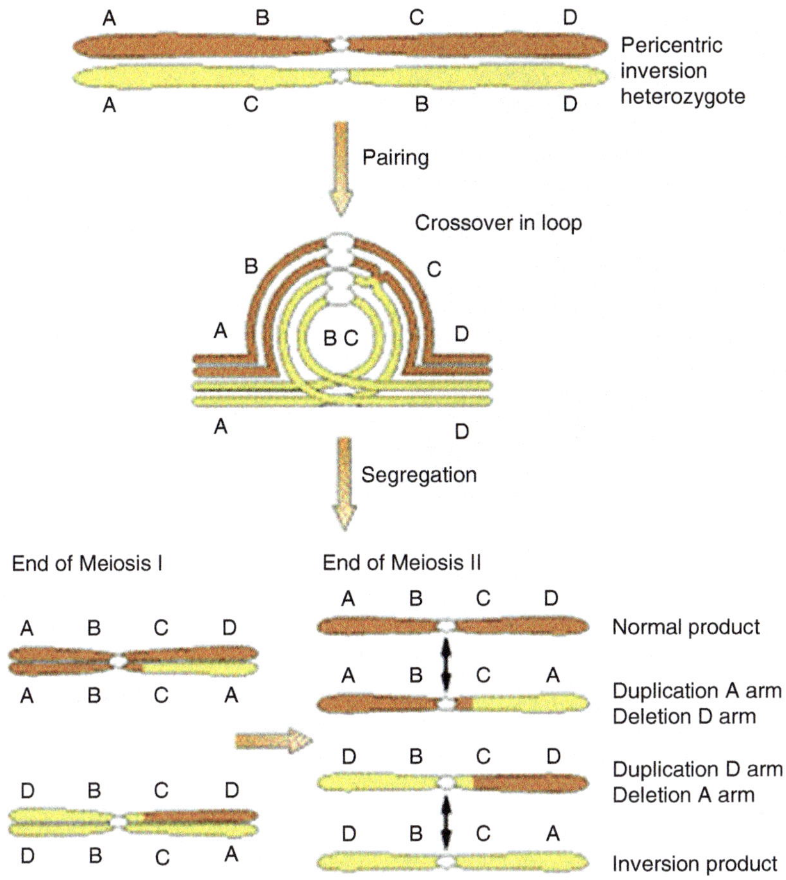

Fig. 8.3 Gamete formation for a pericentric inversion carrier; modified from http:www.fmv.uld.ac.be/genmol/MODGEN/Fig8_20.html. The image depicts the possible gamete formation following one crossing-over event during meiosis. Note the four possible gamete combinations, i.e., 25% normal chromosome, 25% inverted chromosome, and 50% deletion/duplication chromosomes

For reciprocal translocation imbalances one is looking for duplication and/or deletion of chromosomal material [34]. For Robertsonian translocations one is looking for whole chromosome imbalances such as trisomy 13 or trisomy 21 [35].

For pericentric inversions one is looking for duplication deletion imbalances on the chromosome harboring the inversion. While paracentric inversions causing reproductive problems are exceedingly rare, sometimes one can identify the presence of dicentric chromosomes (chromosomes with two centromeres) within day 3 embryos. These dicentric chromosomes contain imbalances and may be the cause of repeat miscarriages [31, 37].

As previously stated, when using FISH to identify structural chromosome aberrations due to reciprocal parental translocations, one cannot tell if the embryo contains the balanced reciprocal translocation or the nontranslocation chromosome product [39]. If one wishes to identify embryos completely free of the translocation, one must use breakpoint DNA clones that span the reciprocal translocation breakpoint in the parent. Our own IVF laboratory shows a 41% clinical pregnancy rate for reciprocal translocations, 35% for

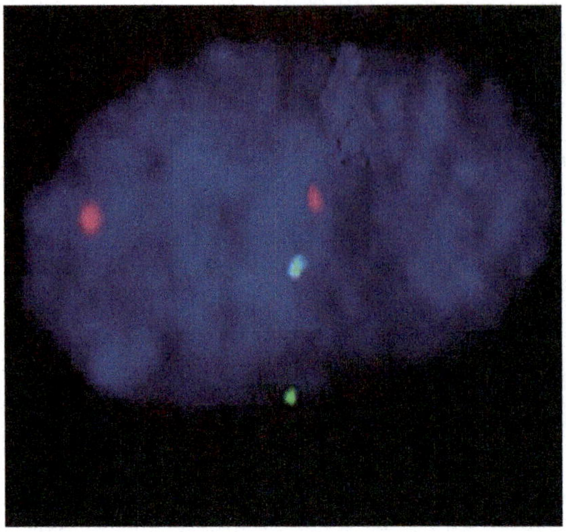

Fig. 8.4 PGD for parental translocation using fluorescence in situ hybridization (FISH): This figure shows a genetically balanced result of a biopsied cell from an embryo of a parent harboring a documented balanced translocation *t*(6p;9q). In this example, FISH probes were used for the subtelomeric regions of 6p and 9q. 6p subtelomeric signals are in red and 9q signals are in green. Because 2 signals for each probe are seen, the embryo must be diploid and genetically balanced for these regions. However, FISH cannot rule out the possibility that the embryo harbors a balanced translocation

Robertsonian translocations, and 33% for inversions. These results are generally consistent with historic data from the ESHRE PGD Consortium [40, 41]. The fact that these pregnancy rates were relatively low was a source of continued frustration for many in the PGD field. For this reason several laboratories, including ours (WGK), have begun using microarrays instead of FISH for evaluation of embryos in patients with documented translocations or inversions with clinical pregnancy rates exceeding 61%. While arrays are not able to detect embryos with balanced translocations, they can detect chromosomal imbalances both related to the parental chromosome aberration and other aneuploidies in all 23 pairs of chromosomes. It is possible that this approach will result in significant improvements in pregnancy rates with array based technology, compared to FISH, in this patient population.

Preimplantation Genetic Screening

Aneuploidy

Ploidy describes the number of copies of each chromosome within an individual nucleus of a cell. Normal diploid cells contain two copies of each autosome (chromosomes 1–22 and 2 sex chromosomes [XX and XY]). In general, monosomies are more lethal than trisomies [5], [42]. Therefore, when testing embryos for numerical chromosome abnormalities (aneuploidy), the only aneuploid conditions associated with a live baby are trisomies for chromosome 13, 18, 21, and sex chromosome aberrations (i.e., XXX, XXY, X, XYY). Aneuploidies for other chromosomes are lethal and are associated with either failed implantation or with spontaneous miscarriage

Chromosomal aneuploidy is the single greatest causal factor in miscarriage [9, 43, 44] and recurrent miscarriage [45]. PGS is the practice of evaluating cells from a developing embryo for the purposes of identifying aneuploidy. PGS was introduced as a technology that was hoped to greatly improve pregnancy efficiency in IVF patients at risk for miscarriage or implantation failure such as couples suffering from RPL or patients with advanced maternal age [21]. However, the practice of PGS for aneuploidy screening is more controversial than the application of PGD for evaluating a specific genetic mutation.

There are many different technologies that are used to determine the ploidy status of embryonic cells for PGS. PGS for aneuploidy was first performed with FISH evaluation for approximately 3–5 chromosomes using a cell taken from the embryo at the cleavage stage. FISH technology then progressed to the evaluation of more chromosome pairs. However, a number of other modalities for conducting genetic analysis for evaluating the ploidy status of embryonic cells have since been introduced. Below is a summary of the most commonly utilized modalities to determine the chromosomal status of embryonic cells for PGS.

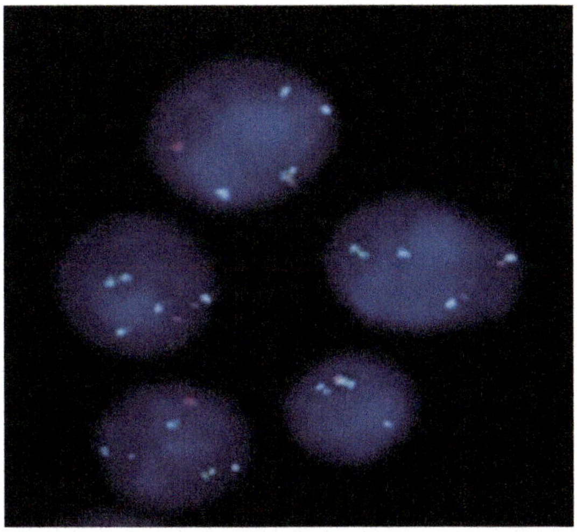

Fig. 8.5 An example of FISH flourochromes as they appear under microscope after DNA hybridization. In this sample, chromosomes 13 (gold), 18 (aqua), 21 (*red*), X (*green*), and Y (*blue*) were evaluated using five flourophores. Two signals are shown for chromosomes 13, 18, and 21. One signal is observed for X and no Y signal was identified

Fluorescent In Situ Hybridization

FISH, or fluorescent in situ hybridization, is a technology that was developed in 1986 in Leiden, Holland. The first application to embryo testing was described in 1992 [46]. FISH is a very robust, accurate molecular cytogenetic technology that uses labeled DNA probes that map to specific loci on individual chromosomes (Fig. 8.5). The actual technique of FISH is conceptually simple. Specifically, luminescent probes are prepared that are specifically designed to hybridize to specific areas of DNA on targeted chromosomes. After this hybridization is complete, the samples are evaluated visually under a microscope and the various flourochromes are observed that correspond to the different hybridization sites. If one flourochrome labeled for a specific chromosome, for example chromosome 21, is observed twice, the sample would be called normal for chromosome 21. However, if the sample had three signals it would be called as trisomy 21 and if the sample had only one signal it would be called monosomy.

Advantages of FISH

One advantage of FISH is that it does not require DNA amplification. This is beneficial for two main reasons. Firstly, amplification errors, both in the form of failed amplification and in contamination, do not exist with FISH. Secondly, FISH testing can be completed within 4–10 h after the receipt of the cells by the PGD laboratory. FISH can also be performed on interphase nuclei and does not require cell synchronization and division to produce metaphase chromosomes for analysis.

Disadvantages of FISH

Despite the above advantages, FISH has significant disadvantages that are increasingly marginalizing its use in PGS. Firstly, FISH is not able to easily test for all 23 chromosomes [47], and more commonly FISH probes for 5–8 chromosomes have been used [48]. While it is possible to test for all 23 pairs of chromosomes using FISH technology, the accuracy and risk for potential misdiagnosis is too great to use this on single cells from embryos. Secondly, FISH probes nearly always hybridize to repetitive DNA sequences on target DNA chromosomes which, in single cells from embryos, leads to "split signals" as one visualizes the fluorescent dots within interphase nuclei. These split signals can lead one to over-call aneuploidy for individual chromosomes within the interphase nuclei of embryonic cells. Currently, most PGS laboratories offer FISH assay for chromosomes associated with first trimester miscarriages.

Comparative Genomic Hybridization (CGH)

Another PGS technology called comparative genomic hybridization or CGH, was originally described in 1992 in order to identify gene amplification's in colon cancer cells [49], CGH was first used to evaluate the chromosomal status of embryos in 1996 [50–52]. CGH on metaphase chromosomes can identify aneuploidy of all 23-chromosome and large structural chromosome aberrations (>10 Mb) [50]. Using this method, one or more cells from an embryo are

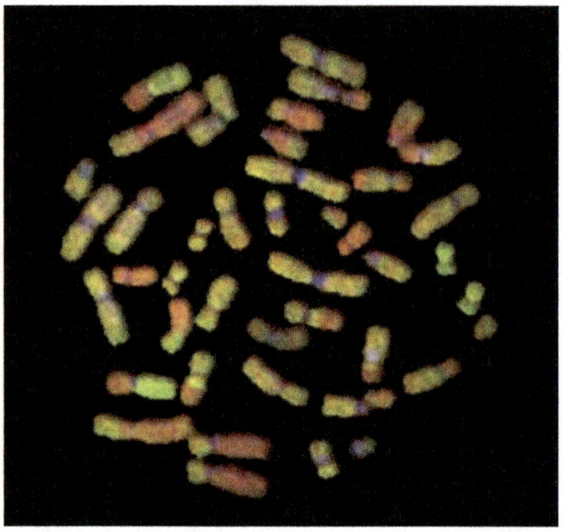

Fig. 8.6 CGH on Metaphase Chromosomes: This figure shows the raw fluorescent image representing a metaphase chromosome spread hybridization in which the red probes have hybridized to the patient chromosomes and the green probes have hybridized to the reference cell chromosomes. A computer readout comparing the ratio of red:green signal intensities between the embryonic and reference sample is then generated that reflects the ploidy status of the embryonic sample

removed and the DNA is amplified using a whole genome amplification protocol. This amplified product is then mixed with an approximately equal concentration of DNA from a known karyotypically normal 46, XY reference sample. Following this, a series of numerous chromosome site-specific flourophores are hybridized to each sample. Following hybridization and stringency washes, approximately 100 metaphase chromosome spreads are analyzed per embryonic sample. In general terms, a computer records a visual image of the embryonic and reference sample and records the intensity of each fluorophore (Fig. 8.6). Therefore, the intensity of each flourophore, corresponding to a specific section of genomic DNA on a specific chromosome, can be compared from the embryonic sample to a known normal sample. In this manner, computer software is able to give an analysis for each marker that states that the embryonic sample is either the same (diploid), twice as strong (trisomic), or half as strong (monosomic).

Advantages of CGH

An advantage of CGH on metaphase chromosomes is that all 23 chromosomes, as well as some large (>10 Mb) duplications and deletions, are able to be identified. Though this technique has some disadvantages, pregnancy rates obtained with CGH on metaphase chromosomes are encouraging and comparable to success rates with other methods of 23 chromosome PGS.

Disadvantages of CGH

A significant disadvantage of CGH on metaphase chromosomes is that the process is laborious and time-consuming. CGH on metaphase chromosomes takes at several days or more to complete and therefore the analysis always requires embryo cryopreservation. Additionally, the process demands DNA amplification which introduces confounders such as failed amplification and erroneous amplification of external DNA introduced through contamination. Unsuccessful amplification has been shown to occur in >10% of blastomeres analyzed [53]. Another disadvantage due to ratio labeling is that CGH can not differentiate triploidy from diploidy.

Microarrays

In the early to mid-2000s several laboratories began developing new technologies to test for all 23 pairs of chromosomes for aneuploidy, while simultaneously testing for structural chromosome aberrations. There are two main types of microarrays available for genetic testing. These are single nucleotide polymorphism (SNP) and CGH arrays. The differences between SNP and CGH are extensive. SNP arrays provide a genotype (i.e., AA, BB, or AB) for each SNP and are more dense than CGH microarrays. CGH arrays use ratio labeling and are less dense than SNP microarrays.

Single Nucleotide Polymorphisms Microarrays

Single nucleotide polymorphisms (SNPs, pronounced snips) are a single nucleotide (A, T, C, or G) change in genomic DNA. These are highly variable within a given species. Because SNPs are by definition single nucleotides, SNP evalua-

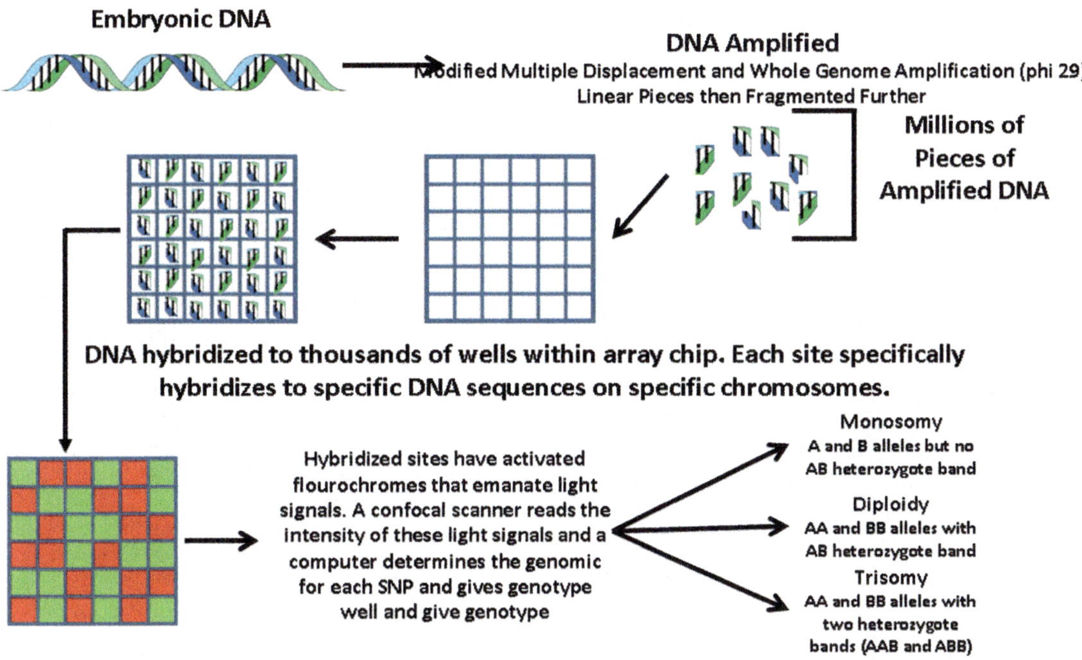

Fig. 8.7 Single nucleotide polymorphism (SNP) arrays: This flow diagram shows the steps involved in performing this technology

tion has many applications. Nearly all SNPs are in noncoding (non-gene) segments of the genome. However, recent research is showing that SNPs previously thought to have no genetic regulatory function may indeed act to activate certain promoters.

SNP microarrays for PGS typically evaluate approximately 300,000 SNPs throughout all 23 chromosomes. Because of this relatively high density of genetic markers, SNP microarrays are also able to detect relatively small chromosomal deletions and duplications within individual chromosomes. For example, our laboratory has documented the ability to detect chromosomal deletions as small is 1.5 Mb (Internal Data).

In SNP arrays for PGS, each array chip is specifically designed with hundreds of thousands of sites [Molecular cytogenetics Illumina]. Each site contains oligonucleotides that are a specific single SNPs on a specific chromosome. DNA from the biopsied cell(s) is amplified millions of times using multiple displacement amplification followed by a whole genome amplification protocol. This amplified DNA is then fragmented into small sections of DNA. The embryonic DNA is then hybridized to specific oligonucleotides within the chip. Following completion of this hybridization process, extraneous material is cleared from the chip through a series of stringency washes. Following these washes immunocytochemistry then adds specific flourophores to specific locations throughout the chip.

Following this, the chip is scanned to determine the fluorescent intensity signal from each site within the chip and translates this to data points. Computer software using extensive bioinformatics then compares this data-set to a known embryonic DNA dataset and generates SNP genotypes for each allele. Simplistically, these genotypes are described in the b allele frequency graph as either an AA, BB, or AB allele for each of these data points and analyzed based on specific

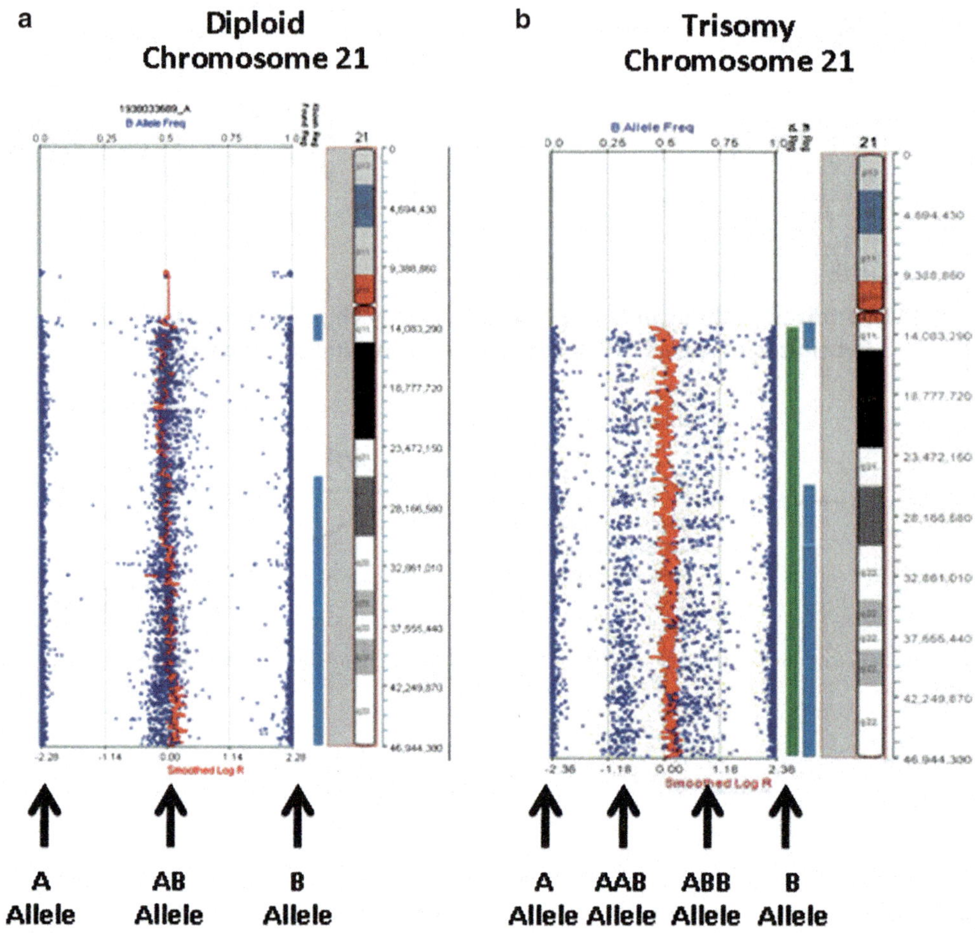

Fig. 8.8 SNP histograms of (**a**) A diploid chromosome 21; and (**b**) A trisomy chromosome 21: Note presence of the A, B, and heterozygote AB band in the diploid sample and the two heterozygote bands (AAB and ABB) associated with the triploid sample. The histograms were produced by KaryoStudio software

proprietary computer algorithms. This data is then reported in a histogram fashion for each chromosome. This computer software generated histogram data is then evaluated by the medical geneticist lab director and the molecular karyotype diagnosis is made (Fig. 8.7).

The organization of the SNP microarray histogram is specific to the ploidy status of the cell. In diploid samples, there is a band on the top and bottom of the histogram depicting SNPs resulting in either the AA or BB alleles (Fig. 8.8a). The center band represents the heterozygote AB band. The DNA copy number is represented by the Log R ratio. In a normal sample, the log R ratio should be approximately 0 or balanced.

In aneuploid results, this pattern is changed. An extra set of genetic material, as in trisomy, results in two heterozygote bands corresponding to AAB and ABB, and an upward shift in the log R ratio, reflecting an increased copy number (Fig. 8.8b). In monosomy, there is simply no heterozygote band coupled with a downward shift in the Log R ratio, reflecting a decreased copy number. The lack of a heterozygote band, also termed the loss of heterozygosity, can also be seen in SNP arrays to diagnose a rare phenomenon called uniparental

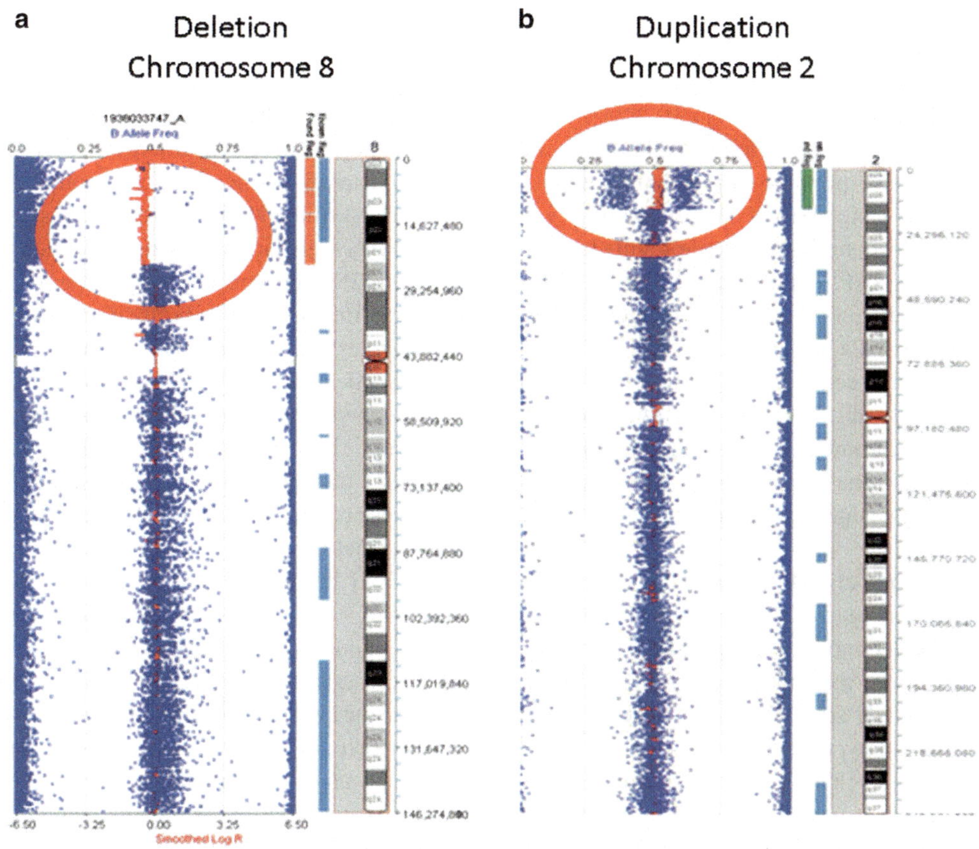

Fig. 8.9 SNP histogram showing examples, in the red circles of (**a**) a deletion of chromosome 8; and (**b**) a duplication of chromosome 2. Note the loss of the heterozygosity (LOH) associated with the deletion and the two heterozygote bands (AAB and ABB) associated with the duplication. The histograms were produced by KaryoStudio software

disomy (UPD). UPD is the presence of two homologous chromosomes from a single parent. Since there is no copy number change, there is no shift in the log R ratio. Clinically significant chromosomal deletions and duplications may also be identified by SNP arrays (Fig. 8.9).

Advantages of SNP Arrays

An advantage of SNP arrays is their ability to evaluate all 23 pairs of chromosomes with a highly dense platform capable of detecting clinically significant deletions and duplications Treff et al 2007, [5, 42]. The high density of the SNP arrays allow detection of many clinically significant deletions and duplications that would likely be missed with a less dense experimental protocol such as CGH arrays, FISH, or real-time PCR [54]. These large duplications and deletions are possibly deleterious to developing embryos, and may represent a cause of early pregnancy loss not detectable on standard karyotypes of products of conception.

Additionally, because SNP arrays provide a genotype for each genetic marker, these microarray platforms can identify triploidy and uniparental disomy (UPD) [55, 56]. As well as the ability to determine the parental origin of the chromosomal aneuploidy and to be able to identify what embryo implanted [57]. Other methodologies, such as 23-chromosome FISH, CGH on metaphase chromosomes, CGH microarrays, real-time PCR, or Bacs-on-a-Bead (described below) do not provide a genotype and cannot identify all triplodies or UPD.

Because SNP arrays actually evaluate specific alleles, it is also possible to test simultaneously some single gene defects in conjunction with PGS. This is accomplished by employing targeted high density SNP evaluation for certain single gene mutations of interest. In the near future, very dense SNPs designed for specific single gene mutations seeded on a 23 chromosome SNP array chip might be able to simultaneously identifiy 23-chromosome aneuploidy, and structural chromosome aberrations along with a specific single gene(s) mutation(s).

Disadvantages of SNP Arrays

One disadvantage of SNP analysis is the high cost of the technology. Array chips for SNPs are more dense and may be as much as twice the cost of CGH array chips.The preparation of SNP array analysis is laborious, often taking 2–3 days of work to amplify and analyze the sample. Therefore, it is impossible for an IVF clinic to do a day-5 biopsy and a day-6 transfer of fresh embryos. In addition, any technique requiring whole genome amplification can lead to allele dropout and/ or preferential amplification of DNA sequences, a possible cause of misdiagnosis.

Comparative Genomic Hybridization Arrays

CGH arrays are in some ways similar to SNP arrays. However, there are a number of significant differences between these two technologies. Firstly, instead of determining genotyping alleles within a sample, CGH array is a comparative ratio assay [52, 58]. In essence, CGH arrays are simply an array form of the CGH on metaphase chromosomes described above. In both CGH on metaphase chromosomes and CGH arrays, DNA is taken from the embryonic sample and mixed with control reference DNA. Both samples are then amplified. In the CGH array construct, the samples are then hybridized onto a CGH microarray array chip.

The CGH array chip is very different from a SNP microarray chip. The CGH array chip is low density (approximately 2,000–3,000 markers) and it uses ratio labeling and not genotyping to identify chromosome abnormalities. CGH arrays use a bacterial artificial chromosome (BAC) DNA or a similar DNA construct. These clones on CGH arrays are larger than the oligonucleotides on the SNP microarrays and permit a shorter DNA amplification and hybridization time. CGH is incapable of detecting many small, clinically significant deletions and duplications that may be diagnosed with SNP arrays. However, some CGH microarray chips are designed to identify small deletions or duplications in subtelomeric sequences and can be used for PGD due to parental reciprocal translocations or pericentric inversions. CGH arrays can also be used to identify embryonic imbalances due to parental Robertsonian translocations. Once the embryo and reference DNA samples have been hybridized onto the CGH array chips, stringency washes as described for SNP arrays are done and the chips are scanned and computer histograms produced for interpretation by the medical geneticist lab director (Figs. 8.10a, b and 8.11).

Advantages of CGH Arrays

CGH arrays have several advantages. Firstly, CGH array platforms are able to complete the entire analysis in as short as 12–15 h. This is a significant advantage over SNP arrays which take approximately 30–40 h to complete the analysis. Running a CGH array for aneuploidy or parental reciprocal translocations, Robertsonian translocations or pericentric inversions can offer IVF clinics the ability to do trophectoderm biopsy and transfer the blastocyst(s) the next day (i.e., a day-5 biopsy and a day-6 transfer). This eliminates the necessity of cryopreserving the biopsied embryos prior to obtaining results.

Disadvantages of CGH Arrays

Disadvantages of the CGH array platform include the less dense genetic evaluation of chromosomes that may not detect some clinically significant deletions and duplications that would be diagnosed with SNP arrays. Additionally,

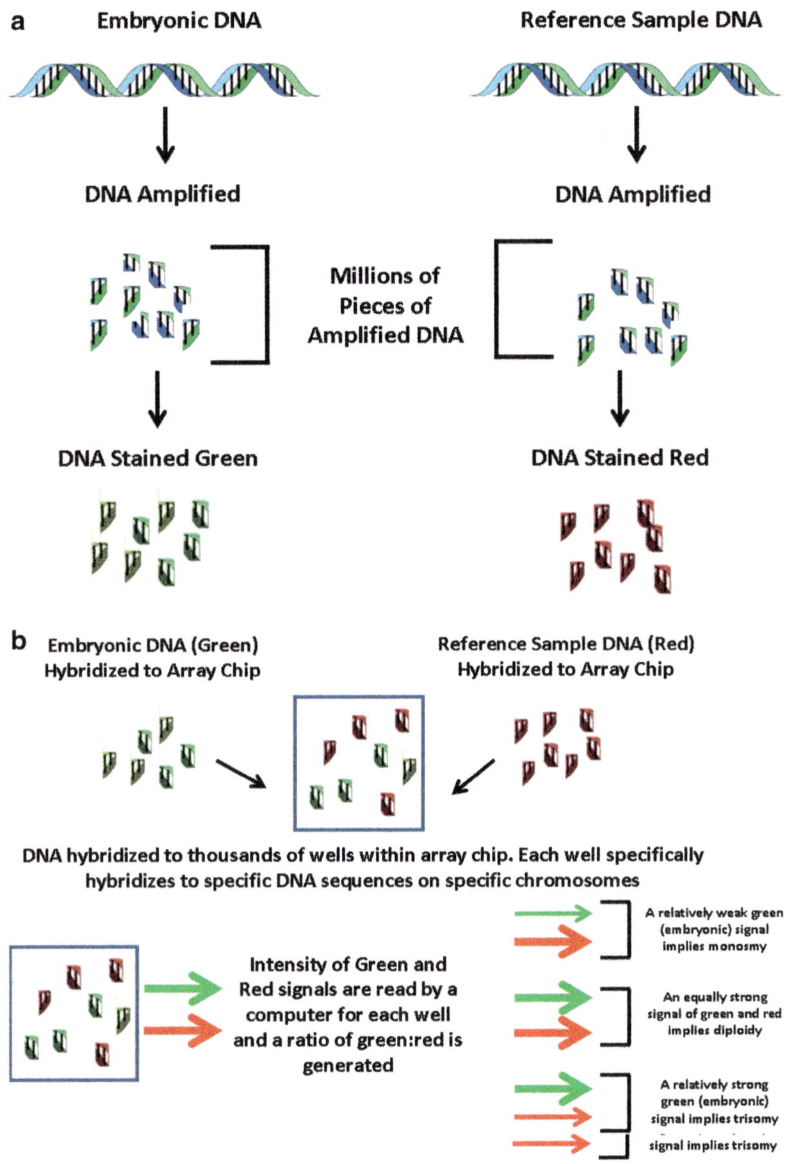

Fig. 8.10 Diagrammatic figure showing the principle of CGH Arrays

because CGH arrays by definition rely on ratio labeling, the technology is not capable of detecting uniform increases in all 23 pairs of chromosomes as is seen in triploid (69, XXX) embryos [55, 56]. However, ratio labeling is capable of detecting triploidy in male (69, XXY) embryos. Additionally, since no genotyping of alleles occurs, one cannot identify UPD or simultaneously detect some single gene mutations. Some other disadvantages specific to metaphase CGH are its inability to identify most clinically significant deletions or duplications. It can detect unbalanced DNA gains or losses at a resolution of 3–10 Mb [59]. Chromosomal microdeletion or duplications that will go undetected using m-CGH (smaller than 3 Mb) can account for about 15% of human genetic disease [60]. In addition since CGH technique detect imbalance

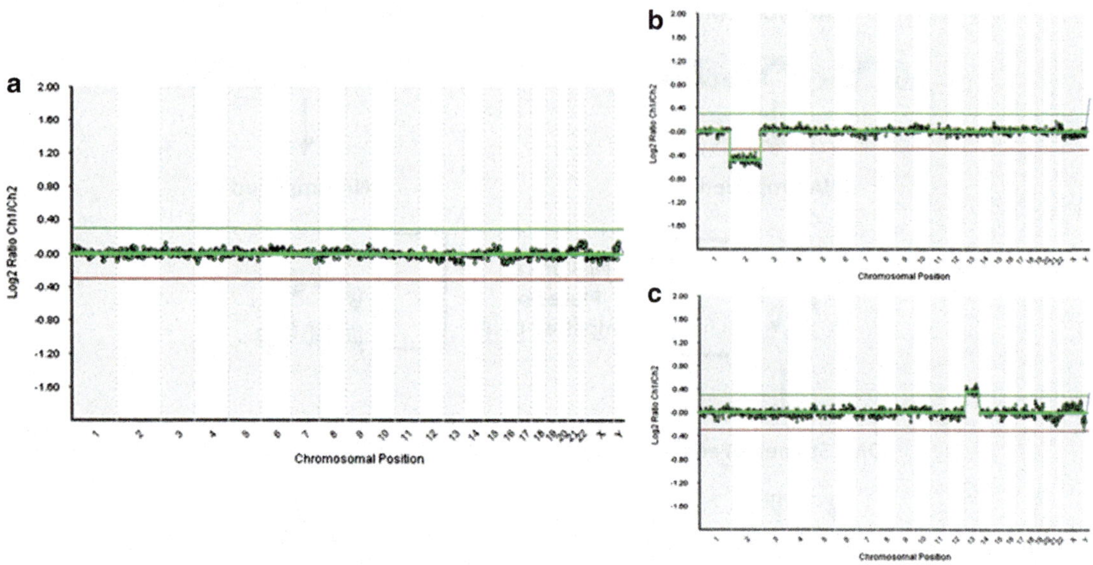

Fig. 8.11 Examples of different samples evaluated by CGH array for PGS: (**a**) A diploid with a relatively equal ratio of *green/red* fluorescence in all 23 pairs of chromosomes; (**b**) A cell monosomic for chromosome 2 with a clear downward deviation of the *plotted line* indicating a relative lack of *green*, as compared to red, signal intensity; (**c**) A cell trisomic for chromosome 13 with a clear upward deviation of the *plotted line* indicating a relative increase of *green*, as compared to *red*, signal intensity

in total DNA content, it cannot detect polyploidies (triploidies, tetraploidies…), inversions, or balanced translocations.

Real-Time PCR

Real-time PCR (RT PCR, or q PCR) is a polymerase chain reaction assay that detects copy number variations along a chromosome and compares this to a control sample [61]. This assay can easily identify aneuploidy for all 23 pairs of chromosomes in a rapid fashion (4–6 h) but it is unable in many cases to also simultaneously identify structural chromosome aberrations. The inability to identify all structural chromosome aberrations is due to the sparsity of alleles detected along each chromosome. Real-time PCR can identify triploidy but not UPD.

Bacs on Beads

This is a technology that binds bac DNA sequences for specific chromosome loci on beads within a microtiter like well reaction chamber. This technology can test for all 23 pairs of chromosomes for aneuploidy as well as the eight most commonly diagnosed microdeletion syndromes (i.e., Miller-Dieker syndrome or Smith-Magenis syndrome) and can complete the analysis in about 24 h Bacs on beads can identify triploidy but not UPD.

DNA Sequencing

Next-generation sequencing is allows us to rapidly sequence our genomes. While this technology holds future promise to identify deleterious DNA variants associated with genetic disease, it also shows geneticists that we all have numerous "variants" that may or may not be associated with disease. Therefore, it is premature to sequence the entire genome of embryos for genetic disorders because one will find thousands of variants of unknown significance. This will lead to the disposal of embryos that are "most likely" normal. One can sequence embryonic DNA for copy number changes (i.e., aneuploidy), clinically significant chromosome deletions or duplications as well as the mitochondrial genome.

A Summary of Error Rates and Expectations

The understanding of error rates is important in order for IVF physicians, geneticists, nurses, and most importantly, the patients, to have realistic expectations about treatment outcome. There are two types of errors. The most common error is an embryo misdiagnosis due to chromosome mosaicism within the embryo. This is where the cell or cells tested are normal but other untested cells are abnormal. As discussed below, the mosaicism rate in day-3 cleavage stage embryos can be as high as ~50% and in blastocysts the discordance between the inner cell mass and trophectoderm appears to be between 5 and 10%. The second type of error is a misdiagnosis on the cell or cells tested. This error rate can vary from laboratory to laboratory but the reported worldwide misdiagnosis rate is approximately 5% [62]

FISH errors for monosomy are mostly due to the DNA probe not hybridizing to the target chromosome within the cell nucleus. All experienced molecular cytogenetics labs should routinely re-hybridize with a different DNA probe to confirm monosomies. Trisomy errors by FISH are due to split fluorescent signals on the repetitive DNA sequences within the nucleus of the embryonic cell. This can lead to an over calling of trisomies. Experienced laboratories recognize this and should have an experienced molecular cytogenetist interpreting the fluorescent signals.

The errors on a single cell or cells for single gene diagnosis, is primarily due to allele drop-out (ADO) (i.e., only one copy of an allele is identified) of one of the gene mutations segregating in their family. Therefore, it is imperative that a form of linkage analysis, that will identify chromosome recombination and confirm the amplification of maternal and paternal chromosomes, also be performed along with gene sequencing, to ensure that a monosomy is not present.

With microarrays there is great redundancy in the number of probes per chromosome analyzed, and therefore the absence of probe signals or the spurious duplication of probe signals in the embryonic DNA are greatly reduced. The main cause of errors using microarrays is poor DNA amplification from the single cell or cells obtained from the embryo. Experienced genetics laboratories using microarrays have established experimental protocols that set minimum thresholds for the determination of successful DNA amplification. These include such things as call rates (the percent of genotyped SNPs) fluorescent intensities and the visualization of the DNA product on electrophoresis gels for SNP arrays. For CGH arrays, labs require a minimum percent of clones hybridized to the target sample, the visualization of the DNA product on electrophoresis gels and an acceptable signal to background fluorescent ratio.

Real-Time PCR or Bacs on Beads have limited numbers of probes that hybridize to individual chromosomes but provide better chromosome coverage than single probe FISH analysis. Artifactual monosomies and trisomies could occur.

Clinical Considerations in Preimplantation Genetic Testing

When Is the Optimal Time to Perform Embryo Biopsy?

Traditionally, PGD and PGS have been performed by taking a single cell from a cleavage stage embryo on day 3 of development. However, other biopsy methods, namely polar body biopsy [14] and trophectoderm biopsy [32, 54, 63–66], are also currently performed. Below is a description of each of these methods.

Polar Body Biopsy: Polar Bodies I and II

Since the majority of de novo aneuploidies come from errors of meiosis, evaluating the polar body of the oocyte prior to fertilization seems a logical place to start (Fig. 8.12). Polar body biopsy is performed prior to fertilization, so has been widely used in Europe where legislation in certain countries prohibits performing a biopsy on an embryo. While this technique is only useful in

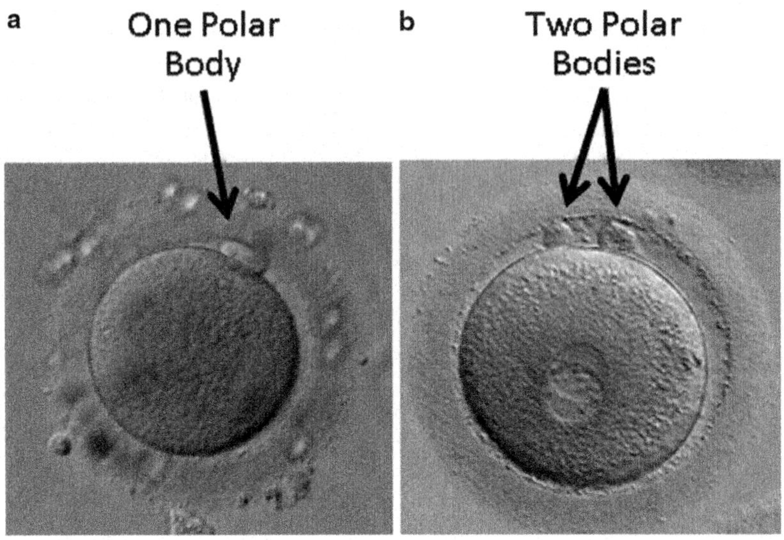

Fig. 8.12 Photographic images showing (**a**) an oocyte with one extruded polar body after ovulation; and (**b**) an oocyte with two polar bodies, 9–22 h after successful fertilization

diagnosing maternally inherited disorders, it is essentially the only method of offering PGS or PGD in some nations [67].

To understand the clinical utility of polar body biopsy, one must understand how polar bodies are derived during meiosis. Shortly before ovulation, the human oocyte possesses a diploid set of chromosomes [67]. At ovulation, this diploid set of chromosomes is split into two haploid sets of chromosomes. One set of chromosomes remains within the oocyte and the other is extruded outside the cell. This extruded set of chromosomes is contained within the 1st polar body. Biopsy of the first polar body should be performed on the day of oocyte retrieval.

At fertilization, each single set of chromosomes within the oocyte again splits into two chromatids [14, 67]. One chromatid remains in the oocyte nucleus and one set is extruded as the second polar body. Because these polar bodies represent a split compliment from the original diploid chromosomes, a gain or loss of chromosomes in the polar body implies a reciprocal loss or gain in the genetic material remaining in the oocyte. Therefore, a monosomy detected in a polar body should predict a trisomy in the genetic material remaining within the oocyte.

Polar body biopsy can be performed either by evaluating the first polar body in isolation prior to fertilization or by taking both polar bodies after fertilization. Recent studies have indicated that evaluating the first polar body in isolation may under-call genetic errors, especially for aneuploidy screening, as up to 50% of meiosis II divisions result in segregation errors [68]. Furthermore, because polar body biopsy by definition only evaluates maternally derived genetic material, the paternal genetic component and mitotic errors are not evaluable.

Advantages of Polar Body Biopsy

Polar body biopsy allows early determination of aneuploidy, maternally derived reciprocal translocation carriers, or maternal single gene carriers either before or after fertilization. Polar body biopsy also has no risk of disturbing the blastomeres that will continue to develop into the inner cell mass and subsequently the fetus or trophectoderm that will develop into the placenta. Therefore, despite the need to create a hole in the zona pellucida, polar body biopsy is, in essence,

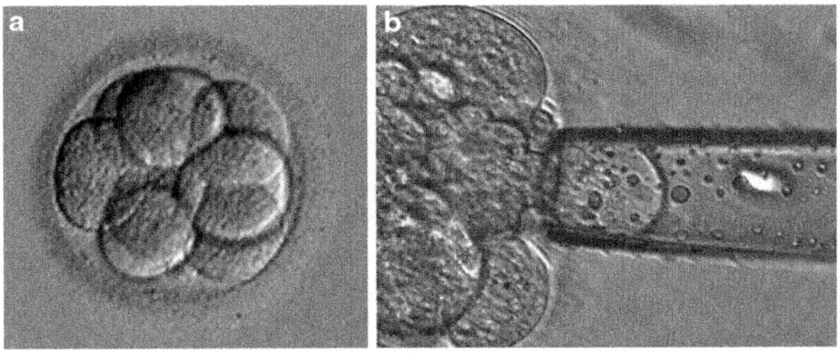

Fig. 8.13 Photographic images of (**a**) An 8-cell stage embryo on day 3; and (**b**) A cleavage-stage embryo undergoing blastomere biopsy

less invasive than other forms of embryo biopsy since it only removes genetic material that is discarded and does not contribute to embryo development..

Disadvantages of Polar Body Biopsy

Polar body biopsy only is capable of evaluating the maternal genetic component of an embryo. Therefore, it cannot detect chromosomal defects or single gene mutations that are paternally derived. Some debate the accuracy of polar body biopsy for aneuploid determination due to the large number of possible segregation patterns seen with polar body screening.

Day 3 Blastomere Biopsy

The most commonly utilized cell biopsied for analysis is a blastomere(s) taken from a cleavage stage embryo on day 3 (day 0 being the day of oocyte retrieval) (Fig. 8.13). At the cleavage stage of development, embryos are comprised of approximately 6–8 totipotent cells [69, 70] Totipotency means that the cells have not differentiated toward a particular cell line, and each cell therefore has the potential to form any part of the embryo or placenta.

Single blastomeres were initially thought to be excellent predictors of the chromosomal status of the embryo as a whole as each blastomere from a cleavage stage embryo should be totipotent and identical. However, this does not take into account the possibility of mitotic errors and mosaicism in the embryo. The major problem with blastomere biopsy, removing a single blastomere and inferring the chromosomal complement of the rest of the embryo based on a single cell is the high rate of aneuploid/euploid mosaicism that exists at this stage of development. Different laboratories have repeatedly demonstrated significant levels of chromosomal mosaicism (up to 50% of embryos) at the cleavage stage [71, 72] This makes biopsy at the cleavage stage problematic, as the biopsied cell will not represent the overall chromosomal makeup of the rest of the embryo in up to 50% of cases. These errors can be both false positive where the cell is abnormal but the majority of the rest of the embryo is normal or false negative where the result of the cell is normal but this does not represent the rest of the embryo which, in fact, is abnormal.

Advantages of Blastomere Biopsy

All PGS or PGD technologies allow completion of the analysis of a day-3 embryo biopsy within 48 h maximum, thereby providing the IVF clinic with a final report on day-5 for embryo transfer.

Disadvantages of Blastomere Biopsy

There are concerns that the act of embryo biopsy at the cleavage stage may be deleterious in and of itself to embryo development. The removal of a cell or cells from a day 3 stage embryo clearly reduces the embryos potential to differentiate to the blastocyst stage. This delay in differentiation may reduce the embryos ability to implant.

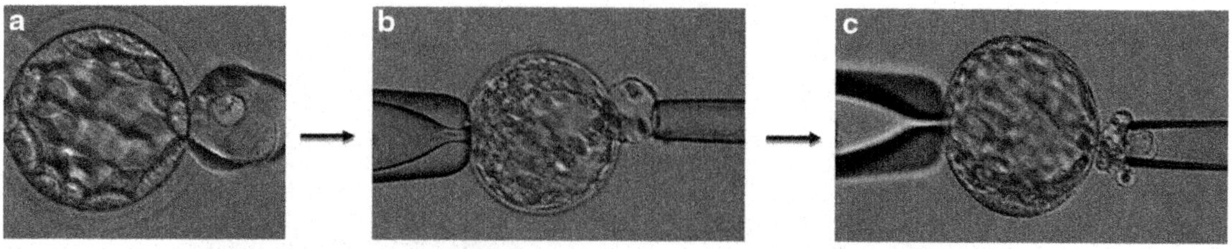

Fig. 8.14 Photographic images showing (**a**) A blastocyst undergoing herniation of TE cells after the application of a laser to breach the zona pellucida; (**b**) and (**c**) The process of obtaining a group of TE cells that will be analyzed for PGS.

Emerging data point to lower pregnancy and live birth rates when embryo biopsy for de novo aneuploidy (PGS) is performed at the cleavage stage [4, 7, 63, 64, 73, 74]. The reasons for this decrease in pregnancy rates may be due to a combination of issues; namely a high rate of chromosomal mosaicism at the cleavage stage, the ability of aneuploid/euploid mosaic embryos to genetically correct themselves during development to the blastocyst stage, and that the embryo biopsy per se may be detrimental to embryo development [47], [75, 76].There is an increasing volume of literature demonstrating the benefits of trophectoderm biopsy rather than the cleavage stage for the reasons outlined below.

Trophectoderm Cells from Differentiated Blastocysts

Four to five days after oocyte fertilization, a normally developing embryo has reached the blastocyst stage. At the blastocyst stage, the embryo is comprised of two distinct cell types:

1. The Inner Cell Mass (ICM), which comprises the mass of cells located within the blastocyst cavity (blastocele) destined to form the fetus
2. The Trophectoderm (TE), which is the population of cells (trophoblast cells) destined to form the placenta.

The blastocyst is comprised of over one hundred cells compared to the 6–8 cells of the cleavage stage embryo 3 days post oocyte retrieval. The configuration of the blastocyst is essentially a fluid filled sphere; with the walls of the sphere comprised of trophophoblasts with a relatively small cadre of cells within the sphere that comprises the ICM. At this point, the embryonic (ICM) cells are pluripotent, destined to go down certain cellular development pathways, rather than the totipotent cells of the cleavage stage embryo. Because the cells of the ICM are pluripotent and already destined to form the embryo, it is not currently possible to biopsy the ICM without taking a significant chance of harming the development of the fetus.

Advantages of Trophectoderm Biopsy

Biopsying TE is possible as these cells are quite numerous and are destined to form the placenta. Thus, TE biopsy (Fig. 8.14) is becoming increasingly popular and widespread. One of the major advantages of TE biopsy is that no part of the developing embryo that forms the fetus (the ICM), is disturbed; rather those cells destined to form the embryonic part of the placenta (the trophectoderm cells) are biopsied. Secondly, recent studies have found that chromosomal mosaicism is far lower at the blastocyst stage compared to the cleavage stage. In a study by our laboratory evaluating all of the cells within blastocysts, there was no chromosomal mosaicism detected, at a threshold of 5% mosaicism, within the ICM and TE cell populations in 42 embryos [47]. However, our data do show that there is approximately a 5–10% discordance between the molecular karyotype of the TE and ICM within a given embryo [47]. Therefore, a TE biopsy may not represent the chromosomal status of the ICM in as many as 5–10% of samples. However, the fact that the placenta and fetus may have discordant karyotypes has been known for some time. Studies evaluating chorionic villus

Table 8.1 PGD and PGS (PGT) Cycle Characteristics and Cancellation Rates Reported to SART 2007–2008 (mean±SD)

	No PGT	Genetic	Aneuploidy	Translocation	Elective sex
Total starts	170, 595	1,246	3,082	483	1,388
Age (year)*	34.9±4.4	33.5±4.2	37.2±3.6	33.5±4.2	34.5±4.1
Oocytes (*n*)	12.6±7.8	16.2±8.6	15.3±8.1	16.7±8.9	15.7±8.6
Embryos transferred (*n*)	2.5±1.0	2.0±0.9	2.0±0.9	1.8±0.8	1.9±0.8
Cancelled Transfers (*n*) (% Cycle Starts)	10,575 (6.2%)	161 (12.9)	532 (17.3)	132 (27.3)	232 (16.7)
Delivery/retrieval (%) (Women ≤42 yo)	35.4	31.6	27.9	24.3	33.4

*Age differs between category, $p<0.0001$
Adapted from Ginsburg et al. [79]

sampling (CVS) have shown that approximately 2% of CVS samples have documented confined placental mosaicism (CPM) [77]. CPM is defined in cases where the fetus at the time of CVS is euploid with aneuploidy documented in the placenta.

Advantage of Trophectoderm Biopsy

A strong argument for TE biopsy over cleavage stage or polar body biopsy is that TE biopsy results in higher pregnancy rates in experienced hands [32, 54, 63–66]. This is likely due to the decreased rate of mosaicism within the ICM and TE cell populations at the blastocyst stage. Additionally, certain forms of 23 chromosome PGS, such as real-time PCR and CGH arrays (see above), are compatible with fresh embryo transfer with TE biopsy.

Disadvantages of TE Biopsy

One disadvantage of TE biopsy is that because the technique has only recently been introduced, many embryologists do not yet have substantial experience with the procedure. A further, albeit perceived, disadvantage of TE biopsy is that SNP microarray evaluation of the biopsied cells typically takes 2–3 days. Because embryos will "hatch" soon after reaching the blastocyst stage, performing a TE biopsy with SNP microarray evaluation has, until recently, necessitated performing embryo cryopreservation and precluded a fresh cycle uterine transfer. However, newer modalities for quickly evaluating the chromosomal ploidy status of cells in just a matter of ~12 h, now makes it possible to offer a fresh transfer with TE biopsy and evaluation of aneuploidy for all 23 pairs of chromosomes.

Clinical Outcomes

Of the 146, 693 IVF/ ICSI cycles reported in the US through the Society for Reproductive Technology (SART) in 2010, 4% or 5,868 involved the use of PGT. This percentage was similar to that in previous years. A SART Writing Group examined the indications for PGT between 2007 and 2008. During that time the use of PGD for single gene defect evaluation and elective sex selection increased, despite the fact that ASRM guidelines discourage the use of PGD for the latter indication. Utilization for PGS decreased and that for translocations dropped slightly.

A high percentage of patients who underwent an IVF cycle and day 3 embryo biopsy with the goal of undergoing PGT, had no embryos transferred (Table 8.1). The SART database codes patients as having PGD or PGT at the time of embryo biopsy, so this study did not include patients who started cycles, but did not produce enough eggs or have enough embryos, or good enough quality embryos to undergo embryo biopsy. Therefore higher percentages of patients likely started an IVF stimulation with the goal of undergoing PGT, but were cancelled prior to biopsy. Overall, 6.2% of infertile IVF patients undergoing standard IVF, who did not undergo embryo biopsy had cycles cancelled after stimulation started, while the percentage of transfers cancelled after embryo biopsy were: 12.9%

Table 8.2 Preimplantation genetic testing data reported to the PGD consortium of ESHRE 1997 to 2007

	Oocyte Retrievals (*n*)	Embryos biopsied (*n*)	Embryos transferred (*n*)/(mean/ET)	Embryo Transfers (*n*)	Cycles with Oocyte Retrieval but no Embryo Transfer (%)	Clincal pregnancy rate per oocyte retrieval/per ET (%)
Single gene	4,733	27, 980	7,035 (1.9)	3,727	21.2	22 29
Structural chromosomal defects	4,253	27,068	4,775 (1.7)	2,731	35.8	17 26
X linked disorders	1,167	7,317	1,598 (1.8)	880	24.6	19 26
Aneuploidy screening	16,086	90,404	21,543 (1.8)	12,071	25.0	19 27
Social Sex selection (elective)	671	4,285	993 (2.0)	492	26.7	21 29

Adapted from Harper et al. [62]

undergoing PGD for genetic testing, 17.3% for PGS (aneuploidy screening), 27.3% for translocations, and 1.7% for elective sex selection. Possible reasons for lack of transfer after biopsy were: no normal embryos available to transfer, all embryos had nondiagnostic test results (uncommon), or all embryos arrested in culture after day 3 biopsy (Table 8.1). It must also be noted that due to the time period of the study biopsies would have been performed on cleavage stage embryos. As in other aspects of IVF, it is very important to set patient expectations based on their age, ovarian reserve, and fact-based estimated likelihood of having normal embryos to transfer.

Recently, ESHRE reported data on 27,000 PGT cycles that reached oocyte retrieval between 1997 and 2007. Sixty one percent of cycles were for aneuploidy screening, 17% for single gene disorders, 16% for chromosomal abnormalities, 4% for sex selection for X linked diseases, and 2% for elective sex selection. Delivery rates per oocyte retrieval and per embryo transfer are shown in Table 8.2. As can be seen, similar to the US data, a high percentage of cycles do not undergo embryo transfer, and clinical pregnancy rates per oocyte retrieval and per embryo transfer are low; patient ages were not given.

The miscarriage rates in patients undergoing PGT vary based on the stage of embryo development at biopsy and the type of PGT testing performed. Miscarriages can be caused by embryo mosaicism, a diagnostic error (i.e., the lab reports the embryo as normal when in fact it and the eventual fetus have an aneuploidy incompatible with continued development), or for other unknown causes. In general, the rates of miscarriage will be higher for couples undergoing day-3 biopsy and PGS due to embryo mosaicism then other types of PGT (such as single gene mutations or translocation imbalances). Overall, the rates of first trimester miscarriage, following 23-chromosome PGS, range between 3% for women under 35 and approximately 20% for women over 40.

Patient Counseling

We encounter situations in clinical practice that result in no embryos undergoing biopsy, for example when the response to ovarian stimulation is poor and there are few embryos, or when embryos on day 3, even if plentiful, are either highly fragmented or slowly cleaving. In such cases it is critical to confer with patients to determine whether they want to cancel the cycle, or in cases of patients undergoing PGS for aneuploidy screening, undergo embryo transfer as in standard IVF, and hope that the process of natural selection will cause abnormal embryos to either fail to implant or miscarry. This is all important information for patients to have before deciding to commit financial resources to PGT, as well as to understanding that even a successful oocyte retrieval and embryo transfer will not result in a high likelihood of delivery.

Single Gene Defects

A tremendous number of diseases related to single gene defects have been identified. It is critical that patients considering undergoing IVF treatment to avoid conception of a child with a single gene defect are aware of what percent of their embryos are likely to be affected. For example, when both partners are carriers of an autosomal recessive (AR) gene, there is a 25% chance that an embryo will be affected, a 50% that it will carry one copy of the abnormal gene, 25% that it will not be a carrier or affected. In autosmal dominant (AD)diseases, all embryos that carry the gene will be affected, so 50% of embryos will be affected. In X lined disorders, ~50% of embryos will be male, of which 50% will be affected, so 25% of embryos will be affected.

Affected embryos are not transferred. The dilemma of whether to transfer AR carrier embryos, which would have the same genetics as one of the parents, must be discussed with the couple prior to initiating PGD. Some couples feel strongly that the gene not be propagated in their family, whereas others want a healthy child and are less concerned about transmission of a gene that will not cause disease in the carrier (e.g., thalassemia trait). In AD conditions, only those without the AD mutation are transferred as the concept of a carrier does not apply.

Translocations

The population incidence of balanced translocations is 1–3/1,000. Among miscarriages ~3% are due to unbalanced translocations. Patients who present for consideration of PGD for balanced translocations typically have had at least 2 but commonly 3 or more SAbs, and in this population the incidence of balanced translocation is ~5% [78] However in a woman of advanced age, the likelihood of her having a balanced translocation will be lower than 5%, because most of her losses are likely to be aneuploid. Interestingly, men with balanced translocations are more likely to be infertile (See Chap. 2 on male) Since the incidence of balanced translocations in the population is low, translocations are the least common indication for PGD (Table 8.1)

Translocations are complex to manage, as the percentage of affected embryos and offspring varies depending on the size of the translocation imbalance. For example, the percentage of viable embryos likely to be identified will vary by the size and nature of the translocation imbalance; for small unbalanced translocations an abnormal offspring will be more likely than a miscarriage. Genetic counseling is therefore absolutely critical before a PGD plan can be made. As can be seen from both SART and ESHRE outcomes data (Tables 8.1 and 8.2), using day 3 biopsy and FISH technology, delivery rates for translocations/structural chromosomal abnormalities have been low.

HLA Matching

Consulting with patients about undergoing HLA matching in order to produce a sibling for a child affected with a lethal or other life-threatening condition may be heart breaking. Often parents have a gravely ill child on a waiting list for a donor for stem cell transplantation. The consultation therefore must include not only genetic counseling about the likelihood of an embryo being a match, but must also include that even when matched embryos are identified and successfully transferred, pregnancy will not necessarily occur. In addition, a plan must also be developed with the couple as to whether healthy, but nonmatching embryos will be frozen for potential future use, or discarded. Psychological support is particularly important for these patients as there are instances when a patient is successfully pregnant, but the ill child does not survive long enough to benefit from the HLA-matched sibling's birth.

Elective Sex Selection

Between 2007 and 2008 the largest increase in PGD utilization in the US was for elective sex selection [79]. The reason for couples or individuals choosing this, however, is not reported to SART, so a percentage of these cycles could have had medical indications such as attempting to avoid male gender so as to lower the risk of having a child with autism, in which males are four times more likely to be autistic than girls. The ASRM discourages elective sex selection [80]. Utilization of elective sex selection is varies from country-to-country in Europe. ART programs vary widely on whether they will perform PGD for elective gender selection. There can be ethical issues for the IVF team if faced with discarding normal embryos which are not of the gender desired by the intended parents.

Aneuploidy Screening/PGS

Although delivery rates with IVF have been increasing steadily despite transferring fewer embryos in each age group (www. sart.org), one exception is for women of advanced maternal age. This is most likely due to an increased risk of meiotic errors in the oocytes leading to aneuploidy. Theoretically selecting embryos by PGS should increase implantation and delivery rates. In 2007 Mastenbroek et al. [81] published a paper in which embryos underwent PGS for aneuploidy using FISH for 8 chromosomes. They concluded that PGS for 8 chromosomes does not improve the likelihood of implantation compared to IVF alone However, there are now 5 randomized clinical trials for advanced maternal age using day 3 embryo biopsy and FISH, showing a lower overall live birth rate than when embryos are not biopsied. Based on available evidence, the Practice Committee of the ASRM and SART concluded in 2008 and again in 2012 that PGS, as currently performed on day 3 embryos, may be associated with an overall lower probability of live birth [1, 8, 40, 41, 82]. A Cochrane review from 2006, updated in 2010, confirmed the conclusions of the ASRM/SART PC in advanced age women and those with prior multiple failed IVF cycles [83]. Despite the early enthusiasm for embryo aneuloidy screening based on the biology of ageing, to select embryos and improve pregnancy rates, the lack of benefit was attributed to the potential harm of embryo biopsy on the developing embryos [84], misdiagnosis due to the well-documented phenomenon of embryo mosaicism [76] and self correction where the abnormal cell(s) were either removed from the embryo at the time of the biopsy or preferentially fail to develop [76]. A study comparing results obtained with FISH and CGH showed up to 25% of "normal embryos" tested by FISH, to be abnormal when tested by CGH because the abnormal chromosome pair (s) was not included in the FISH panel [85].

For PGS to be optimized, our group (WGK) believes that an evaluation of all 23-pairs of chromosomes should be conducted ideally after trophectoderm biopsy. In 2007 PGS was first described evaluating all 23 pairs of chromosomes (autosomes 1–22, X and Y chromosomes) [54, 64]. Since this time, our laboratory along with several other leaders in the field have shifted to recommending that all PGS be performed using technology evaluating all 23 pairs of chromosomes. The clinical accuracy data obtained from 23 chromosome evaluation PGS is significantly superior to FISH PGS [32, 54, 63–66, 86] and some early evidence suggests that clinical pregnancy rates in selected patients might be improved [87].

It must be acknowledged, however, that patients who produce high quality blastocysts are those likely to benefit from the embryo selection that the screening allows; as many women of advanced maternal age also have decreased ovarian reserve, it is unclear what proportion would actually have normal blastocyts to transfer.

PGS is likely less controversial when patients with a history of a prior affected child, or termination of an affected pregnancy e.g., trisomy 21 has lead to significant life trauma. The complicated aspect of the discussion is that such patients are often not infertile, and might conceive readily on their own, and at no cost. Many couples are not comfortable conceiving on their own, undergoing antenatal testing, and then terminating an affected pregnancy. They must be alerted, however, to the high cost and relatively low pregnancy rate per initiated cycle thus far reported in the literature [8].

The specific indications for offering PGS are also not universally agreed upon within the field. Our laboratory (WGK) only recommends PGS testing for aneuploidy for couples with 2 or more first trimester miscarriages, though this position is not currently supported by data from limited randomized trials [8, 82]. All patients offered PGS testing, however, should have extensive genetic counseling prior to undergoing the procedure. The American Society of Reproductive Medicine has published minimum counseling guidelines that should be completed with all patients undergoing preimplantation genetic testing (PGS or PGD) [8]. These include reviewing the risks of IVF, risks of embryo biopsy, briefly reviewing the genetics involved with PGS and PGD procedure proposed, and the limitations of PGD and PGS. Genetic counseling should be done prior to PGT. Once the patient is pregnant antenatal testing with chorionic villus sampling and/ amniocentesis must be discussed, and a strong recommendation for antenatal testing should be included in all PGT consent forms.

Conclusions

The potential capabilities and efficiency of preimplantation genetic testing have dramatically increased in recent years due largely to improvements in the ability to accurately test embryos for single gene defects, structural chromosomal abnormalities, and aneuploidy. Blastocyst biopsy and PGT will likely show higher pregnancy rates, reduced miscarriage rates and more healthy babies versus day-3 biopsy and testing. However, large scale data are lacking. It is anticipated that randomized trials of PGS with trophectoderm biopsy and 23-chromosome testing will be performed in the upcoming years.

Regardless of improvements, patients must be carefully counseled about error rates inherent in all the PGT technologies, as well as outcomes reported to date. Patients must be given accurate information with which to make their treatment decisions, taking into account their age, ovarian reserve, indication for PGT and method of PGT to be employed.

Particularly when PGD is performed to prevent affected children, patients should be strongly counseled to undergo antental testing. As PGS is an evolving field, however, the optimal modality of embryo evaluation for aneuploidy is constantly being reevaluated. It is possible that emerging noninvasive technologies, such as metabolomics and videography, may ultimately be able to predict which embryos will develop into normal fetuses with a high degree of certainty [88, 89]. Regardless of which technologies ultimately are shown to be of greatest benefit, the field of evaluating embryos will certainly be an exciting area of growth in the future.

References

1. ACOG Committee Opinion No. 430: Preimplantation genetic screening for aneuploidy. Obstet Gynecol 2009;113(3):766–7
2. Dequeker E, Ramsden S, Grody WW, Stenzel TT, Barton DE. Quality control in molecular genetic testing. Nat Rev Genet. 2001;2:717–23.
3. Geraedts J, Handyside A, Harper J, Liebaers I, Sermon K, Staessen C, Thornhill A, Vanderfaeillie A, Viville S, ESHRE PGD Consortium Steering Committee. ESHRE Preimplantation Genetic Diagnosis (PGD) Consortium: preliminary assessment of data from January 1997 to September 1998. Hum Reprod. 1999;14:3138–48.
4. Brezina PR, Benner A, Rechitsky S, Kuliev A, Pomerantseva E, Pauling D, Kearns WG. Single-gene testing combined with single nucleotide polymorphism microarray preimplantation genetic diagnosis for aneuploidy: a novel approach in optimizing pregnancy outcome. Fertil Steril. 2011;95(5):1786 e5–8.
5. Brezina PR, Kearns WG. Preimplantation Genetic Screening in the Age of 23-Chromosome Evaluation; Why FISH is no longer an acceptable technology. J Fertil In Vitro. 2011;1:e103.
6. Handyside A, Kontogianni EH, Hardy K, Winston RM. Pregnancies from biopsied human preimplantation embryos sexed by Y-specific DNA amplification. Nature. 1990;344:768–70.
7. Munné S, Lee A, Rosenwaks Z, Grifo J, Cohen J. Diagnosis of major chromosome aneuploidies in human preimplantation embryos. Hum Reprod. 1993; 8:2185–91.
8. Practice Committee of Society for Assisted Reproductive Technology; Practice Committee of American Society for Reproductive Medicine. Preimplantation genetic testing: a Practice Committee opinion. Fertil Steril. 2008;90:S136–43.

9. Hassold T, Chen N, Funkhouser J, Jooss T, Manuel B, Matsuura J, et al. A cytogenetic study of 1000 spontaneous abortions. Ann Hum Genet. 1980;44:151–78.
10. Menasha J, Levy B, Hirschhorn K, Kardon NB. Incidence and spectrum of chromosome abnormalities in spontaneous abortions: new insights from a 12-year study. Genet Med. 2005;7:251–63.
11. Tarin JJ, Handyside AH. Embryo biopsy strategies for preimplantation diagnosis. Fertil Steril. 1993;59: 943–52.
12. Germond M, Nocera D, Senn A, Rink K, Delacrétaz G, Fakan S. Microdissection of mouse and human zona pellucida using a 1.48-microns diode laser beam: efficacy and safety of the procedure. Fertil Steril. 1995;64:604–11.
13. Brezina PR, Benner A, Barker A, Richter K, Cutting GR, Kearns WG. Human embryos with aneuploid cells documented at the cleavage stage undergo genetic correction during differentiation to the blastocyst stage. The 12th International Congress of Human Genetics (The 61st meeting of the American Society of Human Genetics), Montreal, Canada, October 11–15 2011;O-110.
14. Verlinsky Y, Rechitsky S, Verlinsky O, Ivachnenko V, Lifchez A, Kaplan B, et al. Prepregnancy testing for single-gene disorders by polar body analysis. Genet Test. 1999;3:185–90.
15. Treff NR, Scott Jr RT. Methods for comprehensive chromosome screening of oocytes and embryos: capabilities, limitations, and evidence of validity. J Assist Reprod Genet. 2012;29(5):381–90.
16. Verlinsky Y, Cieslak J, Freidine M, Ivakhnenko V, Wolf G, Kovalinskaya L, et al. Pregnancies following preconception diagnosis of common aneuploidies by fluorescent in-situ hybridization. Hum Reprod. 1995;10:1923–7.
17. Laurie AD, Hill AM, Harraway JR, Fellowes AP, Phillipson GT, Benny PS, et al. Preimplantation genetic diagnosis for hemophilia A using indirect linkage analysis and direct genotyping approaches. J Thromb Haemost. 2010;8:783–9.
18. Cirulli ET, Goldstein DB. Uncovering the roles of rare variants in common disease through wholegenome sequencing. Nat Rev Genet. 2010;11:415–25.
19. Hattori M, Yoshioka K, Sakaki Y. High-sensitive fluorescent DNA sequencing and its application for detection and mass-screening of point mutations. Electrophoresis. 1992;13:560–5.
20. Lissens W, Sermon K. Preimplantation genetic diagnosis: current status and new developments. Hum Reprod. 1997;12:1756–61.
21. Harton GL, De Rycke M, Fiorentino F, Moutou C, SenGupta S. Traeger Synodinos J, Harper JC; European Society for Human Reproduction and Embryology (ESHRE) PGD Consortium. ESHRE PGD consortium best practice guidelines for amplification-based PGD. Hum Reprod. 2011;26:33–40.
22. Navidi W, Arnheim N. Using PCR in preimplantation genetic disease diagnosis. Hum Reprod. 1991;6: 836–49.
23. Rechitsky S, Verlinsky O, Amet T, Rechitsky M, Kouliev T, Strom C. Reliability of preimplantation diagnosis for single gene disorders. Mol Cell Endocrinol. 2001;183(1):S65–8.
24. Hussey ND, Davis T, Hall JR, Barry MF, Draper R, Norman RJ. Preimplantation genetic diagnosis for beta-thalassaemia using sequencing of single cell PCR products to detect mutations and polymorphic loci. Mol Hum Reprod. 2002;8:1136–43.
25. Renwick PJ, Lewis CM, Abbs S, Ogilvie CM. Determination of the genetic status of cleavage-stage human embryos by microsatellite marker analysis following multiple displacement amplification. Prenat Diagn. 2007;27:206–15.
26. Renwick PJ, Trussler J, Ostad-Saffari E, Fassihi H, Black C, Braude P, Ogilvie CM, Abbs S. Proof of principle and first cases using preimplantation genetic haplotyping- a paradigm shift for embryo diagnosis. Reprod Biomed Online. 2006;13:110–9.
27. Kuliev A, Rechitsky S, Verlinsky O, Tur-Kaspa I, Kalakoutis G, Angastiniotis M, Verlinsky Y. Preimplantation diagnosis and HLA typing for haemoglobin disorders. Reprod Biomed Online. 2005; 11:362–70.
28. Verlinsky Y, Rechitsky S, Sharapova T, Morris R, Taranissi M, Kuliev A. Preimplantation HLA testing. J Am Med Assoc. 2004;291:2079–85.
29. Brezina P, Zhao Y. Laser Assisted Zona Hatching: What Is the Evidence to Justify its Use? Middle East Fertil Soc J. 2011;16:107–109.
30. Pujol A, Benet J, Staessen C, Van Assche E, Campillo M, Egozcue J, Navarro J. The importance of aneuploidy screening in reciprocal translocation carriers. Reproduction. 2006;131:1025–35.
31. Escudero T, Estop A, Fischer J, Munne S. Preimplantation genetic diagnosis for complex chromosome rearrangements. Am J Med Genet A. 2008; 146A:1662–9.
32. Treff NR, Tai X, Taylor D, Ferry KM, Scott RT. First pregnancies after blastocyst biopsy and rapid 24 chromosome aneuploidy screening allowing a fresh transfer within four hours of biopsy. Fertil Steril. 2010;94:S126.
33. Lim CK, Cho JW, Song IO, Kang IS, Yoon YD, Jun JH. Estimation of chromosomal imbalances in preimplantation embryos from preimplantation genetic diagnosis cycles of reciprocal translocations with or without acrocentric chromosomes. Fertil Steril. 2008;90(6):2144–51.
34. Ko DS, Cho JW, Park SY, Kim JY, Koong MK, Song IO, Kang IS, Lim CK. Clinical outcomes of preimplantation genetic diagnosis (PGD) and analysis of meiotic segregation modes in reciprocal translocation carriers. Am J Med Genet A. 2010;152A:1428–33.

35. Huang J, Lian Y, Qiao J, Chen Y, Ren X, Liu P. Characteristics of embryo development in Robertsonian translocations' preimplantation genetic diagnosis cycles. Prenat Diagn. 2009;29:1167–70.
36. Kuliev A, Verlinsky Y. Current features of preimplantation genetic diagnosis. Reprod Biomed Online. 2002;5:294–9.
37. Treff NR, Northrop LE, Kasabwala K, Su J, Levy B, Scott RT. Single nucleotide polymorphism microarray-based concurrent screening of 24-chromosome aneuploidy and unbalanced translocations in preimplantation human embryos. Fertil Steril. 2011;95:1606–12.
38. Otani T, Roche M, Mizuike M, Colls P, Escudero T, Munné S. Preimplantation genetic diagnosis significantly improves the pregnancy outcome of translocation carriers with a history of recurrent miscarriage and unsuccessful pregnancies. Reprod Biomed Online. 2006;13:869–74.
39. Du L, Brezina PR, Benner AT, Swelstad BB, Gunn M, Kearns WG. The rate of de novo and inherited aneuploidy as determined by 23-chromosome single nucleotide polymorphism microarray (SNP) in embryos generated from parents with known chromosomal translocations. Fertil Steril. 2011;96(3):S221.
40. Harper J, Coonen E, De Rycke M, Fiorentino F, Geraedts J, Vet G, et al. What next for preimplantation genetic screening (PGS)? A position statement from the ESHRE PGD Consortium Steering Committee. Hum Reprod. 2010;25:821–3.
41. Harper JC, Coonen E, De Rycke M, Harton G, Moutou C, Pehlivan T, Traeger-Synodinos J, Van Rij MC, Goossens V. ESHRE PGD Consortium data collection X: cycles from January to December 2007 with pregnancy follow-up to October 2008. Hum Reprod. 2010;25:2685–707.
42. Christianson MS, Brezina PR, Benner AT, Du L, Siegel A, Kearns WG. Chromosomal duplications (≥200 kilobases (KB)) are more common than deletions ≥200 kb in developing human embryos as identified by 23 chromosome single nucleotide polymorphism (SNP) microarray. Fertil Steril. 2011;96:S21–22.
43. Burgoyne PS. Holland k, Stephens R. Incidence of numerical chromosome anomalies in human pregnancy estimation from induced and spontaneous abortion data. Hum Reprod. 1991;6:555–65.
44. Kalousek DK, Pantzar T, Tsai M, Paradice B. Early spontaneous abortion: morphologic and karyotypic findings in 3,912 cases. Birth Defects Orig Artic Ser. 1993;29:53–61.
45. Stephenson MD, Awartani KA, Robinson WP. Cytogenetic analysis of miscarriages from couples with recurrent miscarriage: a case–control study. Hum Reprod. 2002;17:446–51.
46. Griffin DK, Wilton LJ, Handyside AH, Winston RM, Delhanty JD. Dual fluorescent in situ hybridisation for simultaneous detection of X and Y chromosome-specific probes for the sexing of human preimplantation embryonic nuclei. Hum Genet. 1992;89:18–22.
47. Brezina PR, Chipko C, Benner AT, Du L, Christianson MS, Kearns WG. Deletions and duplications identified by 23 chromosome single nucleotide polymorphism (SNP) microarray are associated with aneuploidy. Fertil Steril. 2011;96(4):S21.
48. Jobanputra V, Sobrino A, Kinney A, Kline J. Warburton D. Multiplex interphase FISH as a screen for common aneuploidies in spontaneous abortions Hum Reprod. 2002;17:1166–70.
49. Kallioniemi A, Kallioniemi OP, Sudar D, Rutovitz D, Gray JW, Waldman F, et al. Comparative genomic hybridization for molecular cytogenetic analysis of solid tumors. Science. 1992;258:818–21.
50. Wells D, Levy B. Cytogenetics in reproductive medicine: the contribution of comparative genomic hybridization (CGH). Bioessays. 2003;25:289–300.
51. Wells D, Delhanty J. Evaluating comparative genomic hybridisation (CGH) as a strategy for preimplantation diagnosis of unbalanced chromosome complements. Eur J Hum Genet. 1996;4(1):125.
52. Wells D, Alfarawati S, Fragouli E. Use of comprehensive chromosomal screening for embryo assessment: microarrays and CGH. Mol Hum Reprod. 2008;14:703–10.
53. Harper JC, Sengupta SB. Preimplantation genetic diagnosis: state of the art 2011. Hum Genet. 2012;131:175–86.
54. Treff NR, Su J, Tao X, Levy B, Scott RT. Accurate single cell 24 chromosome aneuploidy screening using whole genome amplification and single nucleotide polymorphism microarrays. Fertil Steril. 2010;94:2017–21.
55. Schaaf CP, Wiszniewska J, Beaudet AL. Copy Number and SNP Arrays in Clinical Diagnostics. Annu Rev Genomics Hum Genet. 2011;12:25–51.
56. Schaaf CP, Wiszniewska J, Beaudet AL. Copy number and SNP arrays in clinical diagnostics. Annu Rev Genomics Hum Genet. 2011;12:25–51.
57. Bisignano A, Wells D, Harton G. Munné S PGD and aneuploidy screening for 24 chromosomes: advantages and disadvantages of competing platforms. Reprod Biomed Online. 2011;23:677–85.
58. Fiegler H, Geigl JB, Langer S, Rigler D, Porter K, Unger K, Carter NP, Speicher MR. High resolution array-CGH analysis of single cells. Nucleic Acids Res. 2007;35:e15.
59. Kirchhoff M, Rose H, Lundsteen C. High resolution comparative genomic hybridisation in clinical cytogenetics. J Med Genet. 2001;38:740–4.
60. Vissers LE, Veltman JA, van Kessel AG, Brunner HG. , Identification of disease genes by whole genome CGH arrays. Hum Mol Genet, 2005; 14 Spec No. 2:R215–23
61. Fiorentino F, Kokkali G, Biricik A, Stavrou D, Ismailoglu B, De Palma R, Arizzi L, Harton G, Sessa

M, Pantos K. PCR-based detection of chromosomal imbalances on embryos: the evolution of PGD for chromosomal translocations. Fertil Steril. 2010;94: 2001–11.

62. Harper JC, Wilton L, Traeger-Synodinos J, Goossens V, Moutou C, SenGupta SB, et al. The ESHRE PGD Consortium: 10 years of data collection. Hum Reprod Update. 2012;18:234–47.
63. Scott RT, Miller KA, Olivares R, Su J, Fratterelli JL, Treff NR. Microarray based 24 chromosome preimplantation genetic diagnosis (mPGD) is highly predictive of the reproductive potential of human embryos: a prospective blinded non-selection trial. Fertil Steril. 2008;90:S22.
64. Kearns WG, Pen R, Benner A, Widra E. Leach. R Comprehensive genetic analyses using a modified whole genome amplification protocol and micro-arrays to identify genetic disorders and determine embryo implantation from single cells Fertil Steril. 2007;88:S237.
65. Benner A, Chipko C, Pen R, Kearns WG. Clinical results on single cells from 470 embryos using 23-chromosome single nucleotide polymorphism (SNP) microarray preimplantation genetic screening (PGS) from 45 patients. Fertil Steril. 2010;94:S123.
66. Benner AT, Brezina PR, Du L, Chipko C, Gunn C, Gunn M, Kearns WG. 23-chromosome single nucleotide polymorphism (SNP) microarray preimplantation genetic screening (PGS) on blastocysts, versus day-3 embryos, results in significantly higher clinical pregnancy rates. Fertil Steril. 2011;963:S221.
67. van der Ven K, Montag M, van der Ven H. Polar body diagnosis - a step in the right direction? Dtsch Arztebl Int. 2008;105:190–6.
68. Fragouli E, Katz-Jaffe M, Alfarawati S, Stevens J, Colls P, Goodall NN, et al. Comprehensive chromosome screening of polar bodies and blastocysts from couples experiencing repeated implantation failure. Fertil Steril. 2010;94:875–87.
69. Goossens V, De Rycke M, De Vos A, Staessen C, Michiels A. VerpoestW, et al. Diagnostic efficiency, embryonic development and clinical outcome after the biopsy of one or two blastomeres for preimplantation genetic diagnosis. Hum Reprod. 2008;23:481–92.
70. De Vos A, Staessen C, De Rycke M. VerpoestW, Haentjens P, Devroey P, Liebaers I. Van de Velde H Impact of cleavage-stage embryo biopsy in view of PGD on human blastocyst implantation: a prospective cohort of single embryo transfers Hum Reprod. 2009;24:2988–96.
71. Munné S, Weier HU, Grifo J, Cohen J. Chromosome mosaicism in human embryos. Biol Reprod. 1994;51: 373–9.
72. Munné S, Weier HU, Grifo J, Cohen J. Chromosome mosaicism in human embryos. Biol Reprod. 1994; 51:373–9.
73. Northrop LE, Treff NR, Levy B, Scott Jr RT. SNP microarray-based 24 chromosome aneuploidy screening demonstrates that cleavage-stage FISH poorly predicts aneuploidy in embryos that develop to morphologically normal blastocysts. Mol Hum Reprod. 2010;16(8):590–600.
74. Treff NR, et al. SNP microarray-based 24 chromosome aneuploidy screening is significantly more consistent than FISH. Mol Hum Reprod. 2010;16: 583–9.
75. Munné S, Velilla E, Colls P. Garcia Bermudez M, Vemuri MC, Steuerwald N, et al. Self-correction of chromosomally abnormal embryos in culture and implications for stem cell production Fertil Steril. 2005;84:1328–34.
76. Barbash-Hazan S, Frumkin T, Malcov M, Yaron Y, Cohen T, Azem F, et al. Preimplantation aneuploid embryos undergo self-correction in correlation with their developmental potential. Fertil Steril. 2009;92: 890–6.
77. Wang BB, Rubin CH, Williams 3rd J. Mosaicism in chorionic villus sampling: an analysis of incidence and chromosomes involved in 2612 consecutive cases. Prenat Diagn. 1993;13:179–90.
78. Jaslow CL, Carney JL, Kutteh WH. Diagnostic factors identified in 1020 women with two versus three or more recurrent pregnancy losses. Fertil Steril. 2010;93:1234–43.
79. Ginsburg ES, Baker VL, Racowsky C, Wantman E, Goldfarb J, Stern JE. Use of preimplantation genetic diagnosis and preimplantation genetic screening in the United States: a Society for Assisted Reproductive Technology Writing Group paper. Fertil Steril. 2011;96:865–8.
80. Ethics Committee of the American Society for Reproductive Medicine. Preconception gender selection for nonmedical reasons. Feritl Steril 2001;75
81. Mastenbroek S, Twisk M, Echten-Arends J, Sikkema-Raddatz B, Korevaar JC, Verhoeve HR, et al. In vitro fertilization with preimplantation genetic screening. N Engl J Med. 2007;357:9–17.
82. Practice Committee of the Society for Assisted Reproductive Technology; Practice Committee of the American Society for Reproductive Medicine. Preimplantation genetic testing: a Practice Committee opinion. Fertil Steril. 2007;88:1497–504.
83. Twisk M, Mastenbroek S, van Wely M, Heineman MJ, Van der Veen F, Repping S. Preimplantation genetic screening for abnormal number of chromosomes (aneuploidies) in in vitro fertilisation or intracytoplasmic sperm injection. Cochrane Database Syst Rev; 2006(1): CD005291.
84. De Vos A, Van Steirteghem A. Aspects of biopsy procedures prior to preimplantation genetic diagnosis. Prenat Diagn. 2001;21:767–80.
85. Wilton L, Voullaire L, Sargeant P, Williamson R, McBain J. Preimplantation aneuploidy screening using comparative genomic hybridization or fluorescence in situ hybridization of embryos from patients with recurrent implantation failure. Fertil Steril. 2003;80:860–8.

86. Hellani A, Abu-Amero K, Azouri J, El-Akoum S. Successful pregnancies after application of array-comparative genomic hybridization in PGS-aneuploidy screening. Reprod Biomed Online. 2008;17:841–7.
87. Scott RT Jr, T.X., Taylor D, Ferry K, Treff N. (2010) A prospective randomized controlled trial demonstrating significantly increased clinical pregnancy rates following 24 chromosome aneuploidy screening: biopsy and analysis on day 5 with fresh
88. Mochida T, Miura Y, Iba Y. & Mio. Y Analysis of compaction initiation in human embryos using time-lapse cinematography Fertil Steril. 2010;94:S88.
89. Yap J, Foo CF, Lee MY, Stanton PG, Dimitriadis E. Proteomic analysis identifies interleukin 11 regulated plasma membrane proteins in human endometrial epithelial cells in vitro. Reprod Biol Endocrinol. 2011;9:73.

9 Embryo Cryopreservation

Matthew D. VerMilyea, Juergen Liebermann, and Michael Tucker

Of First Importance

It can be relatively easy to slip into a state of ignorance when considering the enormity of the achievement of being able to cryopreserve the preimplantation human embryo. From the embryologists' perspective, it is simply considered "business as usual" in the in vitro fertilization laboratory. But to step back and consider the ability to perform this procedure on a regular and consistent basis should perhaps invoke the realization that it has had an impact on mankind that far outweighs the planting of an American flag on the Moon. Not to wax too lyrical, but let us consider only a few centuries ago where we were in appreciation of the reproductive process. Early on, man's curiosity in the formation and development of an organism provoked interest from philosophers and alchemists alike. Some, such as Jan Swammerdam in the mid-1600s, developed the idea of "preformationism," which proposed that the adult is already present in the egg as a miniature form [1]. The alchemist Paracelsus attempted to advance the concept of the "homunculus" (Latin for "little man") with the bogus claim of crafting a creature standing no more than 12 in. tall. This resembled a gnome, a creature said to have betrayed Paracelsus that eventually ran away soon after its creation [2–4]. Later in the 1600s, Antonie van Leeuwenhoek and Nicolas Hartsoeker proposed the appearance of "animalcules" in the sperm of humans suggesting that the sperm was a "little man," which once placed inside the woman would grow and develop into a child. These animalcules became known as "spermists." Some scientists then argued that the only contribution the female made to the next generation of offspring was her womb in which the homunculus grew [1, 5, 6].

Work in the 1700s discredited the idea of preformationism, and revolutionizing experiments conducted by the Italian priest and physiologist Lazaro Spallanzani provided insight into the requirement of physical contact between egg and sperm to create an embryo. Spallanzani was also the first to report that sperm became motionless when subjected to the cooling effects of snow [7, 8]. Suspending the metabolic activities of tissues and cells by cryopreservation was studied thereafter. In the late 1940s the use of glycerol as a permeating solute and cryoprotective additive (CPA) proved to be successful as a protectant of cells at low temperature [9, 10]. Albeit by accident, Chris Polge added an experimental freezing solution to living cells, identified later as glycerol, which resulted in the unexpected survival of his experimentally frozen cells. Soon

M.D. VerMilyea, Ph.D (✉)
Penn Fertility Care, University of Pennsylvania, Philadelphia, PA, 19104, USA
e-mail: matthew.vermilyea@uphs.upenn.edu

J. Liebermann, Ph.D
Fertility Centers of Illinois, Chicago, IL 60610, USA
e-mail: juergen.liebermann@integramed.com

M. Tucker, Ph.D (✉)
IVF Laboratory, Shady Grove Fertility RSC, Rockville, MD 20850, USA
e-mail: Michael.tucker@integramed.com

E.S. Ginsburg and C. Racowsky (eds.), *In Vitro Fertilization: A Comprehensive Guide*,
DOI 10.1007/978-1-4419-9848-4_9, © Springer Science+Business Media New York 2012

after, it was shown that unfertilized mouse oocytes could successfully be preserved in glycerol, thawed, and subsequently fertilized leading to the development of viable embryos [11]. By the early 1970s the reliability of an additional cryoprotectant solution, dimethylsulfoxide (DMSO), resulted in the successful cryopreservation of mouse embryos [12]. The use of glycerol and DMSO as suitable cryoprotectants provided the foundation for which the study of low temperature biology could be further investigated.

The Application of Cryopreservation in IVF

The field of cryobiology experienced increased interest in 1983 following the first successful pregnancy after transfer of a human embryo [13]. In 1984, the first live birth following embryo cryopreservation was reported in Australia, which was followed 2 years later by another such birth in the USA. Embryo cryopreservation and cryostorage is now a routine part of services offered at clinics treating infertility worldwide. According to the 2009 National Summary Report from the Centers for Disease Control and Prevention (CDC), 24,743 frozen embryo transfers from non-donor oocytes were performed in the USA with an average of 2.0 embryos transferred in all patients ≤44 years of age. The percentage of transfers resulting in live births in patients who were ≤40 years old was 35.7%. By comparison, for the 80,429 non-donor oocyte fresh embryo transfers in patients of the same age, an average of 2.2 embryos were transferred and 40.7% of transfers resulted in live births. With improvement of cryopreservation techniques and methods over the last three decades, the process has increasingly complemented standard fresh IVF programs. By improving the cumulative pregnancy rate per oocyte retrieval [14], and by reducing the number of embryos transferred to achieve a successful pregnancy thereby reducing the risk of multiple pregnancies [15], the technology brings two extremely important contributions to the field. Additionally, embryo cryopreservation improves the cost-effectiveness of IVF, and it also provides additional options for infertile couples seeking to conceive.

Equilibrium Cooling ("Slow-Freezing") or Vitrification?

At temperatures below −150°C metabolic activities cease allowing the potential for the stable storage of cells indefinitely. Spermatozoa and oocytes, along with zygotes and multicellular embryos, have been successfully cryopreserved from more than three-dozen mammalian species [16]. As a result, millions of healthy animal offspring have been produced by two cryopreservation strategies that are now routinely practiced in the modern ART laboratory. The two methods are often referred to as "controlled slow-freezing" and "vitrification." Slow-freezing is based on the gradual exposure of relatively low concentrations (~10%) of permeating cryoprotective additives (CPAs—e.g., glycerol or DMSO), followed by slow cooling rates of <1°C/min, and warming rates of ~250°C/min upon thawing. Additional CPAs that have successfully been used alone or in combination for controlled rate freezing include, but are not limited to ethylene glycol, propylene glycol, and non-permeating sucrose, glucose and fructose [17–19]. Following cooling and equilibration, the CPA solution is then seeded, which introduces extracellular freezing. This results in an outward movement of water from the cell and gradual dehydration until the optimal temperature is met at which the internal matrix freezes before the cell(s) is plunged into liquid nitrogen (LN_2) for further storage [20].

Ultra-rapid freezing, or vitrification, is the reversible transition of a liquid into an amorphous noncrystalline glass [21]. The vitrification method, first applied to human embryos by Trounson & Sjoblom in 1988 [22], involved a few minutes' exposure to a medium containing DMSO and sucrose before the embryos were plunged into LN_2 (−196°C); upon warming, high survival rates and further development were achieved. Various methods of vitrification have since been developed requiring the use of high CPA concentrations (20–40%), use of saccharides

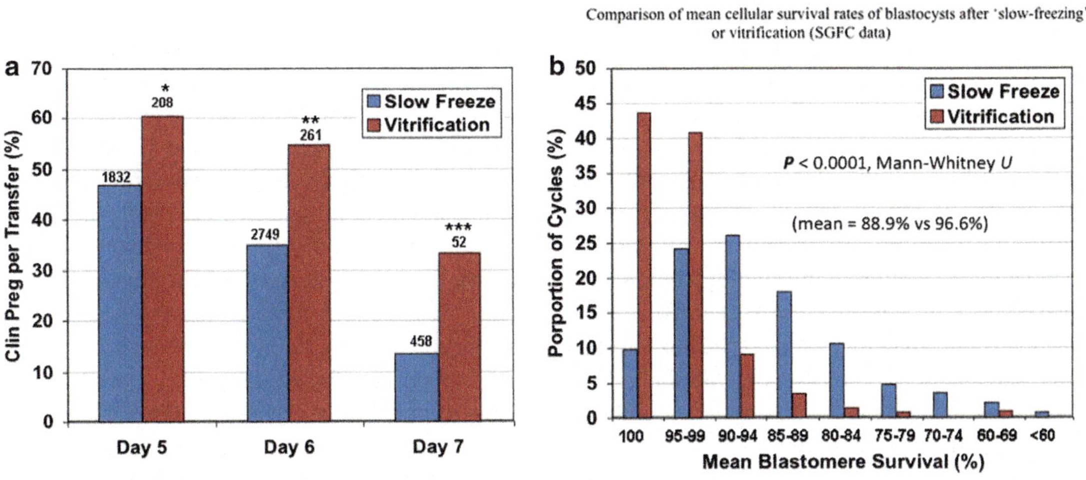

Fig. 9.1 (**a**) Autologous FET pregnancy rates by day of Blastocyst cryopreservation—comparison of "slow-freezing" versus vitrification. Fisher's exact: $*P<0.0002$ day-5, $**P<0.001$ vs. day-6; $***P<0.001$ vs. day-7. (**b**) Comparison of mean cellular survival rates of blastocysts after "slow-freezing" or vitrification. Slow-freeze $n=5{,}901$ survived (6,715 thawed); Vitrification $n=699$ survived (753 warmed). $P<0.001$, Mann–Whitney U (mean 88.9% vs. 96.6%)

as supplements, cooling rates of >1,000°C/min, and very rapid warming rates. Often extremely high cooling rates of >10,000°C/min are used.

The main challenge with vitrification is the use of high concentrations of toxic vitrification solutions (vitrificants), and the potentially damaging effects that these solutions may have on chromosomal integrity [23]. However, recent results achieved with vitrification, especially the cryopreservation of human oocytes and blastocysts, have been very successful clinically. The success of a good vitrification program is dependent upon three factors: the type and quantity of vitrificant used, delivery and dilution of these vitrificants, and optimal cooling and warming rates. Comparisons of results achieved by vitrification with results from standard, slow-cooling methods have almost always demonstrated that vitrification is as good and usually better than standard slow-freezing (Fig. 9.1a, b).

Survival of the Fittest

When cells are immersed in a hypertonic cryoprotectant agent (CPA) they will immediately respond by an efflux of water by osmosis. Given that cell membranes are more permeable to water than to the CPA, an immediate cellular contraction and shrinkage occurs followed by the slow entry of the CPA [24]. Once equilibrium is achieved, the cellular volume is nearly restored and additional cooling to subzero temperatures causes a second wave of osmosis. Several factors are known to be involved in the damage of cells during the freeze and thaw process. In slow controlled-rate freezing/rapid thaw processes, intracellular ice formation and osmotic stresses are key causes of blastomere damage and are of a major concern. Although various protocols have been developed in an attempt to limit such injury, the extent of damage can vary at several stages of embryo development, and no single protocol is likely to be optimized for every cell type. In order significantly to reduce the occurrence of cellular damage, small volume cryopreservation with either a high CPA concentration and very rapid cooling to achieve a state of vitrification or a lower CPA concentration and slow cooling ensuring extracellular ice formation (controlled-rate freezing) is applied.

Experts in the field of assisted reproductive technology have published proposed guidelines in order to establish a global consensus for cryopreservation standardization [25]. Despite many triumphs and developments in the field of cryobiology within the last three decades, variances in methods and opinions still exist. In particular, there is yet to be a general consensus as to the optimal stage of embryo development suitable for cryopreservation to optimize cryo-survival and viability. Nevertheless, all experts would agree that embryo morphology before cryopreservation has been shown to influence the outcome upon thawing with respect to survival and implantation competency. Studies have shown that the cellular symmetry of an embryo, cleavage pattern (synchronous versus asynchronous), percentage of cytoplasmic fragmentation and the mitotic stage of a cell prior to freezing have a dramatic effect on survivability and further development [26–29].

Embryo cryopreservation and frozen embryo transfer outcomes are prone to influences by a number of variables. One such variable is the ability of embryos to survive the freezing and thawing process fully intact. Either cryopreserved by slow-freezing or vitrification, embryo survival rates are key indicators of an efficient cryopreservation program and are routinely calculated to establish benchmarks and to identify potential deviations from protocol. Survivability is determined by the number of embryos that survive post-thaw based on the number of embryos cryopreserved. Embryo viability is commonly identified immediately following the thaw and assessed by morphological evaluation of individual blastomeres or the entire embryo. Some laboratories identify post-thaw embryo competency by culturing the embryo for an extended time or overnight in order to assess further cellular cleavage or re-expansion of the blastocoel cavity.

Zygote (Pronuclear Stage Embryo)

Several reports have indicated that the implantation rate of embryos cryopreserved by slow-freezing at the pronuclear (PN) stage provides better results in comparison to the cleavage stage embryo [30–36]. Damage to the meiotic spindle is not of concern, as the zygote is a single cell and machinery required for cellular division is not at risk of damage. Some would consider the zygote to be at the ideal developmental stage because the pronuclei have completed their centripetal migration [37], nucleoli have begun realignment [38], and entry into the G2 phase has commenced [39]. With the presence or absence of the first cleavage event, assessment of zygote survivability upon thaw is easily identified, as there is no presence of partial survival. The cell is regarded to be either intact or compromised. However, upon examination of previously cryopreserved zygotes, certain factors used for quality scoring and developmental potential were affected by the process and resulted in lower cumulative PN scores [40, 41]. It was especially noted that the proximity of the PN, in concurrence with the orientation and presence of cytoplasmic halos, along with the addition and polarization of nucleolar precursor bodies (NPB), were all disrupted. These disturbances may be partially due to the negative result of thermal depolymerization, caused by the effects of cooling on microtubule organization [42].

Acceptable rates of implantation and clinical pregnancies resulting from embryos derived from frozen–thawed zygotes, prove that PN embryos can recover from minimal injuries caused by the freeze-thaw process. In 2002, the first report of a successful ongoing twin pregnancy after vitrification of PN stage fertilized human oocytes appeared [43], and vitrification of zygotes has now become a routine method in IVF labs around the World [44]. In Germany, for instance, most embryos are cryopreserved as zygotes because local protection laws only allow for the cryopreservation of multicellular embryos in emergency cases. Survival rates have been found to be as high as those reported with slow-freezing, however, it has been reported that a certain percentage of zygotes exhibit poor pronuclear integrity after warming, being associated with poorer outcomes [45]. A small set of data from the clinical application of vitrification for zygotes in the authors' laboratories would suggest that this approach is more than adequate in terms of cryo-survival and live births (Table 9.1).

Table 9.1 Vitrification for zygote cryostorage using EG/DMSO/Sucrose protocol and open carrier system

Zygote warming cycles	17
Number of zygotes stored	168
Number warmed	168
Number survived	163 (97%)
Cleavage	161 (99%)
Number of ETs (day-3/day-5)	17 (7/10)
Embryos transferred (average)	32 (1.9)
Blastocyst surplus to transfer vitrified	48
2PN utilization rate	80/161 (49.5%)
Successful deliveries	9 (53%)
Implantation rate	10/32 (31%)

Data are from Shady Grove Fertility Center (*SGFC*) and Georgia Reproductive Specialists (*GRS*), 2007–2009

Cleavage Stage Embryo

Selection of the best embryo(s) for transfer has been correlated with increased implantation and pregnancy rates [46–48]. Some would argue that freezing at the PN stage does not permit the selection of morphologically superior embryos, and therefore may affect success of fresh and frozen embryo transfer cycle outcomes [33]. Allowing cleavage events to occur, so viability assessments can be based on embryo morphology, can further assess the developmental potential of embryos. It is true that only some cryopreserved embryos remain fully intact after thawing even if the best morphologically appearing embryos were selected for freeze. Multicellular embryos undergoing the freeze/thaw process can be categorized by their blastomere appearance post-thaw. All blastomeres, only some, or none at all may survive with degeneration being identified by darkened cytoplasm or cell disfiguration. In the late 1980s, publications pertaining to Day-2 embryo freezing suggested that pregnancies could be obtained with partially surviving multi-cell embryos, although, a 50% blastomere survival rate was considered to be a minimal threshold for such success [29, 49, 50].

Conflicting reports have demonstrated the importance of transferring only fully intact embryos as implantation rates seemed to be significantly improved compared to embryos which suffered from cell loss [51–54]. Edgar et al. [52] showed that only the loss of two cells from a 4-cell embryo was unfavorable for implantation in a single embryo transfer (SET) study. In addition, Gabrielsen et al. [55] did not identify a negative impact on implantation rates when the embryos were at least >50% intact. For day-3 embryos, several reports conclude similar implantation rates can be obtained for embryos with 1 cell [56, 57] or 1 to 2 cells lost [26, 58] compared to fully intact embryos. The reason for reduced embryo viability as a result of sibling blastomere degeneration remains controversial. It has been proposed that the damaged cells may exert a toxic effect upon their sibling blastomeres within the embryo. Similar to the influences of cytoplasmic fragmentation, this may contribute to the lower implantation rates as compared to the transfer of partially intact embryos [59–61].

The resumption of mitosis can also be considered as a measure of the vitality of an embryo after thawing. Several reports have demonstrated an increase in implantation rates after additional cleavage (of at least one cell) in day-2 embryos compared to those that fail to cleave post-thaw [27, 54, 62, 63]. Implantation rates have also been shown significantly to increase following the successful division of at least two cells [28, 55]. Moreover, this has also been reported to apply exclusively to day-3 embryos [26]. The total number of blastomeres in an embryo, identified immediately before transfer, has also been shown to be an optimistic predictor of better implantation rates. When day-2 frozen embryos were observed to have at least six cells at time of transfer compared to a fewer number of cells, then a higher implantation rate was achieved [54]. A positive correlation has also been established concerning the number of blastomeres in a post-thaw day-3 embryo and clinical pregnancy rates, regardless of the initial number of intact cells [64].

Blastocyst

Worldwide, clinics continue to develop models based on the success of extended culture to the blastocyst stage. Such advances have caused a surge in

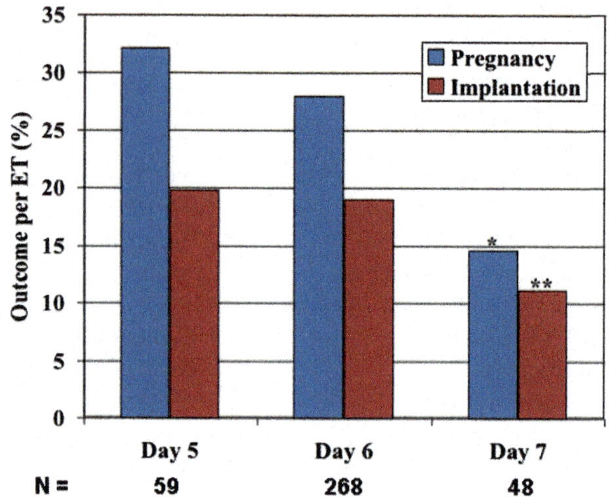

Fig. 9.2 Clinical outcomes of "slow-frozen" blastocysts relative to day of development when cryopreserved. $*P=0.03$ vs. day-5 and 6; $**P=0.05$ vs. day-5 and 6; N=number of transfers in each group

Table 9.2 Distribution of blastocysts vitrified, according to the day of vitrification

Day of development	Day 5	Day 6	Day 7	Total
Blastocysts vitrified (%)	7,115 (47%)	7,645 (50.5%)	377 (2.5%)	15,137

Data are from 4,053 cycles (patient age 33.9±4.9, mean±SD), from the Fertility Centers of Illinois (*FCI*), 2004–2011

the ability to select a single embryo for transfer thereby minimizing the risks associated with multiple pregnancies. Consequently, there is now even more of a requirement for methods and protocols to produce equivalent pregnancy rates following successful cryopreservation of embryos [65, 66].

The blastocyst stage is perceived by many to be the optimal time to cryopreserve embryos, as the greater cell number and further cellular differentiation makes it less vulnerable to negative effects caused by the freeze-thaw process [65]; that, and the fact that this stage of development represents a self-selected cohort of higher potential viability [67]. With the ever-increasing production of mid-to-fully expanded and hatched blastocysts on the fifth, sixth, and seventh day of embryo culture, it is imperative that blastocysts are of good quality prior to undergoing any cryopreservation method commonly used in assisted reproductive technologies (ART). It is commonly accepted that blastocysts which exhibit a clear presence of a well-defined inner cell mass (ICM), and an adequate total cell count are of better quality and deemed more potentially viable by morphological assessment than those with a poorly defined ICM and few trophectoderm cells.

Many studies have shown that the time an embryo takes to achieve the blastocyst stage is a positive indicator of viability [68–70]. Arguably, others suggest that embryo viability is determined more by the stage of blastocyst development [71] and not dependent upon the time spent in culture at which the embryo reaches a certain morphological stage. Nevertheless, both theories are often applied when selecting blastocysts for cryopreservation. Data suggest that expanded blastocysts show no significant differences in viability, implantation potential, or pregnancy outcome when frozen on day 5 versus day 6 (Fig. 9.2) [72]. However, the implantation and pregnancy rates for expanded day-7 blastocysts are lower than that of day-6, but much higher than previously reported day-7 fresh embryo transfer rates. These data reinforce the importance of obtaining a developmentally competent expanded blastocyst prior to the freezing process to ensure viability potential post-thaw.

A body of data [67] (Tables 9.1–9.4) from a large blastocyst vitrification program refutes the

Table 9.3 Clinical outcomes from blastocyst vitrification

Variable	Values
Patient age (years)	35.0±5.0
Warming cycles	2,883
Vitrified embryos transfers (VET)	2,865
Blastocysts warmed	5,496
Blastocysts survived (%)	5,355 (97.4)
Blastocysts transferred	5,269
Mean # blastocysts transferred	1.8
Implantations (%)	1,620 (30.7)
Initiated pregnancy/warm (%)	1,417 (49.2)
Initiated pregnancy/VET (%)	1,417 (49.5)
Clinical pregnancy/warm (%)	1,284 (44.5)
Clinical pregnancy/VET (%)	1,284 (44.8)
Ongoing/Del. pregnancies/VET (%)	1,000 (35.0)
Livebirths	935 (458 boys and 477 girls)

Data are from all blastocyst vitrifications performed at the Fertility Centers of Illinois (*FCI*), 2004–2011
Values are numbers unless otherwise described

Table 9.4 Clinical outcomes from blastocyst vitrification according to day of development when vitrified

Day of development	Day 5	Day 6
Patient age (years)	34.8±5.1	35.2±5.0
Warming cycles	1,498	1,385
Vitrified embryo transfers (VET)	1,495	1,370
Blastocysts warmed	2,903	2,593
Blastocysts survived (%)	2,830 (97.5)	2,525 (97.4)
Blastocysts transferred	2,772	2,497
Mean # blastocysts transferred	1.9	1.8
Implantations (%)	965 (34.8)[a]	655 (26.2)[a]
Positive pregnancy/warm (%)	828 (55.3)[b]	589 (42.5)[b]
Positive pregnancy/VET (%)	828 (55.4)[c]	589 (43.0)[c]
Clinical pregnancy/warm (%)	717 (47.9)[d]	513 (37.0)[d]
Clinical pregnancy/VET (%)	717 (48.0)[e]	513 (37.5)[e]
Ongoing/del pregs/VET (%)	581 (38.9)[f]	419 (30.6)[f]
Livebirths	547	388

Data are from the Fertility Centers of Illinois (*FCI*), 2004–2011
Values are numbers unless otherwise described
$^{a,f}P<0.05$; $^{b,c,d,e}P<0.01$

Table 9.5 Clinical outcomes with or without artificial collapsing of Day 6 blastocysts before vitrification

Day of development	Day 6 without AC	Day 6 with AC
Patient age (years)	35.4±5.0	35.2±5.8
Warmed cycles	523	65
Vitrified embryo transfers (VET)	519	65
Mean # blastocysts transferred	1.8	1.6
Implantation rate (%)	26.5	45.9
Initial pregnancy/VET (%)	44.1	66.1
Clinical pregnancy/VET (%)	38.3	60.0
Ongoing/Del. pregnancies/VET (%)	33.1	53.8

AC artificial collapsing
Data are from vitrification using an aseptic, "closed carrier" system at the Fertility Centers of Illinois (*FCI*) during a 10-month period in 2011

comparable implantation of blastocysts cryopreserved on day-5 or -6, which may be overcome potentially by artificial collapse of the blastocoele prior to vitrification in day-6 blastocysts (Table 9.5). However, others consider that blastocoelic collapse is necessary pre-vitrification whatever the day the blastocyst forms [71, 73].

Frozen–thawed blastocysts undergo multiple morphological changes that include the collapse of the blastocoelic cavity along with cellular lysis and degeneration. Morphological assessments of blastocysts post-thaw are also necessary to estimate the survivability of individual cells and the embryo in its entirety (Fig. 9.3). Previous studies have demonstrated the clinical significance of variation in the proportion of blastomeres that survive the cryopreservation process. By visual examination of the extent and locale of cellular degeneration, a skilled embryologist can estimate the viability percentage of a freeze-thaw blastocyst. This estimate of total embryo survivability is shown to correlate with the implantation potential of the given embryo. Studies show that the probability of implantation is relatively high when the majority, if not all, cells survive. However, implantation potential begins to drop steadily as cell survival declines below 95%. When fewer than 80% of cells survive, implantation potential appears minimal [74] (Fig. 9.4).

Whatever the approach to cryopreservation, the objective of a successful blastocyst cryostorage program should be to maximize the potential viability of embryos transferred whilst reducing the number of embryos needing to be thawed in order to produce a pregnancy. By selecting

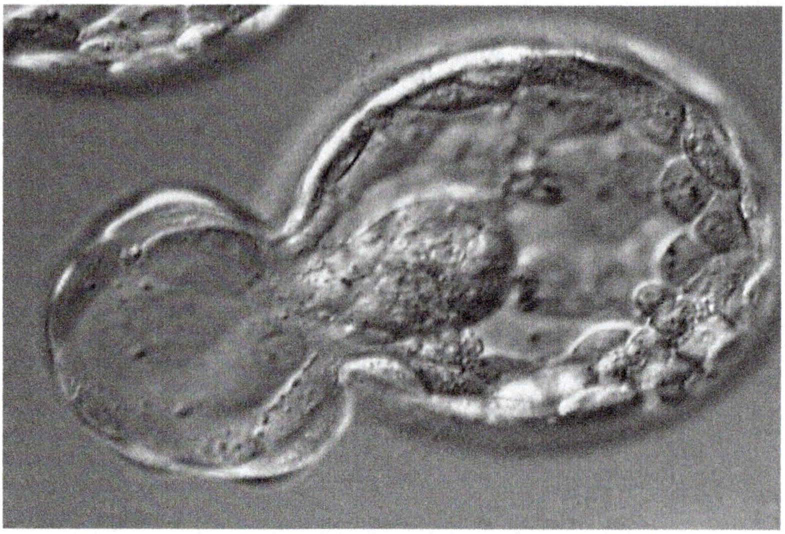

Fig. 9.3 Hatching blastocyst post-vitrification

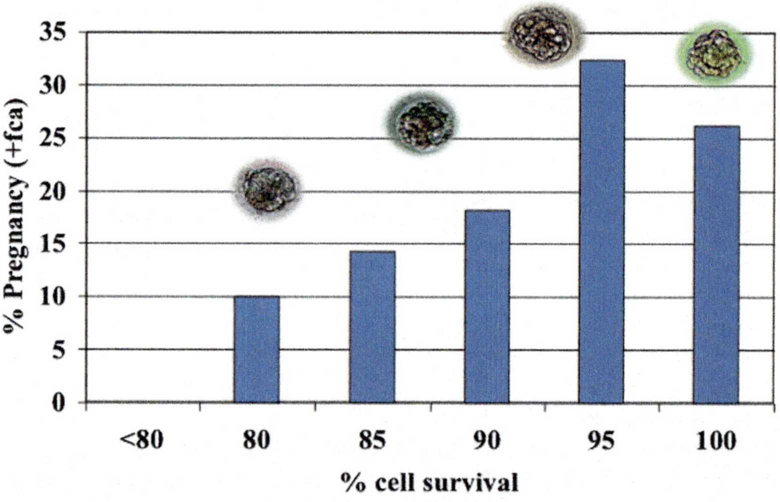

Fig. 9.4 "Slow-freeze" blastocysts correlation of percentage cellular survival and successful implantation. $R^2=0.081$, $P=0.0001$. R^2 statistic measures the goodness-of-fit of trend

embryos which fulfill morphological criteria that are not dependent upon their day of development, along with accurate quality estimations of freeze/thaw damage, one can greatly improve the clinical outcomes following transfer of embryos post-cryopreservation. As technology continues to develop in the field of cryobiology, its purpose in ART becomes of greater relevance. With the introduction and increased application of newer techniques such as vitrification in the ART laboratory, we routinely seem to see close to a doubling of the survival rates of blastocysts when compared to blastocysts frozen by conventional slow-rate freezing (Fig. 9.1a, b). Nevertheless it is critical that we continue to investigate and reach a wider consensus in the industry that may enable us to reach yet closer to perfect survivability in the future.

Cryopreservation Benefits

To be able to put surplus embryos from a fresh oocyte retrieval "on ice," and to do so in a consistent and reliable fashion has been a traditional benefit of the embryo cryopreservation process;

which, with improvement in cryo-survival and implantation rates, has taken on an increasing role to encourage elective single embryo transfer both fresh and post-thaw [75]. Additionally, a variety of other advantages exist that pivot around the use of embryo cryopreservation which rely entirely upon the effectiveness of the technology through what might be referred to as a "freeze all" strategy. "Freeze all" cycles may be undertaken for endometrial reasons; following trophectoderm biopsy to allow for chromosomal/genetic testing; fertility preservation; and in emergency circumstances where either personal or environmental catastrophe may dictate putting embryo transfer and/or pregnancy on hold.

Intrinsic to superovulation therapy is the risk for severe ovarian hyperstimulation syndrome (OHSS). At present, there is no consensus regarding the best strategy to prevent OHSS, however options for prevention do exist, including the elective cryopreservation of all embryos and postponement of embryo transfer [76, 77]. In a 2002 survey of applicable ways to prevent OHSS, the medical decision to freeze-all embryos was decided upon in one-third of OHSS cases [78]. The cryopreservation of all produced embryos in cases at risk of OHSS has been instigated with varied and inconsistent results. However, different cryopreservation techniques and protocols may be to blame for such variability [79, 80]. Some argue that if adopted as a standard emergency procedure for patients at risk of developing severe OHSS, highly efficient embryo vitrification protocols can reduce, if not completely eliminate, this risk and conserve pregnancy potential in the form of stored embryos for later use [81].

Currently, morphologic and developmental characteristics are the most proven tools for embryo selection, although the implantation potential of embryos produced in vitro remains relatively low. A study in 2007 showed that chromosomal anomalies were prevalent in 6,000 IVF produced embryos, and these abnormalities were not necessarily dependent on maternal age or embryo morphology [82]. Preimplantation genetic diagnosis (PGD) is utilized in many ART clinics for the analysis of single gene disorders, and additionally molecular karyotyping of embryos has become increasingly applied (preimplantation genetic screening—PGS). Many laboratories now routinely conduct blastocyst biopsy followed by vitrification, prior to analysis and transfer of embryos in a subsequent frozen embryo transfer cycle. This allows analysis to be completed whilst not compromising the synchrony of embryo transfer and implantation timing [83, 84]. Optimization of vitrification techniques combined with rigorous embryo morphology assessments has allowed ART clinics to implement a blastocyst-based single embryo transfer model to maximize cumulative pregnancy rates following advanced genetic testing, whether for genetic disorders or for aneuploidy screening.

Fertility preservation through embryo banking [85] prior to chemotherapy is an increasingly utilized approach for women in a committed relationship. While cryo-stored embryos may present a considerable risk to the laboratory in the event of a natural disaster, embryo cryopreservation may actually be used as a means to deal with an otherwise assumed loss of all embryos in culture. Since cryo-stored embryos need to be protected and possibly removed from the site of the disaster [86, 87], a converse consideration is that in the event of an impending disaster, all embryos can be cryopreserved securely on site, or be transported away from the laboratory for future use. This should be an essential consideration in the disaster plan of all IVF clinics. On a more personal level, an individual couple who may experience a catastrophe of their own during an IVF cycle, may wish to adopt an embryo "freeze all" policy to enable them to deal with more pressing concerns, delaying embryo transfer till a later time when more convenient.

Safety Issues

Contamination Risks

The aseptic cryopreservation and storage of embryos are often disregarded due to the exhaustive microbiological monitoring of the culture environment in which germplasm is processed and embryos are produced. The storage of such tissues is not often considered to be susceptible to the risks of potential contamination; however, it may be of concern to regulatory authorities in the prevention of possible disease transmission during ART, especially by embryo transfer. Nevertheless, studies have shown that the risk of pathogen contamination of both semen and embryos are present and both are at risk of infection especially when liquid nitrogen (LN_2) is used [88–90]. In addition, contaminating microorganisms have been shown to remain viable for an extended period of time and able to withstand the subzero temperatures of LN_2 [91].

Further, when cryopreserved products are kept together during storage, the risk of cross-contamination might increase due to defective vessels that may crack, leak, or lose their hermetic seals thus exposing the contents to possible contaminants. It is important to inspect these storage receptacles carefully and to follow the manufacturers' protocols for use and storage. The storage dewar itself can also pose risk of microbial contamination to the long-term cryopreservation of samples. Ice accumulations that form in the atmosphere and fall into an open dewar, along with crystal formation on cold surfaces of material storage vessels (straws, cryovials, etc.) can accumulate and trap bacteria, fungal spores and laboratory debris present within the LN_2 [92].

These concerns have been highlighted in recent years due to the increased use of direct exposure of embryos to LN_2 in the interests of increasing the cooling rates of embryos to improve consistency of vitrification [67]. There exists then, an ongoing debate about the use of "open" versus "closed" carriers for ultra-rapid cooling by vitrification, based on the assumption that there is a potential risk of disease transmission via contaminated LN_2. Although suppliers of LN_2 may certify the level of purity of their product and cleansing methods are in place during production and delivery, there remains a risk of contamination. Recent methods that have been applied for the decontamination of LN_2 by filtration and UV irradiation have been shown to be a practical and easy method to insure that contamination risks can be minimized [93]. Since UV radiation disables the growth of all microorganisms [94], this method of disinfection may prove to be key in the assurance that material is stored safely in liquid nitrogen for future use in ART procedures.

The vapor phase of liquid nitrogen ($VPLN_2$) has also been proposed as an alternative for the safe storage of cryopreserved material, including human semen and oocytes [95, 96]. Difficulties may exist, however, during the prolonged storage of material in vapor phase refrigerators because of possible fluctuations in temperature. Dry-shippers, or dewars that do not contain LN_2, are deemed "non-hazardous" and are usually not subject to strict regulation when transported by air. That such dry-shipping dewars are efficient at maintaining temperatures below −150°C for up to 14 days does suggest that $VPLN_2$ storage and transportation may not be so problematic. However, the length of cryo-storage over months or even years presents many more opportunities for significant fluctuations in temperature to occur to jeopardize the viability of vitrified embryos.

Cryotanks do require periodic decontamination by means of an effective disinfectant that will rid the container of a potential cross-contamination risk. Any agent that does not react with aluminum or stainless steel is recommended by the manufacturers. This may include a 1:9 (chlorine bleach to water ratio) or a mild soap solution, sprayed into the inner vessel and onto the cryovial racking devices, making sure that after exposure to the disinfectant (15–30 min) all components are rinsed thoroughly and residual cleaner is completely removed [97]. Bielanski [97] continues the potential concerns for cross-contamination by stating that there are no known available data regarding the efficacy of disinfectants for LN_2 cryotank and dewar decontamination. All this said, it is possible that in the grand scheme of things contamination during cryostorage of human embryos may be being highly overstated as a "real-world" risk. Very recently, a report considering just such potential risks suggests that this may be the case [98], thereby mirroring the historic absence of reports of contamination from decades of cryostorage of human embryos.

Chain of Custody Issues

More mundane considerations related to embryo cryopreservation are those that confirm "chain of custody" with respect to embryo ownership. This is the process that guarantees that a chosen embryo that is cryo-stored for a specific couple is effectively returned to them post-warming/thaw to attempt pregnancy. When genetic screening of embryos is involved, not only is assurance of ownership key but also the retrieval from cryostorage of the correct embryo that has had successful diagnosis. This sounds simple, but it requires foolproof labeling that will not be shed during storage, nor lose its legibility, in addition to a cryo-inventory system that has checks and verification processes to make sure that all is present and correct. Enough said, but when it comes to real-world risk, this is an area of particular concern regarding legal liability within the ART industry. With the ever growing relevance of embryo cryopreservation to facilitate and enhance clinical IVF outcomes, the dependence on this technology to put all or some embryos "on hold" has to be undertaken in a manner that is near seamless, and which provides an infallible level of performance when it comes to assuring continuity of genetic material.

Tank Storage and Disposition Issues

It seems almost superfluous to mention that maintenance of the cryo-storage environment itself is paramount to a successful cryopreservation program. Daily QC logs to ascertain appropriate level of LN_2 in all storage dewars, in addition to some form of effective remote monitoring for these storage tanks must be in place to enable constant oversight of this precious human material. The precise wording and legally binding nature of all consents and permits signed by couples prior to cryostorage must be comprehensive and address all eventualities, including but not limited to death of either or both partner "owners"; separation and divorce; donation for reproductive use or research; discard; as well as accidental loss of embryos during cryostorage.

Cryopreserved Embryo Transfer

Current randomized trials do not show significant differences in implantation and pregnancy rates when comparing replacement of cryopreserved embryos in natural cycles or those when the endometrium is prepared by GnRH agonist plus estradiol and progesterone, or estradiol and progesterone without a GnRH agonist. Outcomes with various formulations and routes of delivery of estradiol and progesterone do not appear different. hCG administration during natural cycles results in lower pregnancy rates [100, 101]. Figure 9.5 and Table 9.6 indicate schemas for endometrial preparation and natural cycle replacement options for cryopreserved embryos.

In Conclusion

By drawing upon centuries of study into cellular cryopreservation, the first pregnancies from frozen–thawed embryos in humans occurred in the early 1980s. Since that time, embryo cryopreservation has evolved into one of the keystones in the overall picture of infertility treatment. With over half a million babies born following embryo cryopreservation, this technology has become a well-established and widely used routine procedure in the field of ART that allows important expansion of therapeutic strategies when IVF is used to treat infertility. Many of the potential dangers of using low temperature cryostorage, such as deleterious crystallization of water within cells leading to injurious physical and chemical events, have been largely overcome by more recent approaches, most notably vitrification. When performed appropriately, vitrification is able to achieve arrest of all cellular metabolism with maintenance of structural and genetic integrity, yielding high rates of cell survival post-warming in a consistent and reliable fashion.

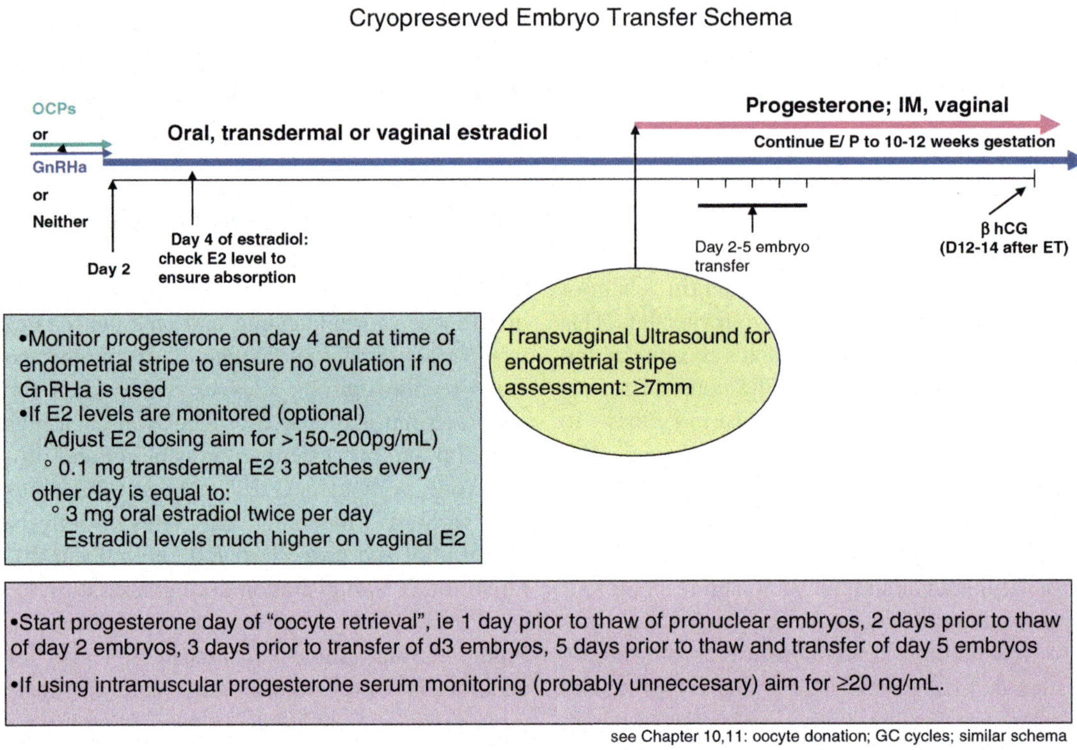

Fig. 9.5 Schema for replacement of cryopreserved embryos into a prepared endometrium

Table 9.6 Schema for replacement of cryopreserved embryos in a natural cycle

Cycle day	Day of thaw (based on day of cryopreservation)	Progesterone (optional)
LH surge[a]		
Surge +1[b] (day of ovulation)		
Surge +2	Pronuclear embryos	Half dose
Surge +3	Day 2 embryos	Full dose
Surge +4	Day 3 embryos	Full dose
Surge +5		Full dose
Surge +6	Day 5 embryos	Full dose
Surge +7	Day 6 embryos	Full dose

[a]Urinary or blood testing
[b]Confirm ovulation with serum progesterone 24–48 h post-LH surge

While not ideal, on certain occasions it becomes necessary to carry out re-cryopreservation of embryos, which may occur following thawing of earlier stage embryos which yields too many embryos for transfer, when transfer fails, or perhaps to facilitate chromosomal screening of a previously cryopreserved embryo. This strategy is feasible and will yield pregnancies [99]; and as such this may serve as an appropriate endnote to this chapter to underscore the increasing robustness of the technology of embryo cryopreservation. ART in general, and IVF therapy in particular, has been enormously enhanced by embryo cryopreservation in a variety of ways, all of which are focused ultimately on good patient care, and provision of healthy offspring.

References

1. Rossi P. The birth of modern science. Oxford: Blackwell; 2001.
2. Pagel W. Paracelsus: an introduction to philosophical medicine in the era of the Renaissance. Basel: Karger; 1982.
3. Grell OP. Paracelsus: the man and his reputation. Leiden: Brill; 1998.

4. Debus AG. The chemical philosophy Paracelsian science and medicine in the sixteenth and seventeenth centuries; two volumes bound as one. Mineola: Dover Publication; 2002.
5. Hill KA. Hartsoeker's homonculus: A corrective note. J Hist Behav Sci. 1985;21(2):178–9. Available at: http://dx.doi.org/10.1002/1520-6696(198504)21:2<178::AID-JHBS2300210208>3.0.CO;2-T.
6. Dobell C. Antony Van Leeuwenhoek and His "little Animals". 1932.
7. Spallanzani L, Bonnet C. Dissertations relative to the natural history of animals and vegetables. J. Murray; 1784.
8. Spallanzani L. An essay on animal reproductions. T. Becket, PA de Hondt; 1769.
9. Polge C, Smith AU, Parkes AS. Revival of spermatozoa after vitrification and dehydration at low temperatures. Nature. 1949;164(4172):666.
10. Smith AU. Biological effects of freezing and supercooling Issue 9 of Monographs (Physiological Society (Great Britain)), Physiological Society (Great Britain). Issue 9 of Monographs of the Physiological Society. Williams & Wilkins; 1961:462.
11. Sherman JK, Lin TP. Effect of glycerol and low temperature on survival of unfertilized mouse eggs. Nature. 1958;181(4611):785–6.
12. Whittingham DG, Leibo SP, Mazur P. Survival of mouse embryos frozen to-196 and-269°C. Science. 1972;178(4059):411–4.
13. Trounson A, Mohr L. Human pregnancy following cryopreservation, thawing and transfer of an eight-cell embryo. Nature. 1983;305(5936):707–9.
14. Bergh C, Josefsson B, Nilsson L, Hamberger L. The success rate in a Swedish in-vitro fertilization unit: a cohort study. Acta Obstet Gynecol Scand. 1995;74(6):446–50.
15. Tiitinen A, Halttunen M, Härkki P, Vuoristo P, Hyden-Granskog C. Elective single embryo transfer: the value of cryopreservation. Hum Reprod. 2001;16(6):1140–4.
16. Saragusty J, Arav A. Current progress in oocyte and embryo cryopreservation by slow freezing and vitrification. Reproduction. 2011;141(1):1–19.
17. Leibo SP, Pool TB. The principal variables of cryopreservation: solutions, temperatures, and rate changes. Fertil Steril. 2011;96(2):269–76.
18. Barceló-Fimbres M, Seidel GE. Effects of either glucose or fructose and metabolic regulators on bovine embryo development and lipid accumulation in vitro. Mol Reprod Dev. 2007;74(11):1406–18.
19. Chen SU, Lien YR, Chen HF, Chang LJ, Tsai YY, Yang YS. Observational clinical follow-up of oocyte cryopreservation using a slow-freezing method with 1,2-propanediol plus sucrose followed by ICSI. Hum Reprod. 2005;20(7):1975–80.
20. Mazur P. Kinetics of water loss from cells at subzero temperatures and the likelihood of intracellular freezing. J Gen Physiol. 1963;47:347–69.
21. Rall WF, Fahy GM. Ice-free cryopreservation of mouse embryos at- 196 C by vitrification. Nature. 1985;313(6003):573–5.
22. Trounson A, Sjöblom P. Cleavage and development of human embryos in vitro after ultrarapid freezing and thawing. Fertil Steril. 1988;50(2):373–6.
23. Liebermann J, Nawroth F, Isachenko V, Isachenko E, Rahimi G, Tucker MJ. The potential importance of vitrification in reproductive medicine. Biol Reprod. 2002;67:1671–80.
24. Schneider U, Mazur P. Osmotic consequences of cryoprotectant permeability and its relation to the survival of frozen-thawed embryos. Theriogenology. 1984;21(1):68–79.
25. Alpha Istanbul Consensus Meeting Nov 2011: Cryo KPIs and Benchmarks. *Reprod BioMed Online*. 2012:pending
26. Solé M, Santaló J, Rodríguez I, et al. Correlation between embryological factors and pregnancy rate: development of an embryo score in a cryopreservation programme. J Assist Reprod Genet. 2011; 28(2):129–36.
27. Salumets A, Suikkari AM, Mäkinen S, Karro H, Roos A, Tuuri T. Frozen embryo transfers: implications of clinical and embryological factors on the pregnancy outcome. Hum Reprod. 2006;21(9):2368–74.
28. Edgar DH, Archer J, McBain J, Bourne H. Embryonic factors affecting outcome from single cryopreserved embryo transfer. Reprod Biomed Online. 2007;14(6):718–23.
29. Hartshorne GM, Wick K, Elder K, Dyson H. Effect of cell number at freezing upon survival and viability of cleaving embryos generated from stimulated IVF cycles. Hum Reprod. 1990;5(7):857–61.
30. Camus M, Van den Abbeel E, Van Waesberghe L, Wisanto A, Devroey P, Van Steirteghem AC. Human embryo viability after freezing with dimethylsulfoxide as a cryoprotectant. Fertil Steril. 1989;51(3):460–5.
31. Lassalle B, Testart J, Renard JP. Human embryo features that influence the success of cryopreservation with the use of 1,2 propanediol. Fertil Steril. 1985;44(5):645–51.
32. Fugger EF, Bustillo M, Dorfmann AD, Schulman JD. Human preimplantation embryo cryopreservation: selected aspects. Hum Reprod. 1991;6(1): 131–5.
33. Horne G, Critchlow JD, Newman MC, Edozien L, Matson PL, Lieberman BA. A prospective evaluation of cryopreservation strategies in a two-embryo transfer programme. Hum Reprod. 1997;12(3): 542–7.
34. Veeck LL, Amundson CH, Brothman LJ, et al. Significantly enhanced pregnancy rates per cycle through cryopreservation and thaw of pronuclear stage oocytes. Fertil Steril. 1993;59(6):1202–7.
35. Veeck LL. Freezing of preembryos: early versus late stages. J Assist Reprod Genet. 1993;10(3):181–5.

36. Senn A, Vozzi C, Chanson A, De Grandi P, Germond M. Prospective randomized study of two cryopreservation policies avoiding embryo selection: the pronucleate stage leads to a higher cumulative delivery rate than the early cleavage stage. Fertil Steril. 2000;74(5):946–52.
37. Payne D, Flaherty SP, Barry MF, Matthews CD. Preliminary observations on polar body extrusion and pronuclear formation in human oocytes using time-lapse video cinematography. Hum Reprod. 1997;12(3):532–41.
38. Wright G, Wiker S, Elsner C, et al. Observations on the morphology of pronuclei and nucleoli in human zygotes and implications for cryopreservation. Hum Reprod. 1990;5(1):109–15.
39. Balakier H, MacLusky NJ, Casper RF. Characterization of the first cell cycle in human zygotes: implications for cryopreservation. Fertil Steril. 1993;59(2):359–65.
40. Scott L. Pronuclear scoring as a predictor of embryo development. Reprod Biomed Online. 2003;6(2):201–14.
41. Senn A, Urner F, Chanson A, Primi MP, Wirthner D, Germond M. Morphological scoring of human pronuclear zygotes for prediction of pregnancy outcome. Hum Reprod. 2006;21(1):234–9.
42. Mandelbaum J, Anastasiou O, Lévy R, Guérin JF, de Larouzière V, Antoine JM. Effects of cryopreservation on the meiotic spindle of human oocytes. Eur J Obstet Gynecol Reprod Biol. 2004;113 Suppl 1:S17–23.
43. Jelinkova L, Selman HA, Arav A, Strehler E, Reeka N, Sterzik K. Twin pregnancy after vitrification of 2-pronuclei human embryos. Fertil Steril. 2002;77(2):412–4.
44. Al-Hasani S, Ozmen B, Koutlaki N, Schoepper B, Diedrich K, Schultze-Mosgau A. Three years of routine vitrification of human zygotes: is it still fair to advocate slow-rate freezing? Reprod Biomed Online. 2007;14(3):288–93.
45. Isachenko V, Todorov P, Dimitrov Y, Isachenko E. Integrity rate of pronuclei after cryopreservation of pronuclear-zygotes as a criteria for subsequent embryo development and pregnancy. Hum Reprod. 2008;23(4):819–26.
46. Shulman A, Ben-Nun I, Ghetler Y, Kaneti H, Shilon M, Beyth Y. Relationship between embryo morphology and implantation rate after in vitro fertilization treatment in conception cycles. Fertil Steril. 1993;60(1):123–6.
47. Staessen C, Camus M, Bollen N, Devroey P, Van Steirteghem AC. The relationship between embryo quality and the occurrence of multiple pregnancies. Fertil Steril. 1992;57(3):626–30.
48. Ziebe S, Petersen K, Lindenberg S, Andersen AG, Gabrielsen A, Andersen AN. Embryo morphology or cleavage stage: how to select the best embryos for transfer after in-vitro fertilization. Hum Reprod. 1997;12(7):1545–9.
49. Testart J, Lassalle B, Belaisch-Allart J, et al. Human embryo freezing. Ann N Y Acad Sci. 1988;541:532–40.
50. Veiga A, Calderon G, Barri PN, Coroleu B. Pregnancy after the replacement of a frozen-thawed embryo with less than 50% intact blastomeres. Hum Reprod. 1987;2(4):321–3.
51. Van den Abbeel E, Camus M, Van Waesberghe L, Devroey P, Van Steirteghem AC. Viability of partially damaged human embryos after cryopreservation. Hum Reprod. 1997;12(9):2006–10.
52. Edgar DH, Bourne H, Speirs AL, McBain JC. A quantitative analysis of the impact of cryopreservation on the implantation potential of human early cleavage stage embryos. Hum Reprod. 2000;15(1):175–9.
53. Burns WN, Gaudet TW, Martin MB, et al. Survival of cryopreservation and thawing with all blastomeres intact identifies multicell embryos with superior frozen embryo transfer outcome. Fertil Steril. 1999;72(3):527–32.
54. Guerif F, Bidault R, Cadoret V, Couet ML, Lansac J, Royere D. Parameters guiding selection of best embryos for transfer after cryopreservation: a reappraisal. Hum Reprod. 2002;17(5):1321–6.
55. Gabrielsen A, Fedder J, Agerholm I. Parameters predicting the implantation rate of thawed IVF/ICSI embryos: a retrospective study. Reprod Biomed Online. 2006;12(1):70–6.
56. Pal L, Kovacs P, Witt B, Jindal S, Santoro N, Barad D. Post-thaw blastomere survival is predictive of the success of frozen-thawed embryo transfer cycles. Fertil Steril. 2004;82(4):821–6.
57. Tang R, Catt J, Howlett D. Towards defining parameters for a successful single embryo transfer in frozen cycles. Hum Reprod. 2006;21(5):1179–83.
58. Zheng X, Liu P, Chen G, Qiao J, Wu Y, Fan M. Viability of frozen-thawed human embryos with one-two blastomeres lysis. J Assist Reprod Genet. 2008;25(7):281–5.
59. Alikani M, Cohen J, Tomkin G, Garrisi GJ, Mack C, Scott RT. Human embryo fragmentation in vitro and its implications for pregnancy and implantation. Fertil Steril. 1999;71(5):836–42.
60. Alikani M, Olivennes F, Cohen J. Microsurgical correction of partially degenerate mouse embryos promotes hatching and restores their viability. Hum Reprod. 1993;8(10):1723–8.
61. Rienzi L, Nagy ZP, Ubaldi F, et al. Laser-assisted removal of necrotic blastomeres from cryopreserved embryos that were partially damaged. Fertil Steril. 2002;77(6):1196–201.
62. Van der Elst J, Van den Abbeel E, Vitrier S, Camus M, Devroey P, Van Steirteghem AC. Selective transfer of cryopreserved human embryos with further cleavage after thawing increases delivery and implantation rates. Hum Reprod. 1997;12(7):1513–21.
63. Ziebe S, Bech B, Petersen K, Mikkelsen AL, Gabrielsen A, Andersen AN. Resumption of mitosis

during post-thaw culture: a key parameter in selecting the right embryos for transfer. Hum Reprod. 1998;13(1):178–81.
64. Zhang S, Lu C, Lin G, Gong F, Lu G. The number of blastomeres in post-thawing embryos affects the rates of pregnancy and delivery in freeze-embryo-transfer cycles. J Assist Reprod Genet. 2009;26(11–12):569–73.
65. Veeck LL, Bodine R, Clarke RN, et al. High pregnancy rates can be achieved after freezing and thawing human blastocysts. Fertil Steril. 2004;82(5):1418–27.
66. Choi DH, Chung HM, Lim JM, Ko JJ, Yoon TK, Cha KY. Pregnancy and delivery of healthy infants developed from vitrified blastocysts in an IVF-ET program. Fertil Steril. 2000;74(4):838–9.
67. Liebermann J, Tucker MJ. Comparison of vitrification versus conventional cryopreservation of day 5 and day 6 blastocysts during clinical application. Fertil Steril. 2006;86:20–6.
68. Shapiro BS, Daneshmand ST, Garner FC, Aguirre M, Ross R. Contrasting patterns in in vitro fertilization pregnancy rates among fresh autologous, fresh oocyte donor, and cryopreserved cycles with the use of day 5 or day 6 blastocysts may reflect differences in embryo-endometrium synchrony. Fertil Steril. 2008;89(1):20–6.
69. Shapiro BS, Richter KS, Harris DC, Daneshmand ST. A comparison of day 5 and day 6 blastocyst transfers. Fertil Steril. 2001;75(6):1126–30.
70. Wilson M, Hartke K, Kiehl M, Rodgers J, Brabec C, Lyles R. Transfer of blastocysts and morulae on day 5. Fertil Steril. 2004;82(2):327–33.
71. Vanderzwalmen P, Bertin G, Debauche C, et al. Births after vitrification at morula and blastocyst stages: effect of artificial reduction of the blastocoelic cavity before vitrification. Hum Reprod. 2002;17(3):744–51.
72. Richter KS, Shipley SK, McVearry I, Tucker MJ, Widra EA. Cryopreserved embryo transfers suggest that endometrial receptivity may contribute to reduced success rates of later developing embryos. Fertil Steril. 2006;86(4):862–6.
73. Mukaida T, Oka C, Goto T, Takahashi K. Artificial shrinkage of blastocoeles using either a microneedle or a laser pulse prior to the cooling steps of vitrification improves survival rate and pregnancy outcome of vitrified human blastocysts. Hum Reprod. 2006;21:3246–52.
74. Shipley SK, Richter KS, Tucker MJ, Stillman RJ. P-532: Single embryo transfer of frozen-thawed blastocysts: Proportion of cells surviving the cryopreservation process is indicative of implantation potential. Fertil Steril. 2006;86(3):S332.
75. Stillman RJ, Richter KS, Banks NK, Graham JR. Elective single embryo transfer: a six year progressive implementation of 784 single blastocyst transfers and the influence of payment on patient choice. Fertil Steril. 2009;92:1895–906.
76. Delvigne A, Rozenberg S. Preventive attitude of physicians to avoid OHSS in IVF patients. Hum Reprod. 2001;16(12):2491–5.
77. Amso NN, Ahuja KK, Morris N, Shaw RW. The management of predicted ovarian hyperstimulation involving gonadotropin-releasing hormone analog with elective cryopreservation of all pre-embryos. Fertil Steril. 1990;53(6):1087–90.
78. D'Angelo A, Amso NN. Embryo freezing for preventing ovarian hyperstimulation syndrome: a Cochrane review. Hum Reprod. 2002;17(11):2787–94.
79. Queenan JT, Veeck LL, Toner JP, Oehninger S, Muasher SJ. Cryopreservation of all prezygotes in patients at risk of severe hyperstimulation does not eliminate the syndrome, but the chances of pregnancy are excellent with subsequent frozen-thaw transfers. Hum Reprod. 1997;12(7):1573–6.
80. Awonuga AO, Pittrof RJ, Zaidi J, Dean N, Jacobs HS, Tan SL. Elective cryopreservation of all embryos in women at risk of developing ovarian hyperstimulation syndrome may not prevent the condition but reduces the live birth rate. J Assist Reprod Genet. 1996;13(5):401–6.
81. Selman H, Brusco GF, Fiorini F, Barnocchi N, Mariani M, El-Danasouri I. Vitrification is a highly efficient method to cryopreserve human embryos in in vitro fertilization patients at high risk of developing ovarian hyperstimulation syndrome. Fertil Steril. 2009;91(4 Suppl):1611–3.
82. Munné S, Chen S, Colls P, et al. Maternal age, morphology, development and chromosome abnormalities in over 6000 cleavage-stage embryos. Reprod Biomed Online. 2007;14(5):628–34.
83. Wells D, Fragouli E, Stevens J, Munne S, Schoolcraft WB, Katz-Jaffe MG. High pregnancy rate after comprehensive chromosomal screening of blastocysts. Fertil Steril. 2008;90:S80.
84. Magli MC, Gianaroli L, Grieco N, Cefalù E, Ruvolo G, Ferraretti AP. Cryopreservation of biopsied embryos at the blastocyst stage. Hum Reprod. 2006;21(10):2656–60.
85. Rossi BV, Ashby RK, Srouji SS. Embryo banking between induction and consolidation chemotherapy in women with leukemia. Fertil Steril. 2011;96(6):1412–4.
86. Dickey RP, Lu PY, Sartor BM, Dunaway HE, Pyrzak R, Klumpp AM. Steps taken to protect and rescue cryopreserved embryos during Hurricane Katrina. Fertil Steril. 2006;86(3):732–4.
87. Ishihara O, Yoshimura Y. Damages at Japanese assisted reproductive technology clinics by the Great Eastern Japan Earthquake of 2011. Fertil Steril. 2011;95:2568–70.
88. Tedder RS, Zuckerman MA, Goldstone AH, et al. Hepatitis B transmission from contaminated cryopreservation tank. Lancet. 1995;346(8968):137–40.
89. Bielanski A, Vajta G. Risk of contamination of germplasm during cryopreservation and cryobanking in IVF units. Hum Reprod. 2009;24(10):2457–67.

90. Stringfellow DA, Givens MD, Waldrop JG. Biosecurity issues associated with current and emerging embryo technologies. Reprod Fertil Dev. 2004;16(1–2):93–102.
91. Bielanski A, Bergeron H, Lau PC, Devenish J. Microbial contamination of embryos and semen during long term banking in liquid nitrogen. Cryobiology. 2003;46(2):146–52.
92. Morris GJ. The origin, ultrastructure, and microbiology of the sediment accumulating in liquid nitrogen storage vessels. Cryobiology. 2005;50(3):231–8.
93. Parmegiani L, Accorsi A, Cognigni GE, Bernardi S, Troilo E, Filicori M. Sterilization of liquid nitrogen with ultraviolet irradiation for safe vitrification of human oocytes or embryos. Fertil Steril. 2010;94(4): 1525–8.
94. Srikanth B. The basic benefits of ultraviolet technology. *Water Conditioning Purification.* 1995(Dec):26-27.[http://aquvair.com/Basic%20Benefits%20of%20UV%20-WCP%20Reprint.pdf].
95. Clarke GN. Sperm cryopreservation: is there a significant risk of cross-contamination? Hum Reprod. 1999;14(12):2941–3.
96. Cobo A, Romero JL, Pérez S, de los Santos MJ, Meseguer M, Remohí J. Storage of human oocytes in the vapor phase of nitrogen. Fertil Steril. 2010; 94(5):1903–7.
97. Bielanski A. A review of the risk of contamination of semen and embryos during cryopreservation and measures to limit cross-contamination during banking to prevent disease transmission in ET practices. Theriogenology. 2012;77(3):467–82.
98. Cobo A, Bellver J, Jose de los Santos M, Remohi J. Viral screening of spent culture media and liquid nitrogen samples of oocytes and embryos from hepatitis B, hepatitis C, and human immunodeficiency virus chronically infected women undergoing in vitro fertilization cycles. Fertil Steril. 2012;97:74–8.
99. Koch J, Costello MF, Chapman MG, Kilani S. Twice-frozen embryos are no detriment to pregnancy success: a retrospective comparative study. Fertil Steril. 2011;96:58–62.
100. Ghobara T, Vandekerckhove P. Cycle regimens for frozen-thawed embryo transfer. Cochrane Database Syst Rev. 2008;23:CD003414.
101. Glujovsky D, Pesce R, Fiszbajn G, Sueldo C, Hart RJ, Ciapponi A. Endometrial preparation for women undergoing embryo transfer with frozen embryos or embryos derived from donor oocytes. Cochrane Database Syst Rev. 2010; (1):CD006359.

Oocyte Donation

10

Joshua U. Klein and Mark V. Sauer

The History of Oocyte Donation

Over the past three decades, oocyte donation (OD) has developed into a practical and highly effective treatment option used in the routine armamentarium of the modern reproductive endocrinologist. Refinements in the method of oocyte donation may be viewed as a relative completion of the process of "creative deconstruction" that the advent of assisted reproductive technology has wreaked on more traditional notions of procreation. Not only is there no longer a requirement for an intimate relationship, or even a sexual act, between a man and a woman in order to achieve a pregnancy; and not only can a pregnancy be initiated outside the natural environment of the female reproductive tract; but when oocyte donation is practiced, the entire conception process can occur essentially independent of the genetic "father" and "mother," as long as there is a receptive uterus available for implantation when the process is complete.

When considered from this philosophical perspective, oocyte donation actually "unlinks" the conceptual components of human reproduction: the agents of conception (i.e., the sources of the gametes) are no longer necessarily connected in any way to the agent of gestation and birth. The profundity of this separation cannot be overstated; in fact, the early history of oocyte donation reflects the transition that was necessary for such a radical departure to occur.

The earliest precursor to modern oocyte donation is actually more aptly referred to as embryo donation, in that fertilization of the oocyte actually occurred in vivo, and the embryo, rather than the egg, was the entity being donated. In 1890, Walter Heape reported the transfer of embryos from an Angora doe rabbit to a synchronized Belgian hare recipient, resulting in the birth of healthy offspring [1]. Using the technique of uterine lavage to retrieve early embryos, Heape's basic approach was subsequently applied to multiple mammalian species through the course of the twentieth century, with the first successful bovine embryo transfer reported in 1951 [2]. Embryo donation became popular amongst cattle breeders in the 1970s, and by 1990 almost 19,000 calves were born annually in the USA as a result of this technique [3]. Today, embryo donation is still regularly employed for breeding endangered species and in commercial animal husbandry.

Steptoe and Edwards' first successful IVF in 1978 generated excitement and interest in all aspects of human fertility, and soon thereafter researchers at the Harbor-UCLA Medical Center

J.U. Klein, M.D.
Division of Reproductive Endocrinology and Infertility, Department of Obstetrics and Gynecology, New York Presbyterian Hospital, Columbia University Medical Center, New York, NY 10032, USA
e-mail: juk2103@columbia.edu

M.V. Sauer, M.D. (✉)
Center for Women's Reproductive Care, Columbia University Medical Center, New York, NY 10019, USA
e-mail: mvs9@columbia.edu

E.S. Ginsburg and C. Racowsky (eds.), *In Vitro Fertilization: A Comprehensive Guide*,
DOI 10.1007/978-1-4419-9848-4_10, © Springer Science+Business Media New York 2012

in Los Angeles, directed their attention and efforts to using embryo donation for the treatment of infertility in humans. Years of work went into developing a catheter capable of performing uterine lavage and embryo recovery, and in 1983, Buster et al. performed artificial insemination upon a fertile woman and successfully recovered the in vivo-fertilized ovum; the recovered blastocyst was then transferred to the uterus of a synchronized ovulatory infertile recipient resulting in pregnancy [4]. The first live birth from this approach was reported the following year [5].

While the California group was breaking new ground by separating the embryo from its intended implantation site, an independent group at Monash University in Australia was concomitantly applying standard IVF technology to oocyte donation by experimenting with oocytes retrieved laparoscopically from an infertile woman who also agreed to act as an egg donor. Following retrieval of her eggs one oocyte was donated to an infertile couple for their use. The donated oocyte was fertilized in vitro, and subsequently a single embryo was transferred to the infertile recipient. This group too reported its first pregnancy in 1983 [6] and first live birth in 1984 [7].

In the early 1980s, oocyte donation was heralded as a miracle cure for women with otherwise intractable infertility due to ovarian failure, but it should be remembered that peri-menopausal and menopausal women were not initially considered appropriate candidates for this treatment. The earliest OD investigators did pioneer the successful establishment and maintenance of pregnancy in patients with premature ovarian failure [7]; however, the idea that reproductive capacity could actually be extended beyond "natural" or "normal" ovarian failure (i.e., menopause) was not considered seriously or pursued in earnest until several years later [8, 9].

In addition to expanding the indications for OD to women with "normal" ovarian failure, advances in related fields have continued to accrue and enlarge the candidate population for OD. For example, advances in clinical and molecular genetics have led couples to use OD to avoid transmitting heritable diseases to offspring [10]; better understanding of the biology of ovarian aging and oocyte quality, in conjunction with an improvement in "standard" (non-donor-oocyte) IVF have led to more couples using OD for consistently poor embryo quality and repetitive IVF failure; and change in social mores has led to using OD in lesbian couples who share in the creation of their child by having one partner donate the oocytes, while the other carries the fetus, and for same sex male couples using a gestational carrier to create a child.

While the focus of research in OD has always been primarily upon achieving pregnancy in the recipients, as the field has matured several other areas of interest have attracted attention from clinicians and researchers. These include studies of donors and their attitudes, experiences, and motivations; obstetric and pediatric studies of OD offspring; ethical discussions regarding compensation and eligibility; and many others. Other future directions for research in this field include promising new areas of inquiry such as in vitro maturation of unstimulated oocyte donors; oocyte cryopreservation and the possibility of "donor egg banks"; and the newest developments with regard to using gametes from oocyte donors to produce programmable stem cells for research application in various diseases.

Epidemiology

In 1995, 4,783 OD cycles were performed, representing approximately 8% of all ART cycles in the USA. According to the most recent published CDC data (2009), the absolute number of OD cycles has increased almost fourfold to 17,697 cycles. Furthermore, when considered as a proportion of all ART being performed, donor eggs were used in approximately 12% of ART cycles performed in the USA in 2009; this represents approximately a 50% increase from 1995.

As one might expect, the growth in OD cycles is largely a reflection of the evolving indications for OD, specifically the increased number of women of advanced reproductive age seeking fertility treatment. Whereas amongst women age <35 years, fewer than 5% of ART cycles involve

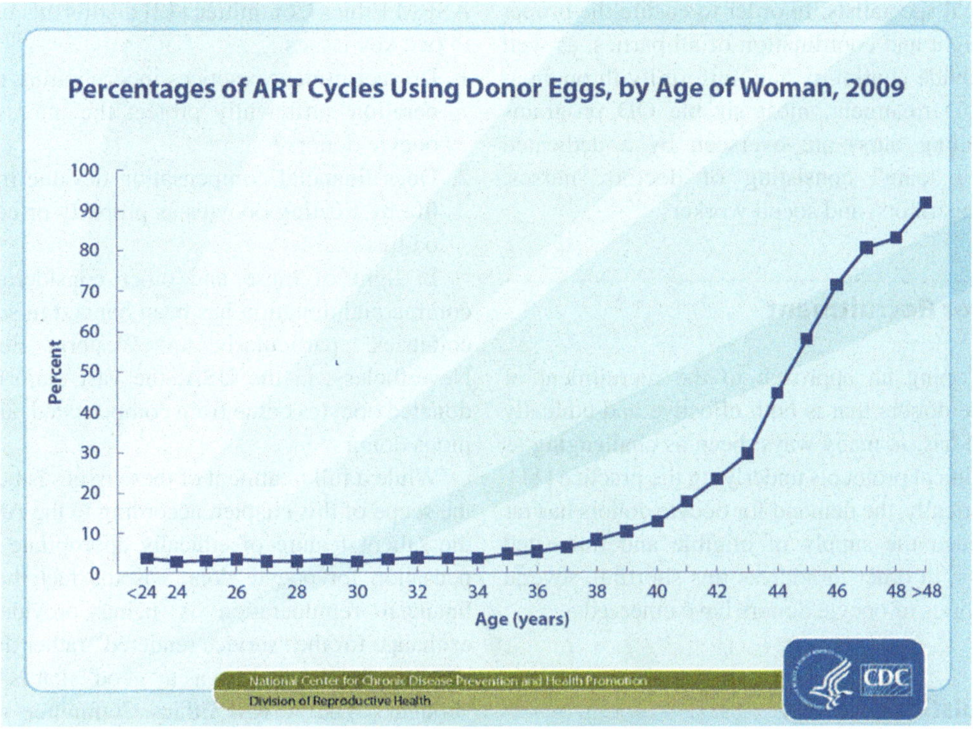

Fig. 10.1 Percentages of ART cycles using donor eggs, by age of woman, 2009

the use of donor oocytes, the vast majority of women 45 years and older who undergo ART use oocyte donation (see Fig. 10.1). While data regarding indications for OD are limited, it is highly likely DOR was the primary indication in most of these cases.

Practical Implementation

The management of clinical OD is complex and requires a great deal of clinical and organizational coordination amongst multiple parties. In order to achieve successful outcomes, several following steps must be collaboratively accomplished.

1. Medical screening and clearance of the OD recipient
2. Recruitment and screening of potential oocyte donors
3. Identification and matching of an appropriate donor to the OD recipient
4. Synchronization and manipulation of the donor and recipient cycles, including
   (a) Downregulation of the donor's hypothalamic–pituitary–gonadal axis
   (b) Downregulation of the recipient's hypothalamic–pituitary–gonadal axis
   (c) Controlled ovarian hyperstimulation (COH) of the donor
   (d) Endometrial preparation of the recipient
5. Oocyte retrieval
6. Insemination or ICSI of donated eggs with partner or donor sperm
7. Embryo culture, preferably to the blastocyst stage if possible
8. Embryo transfer to recipient; cryopreservation of supernumerary embryos
9. Endometrial/luteal support and pregnancy monitoring in recipient

The parties responsible for the coordinated completion of these steps include, at a minimum, the OD recipient, the oocyte donor, and the reproductive endocrinology and embryology team; typically, however, various other parties are also involved including social workers, psychologists, a donor agency, sperm bank, and other consulting medical specialists. In order to ensure the proper oversight and coordination of all parties, as well as provide continuity and uniformity throughout the OD treatment, most sizable OD programs (including ours) are overseen by a dedicated "donor team" consisting of doctors, nurses, administrators, and social workers.

Donor Recruitment

Developing an approach to the recruitment of oocyte donors that is both effective and ethically sound has, in many ways, been as challenging as the clinical protocols underlying the practice [11]. Historically, the demand for oocyte donors has far exceeded the supply of eligible and interested donors; in order to address this shortfall, several categories of oocyte donors have emerged.

Altruistic Donation

The sympathy and compassion aroused by the plight of an infertile couple motivates some women to volunteer for oocyte donation for purely altruistic reasons. While some altruistic donors would be willing to donate eggs to a couple unknown to them (i.e., altruistic anonymous donation), most altruistic donation occurs in the setting of "known donation," i.e., when an infertile couple asks a friend or relative to consider a "directed donation" on their behalf. While in many ways altruistic donation relieves some of the ethical problems raised by donor compensation (see below), it also can raise unique emotional and psychological challenges that might complicate the human experience of OD in the long term (e.g., a donor who donates successfully to her sister and brother-in-law but later in life struggles with infertility herself).

Commercial/Anonymous Donation

The notion of providing a financial incentive to oocyte donors has long invoked discomfort amongst ethicists and lay people alike. The ASRM Ethics Committee [12] distills this unease to two key issues.

1. Do recruitment practices incorporating remuneration sufficiently protect the interests of oocyte donors?
2. Does financial compensation devalue human life by treating oocytes as property or commodities?

In light of these and other considerations, commercial donation has been banned in several countries, particularly in Western Europe. Nevertheless, in the USA, the vast majority of donated oocytes come from compensated, anonymous donors.

While a full treatment of these issues is beyond the scope of this chapter, according to the ASRM, the salient feature of ethically appropriate compensation for oocyte donors is the fact that the financial remuneration is being provided in exchange for the "service rendered" rather than as payment for the oocytes as a "good" that is being "bought." The ASRM Ethics Committee states: "Compensation should be structured to acknowledge the time, inconvenience, and discomfort associated with screening, ovarian stimulation, and oocyte retrieval. Compensation should not vary according to the planned use of the oocytes, the number or quality of oocytes retrieved, the number or outcome of prior donation cycles, or the donor's ethnic or other personal characteristics" [12]. Furthermore, in order to minimize the potential for exploitation of financially vulnerable donors, the amount of compensation should reflect the significance of oocyte donation but not be so high as to represent undue inducement. Payments to donors in excess of $5,000 require "justification" and compensation exceeding $10,000 is considered "not appropriate." A 2006 SART survey revealed a national average of $4,217, with compensation being the highest in the East/Northeast at an average of $5,018 per cycle [13]. Currently in New York City, the standard compensation for oocyte donors at large programs has risen to $8,000 per cycle.

With regard to actually recruiting candidates for oocyte donation, most ART clinics solicit interest using traditional print and digital advertising. An additional level of commercial interest has crept into the process of OD as many "egg donor agencies" have been created to help couples locate an appropriate donor, and more generally, to help navigate the practical and legal intricacies of egg donation in exchange for a fee. Recognizing this, the ASRM and SART have established a "registry" of egg donor agencies that have signed an agreement to abide by the ASRM and SART guidelines regarding ethical and appropriate practices in egg donation. A list of these agencies is maintained online at http://www.asrm.org/Egg_Donor_Agencies/.

Egg Sharing

Despite the ethical framework supported by a policy of standardized, regulated compensation for oocyte donation "services" rather than the explicit "sale" of the eggs themselves, an alternative model of oocyte donation was developed in the 1990s and continues to be practiced in many programs in the USA and abroad. An "egg sharing" arrangement is one in which an infertile patient undergoing ART for her own benefit agrees to "donate" some proportion (usually half) of the oocytes retrieved to an anonymous recipient in exchange for some financial incentive or discount on the fees for her care. Such an approach eliminates the need to recruit healthy donors and subject them to the short-term and long-term risks of oocyte donation, and also removes the explicit exchange of money for gametes.

From an ethical standpoint, while egg sharing does seem to present some potential benefits, the relative merits of these advantages are arguable [11]. Egg sharing generates different, but similarly troublesome, ethical concerns, e.g., the potential for exploitation when a presumably vulnerable infertile patient is being asked to consent to donate some of her eggs. Furthermore, data are limited regarding the impact of egg sharing on the clinical outcomes of both donor and recipient; almost all studies in the literature are retrospective and lacking appropriate control groups. One of the larger and better-designed studies showed that while pregnancy rates were comparable between "shared" and "exclusive" cycles, the possibility of having excess embryos available for cryopreservation was significantly reduced in the shared cycles [14]. All in all, when compared with traditional commercial egg donation, egg sharing presents a different, but similarly complicated, mix of advantages and disadvantages to the donor, recipient, and providers.

Donor Screening

Identifying and securing a suitable oocyte donor can be challenging. Multiple requirements must be met before a particular individual can be deemed an appropriate candidate for OD. A large proportion of women who express interest in OD and initiate the screening process will ultimately be disqualified from proceeding due to a variety of factors. In one report, only 1 in 25 women who initiated screening ultimately went on to complete an OD cycle [15]. Issues that require consideration and assessment can be conceptually categorized into "donor-centric" vs. "recipient-centric."

Donor-Centric Screening

From a donor-centric perspective, protecting the safety and well-being of the donor is paramount. Therefore, it is important that the donor be physically capable of tolerating the OD treatment protocol, including controlled ovarian hyperstimulation (COH) and oocyte retrieval under anesthesia, without incurring undue risk of complication or harm. Women with significant preexisting medical disease or risk factors, such as obesity, diabetes, hypertension, immunologic and/or allergic disease, are suboptimal candidates for oocyte donation. A full medical history and thorough physical examination are necessary in order to make this determination. Potential donors with chronic medical illness not only are at higher risk themselves but also may transmit undesirable traits to offspring; these women should therefore be disqualified as anonymous donors.

Additionally, the donor must convincingly demonstrate the ability to provide informed consent to participate in OD. Women who have underlying intellectual or (more commonly) psychological impediments to a thorough understanding of the risks and implications, medical and emotional, from both a short- and long-term perspective, should be discouraged or disqualified from participating. In this regard, a social worker or other mental health professional is often better qualified to perform the initial assessment than the reproductive endocrinologist or other members of the medical team. In a related vein, although not required by the ASRM or the FDA, some large OD programs (including ours) perform routine urine toxicology screening for all potential OD candidates [16]. Management of positive results must be individualized; at a minimum, repeat testing is required before proceeding with further consideration for OD in any woman who tests positive.

Table 10.1 Required screening for donors

Test
CBC
Blood type
HIV 1 and HIV 2[a]
RPR[a]
Hepatitis B Surface Antigen[a]
Hepatitis B Core Antibody[a]
Hepatitis C[a]
Pap smear
Cervical or urine DNA screen for gonorrhea and chlamydia[a]
Ovarian reserve testing (e.g., anti-mullerian hormone)
Urine toxicology panel
Cystic Fibrosis
Fragile X
Spinal muscular atrophy
Other genetic testing depending on ethnicity (e.g., hemoglobin electrophoresis, Tay-Sachs, etc.)

[a]Indicates FDA required screening donor undergoing treatment in the USA; testing must be performed by FDA approved methodologies

Recipient-Centric Screening

From a recipient-centric perspective, two fundamental considerations come into play. The first is the medical suitability of the OD candidate to provide oocytes that will lead to a healthy pregnancy. Age is an important limiting factor here, given the association between female age and reproductive potential. The ASRM recommends limiting OD to donors aged 21–34 years; if a donor is 35 years or older, the potential for diminished chances of success should be discussed with the recipient [17]. Furthermore, many clinics generally limit anonymous OD to donors no older than age 30 years; in general, there is reliable data supporting the inverse relationship between donor age and OD outcomes, possibly even for donors in their twenties [18, 19]. In the case of known (as opposed to anonymous) donation, when the recipient intends to use oocytes from a friend, relative, or significant other, most programs will often be more lenient with regard to donor age, although again, informed consent is crucial. In addition to age, a reproductive and/or gynecologic history and physical exam are important screening tools for identifying polycystic ovarian disease or other disorders likely to impact the likelihood of successful donation.

Another major area relevant to the recipient-centric perspective is the potential for transmission of infectious disease. At present, fully definitive exclusion of infectious disease is impossible in the setting of OD, due to the fact that a true quarantine period would be necessary to identify the presence of infectious diseases at the time of oocyte retrieval, but this is impossible without invoking oocyte cryopreservation. The safety and efficacy of oocyte cryopreservation has been rapidly advancing in the past few years, and the ASRM no longer considers the technology experimental [20]. However, more widespread clinic-specific data are deemed necessary before establishment of universal oocyte donor banks.

In light of this issue, the FDA and ASRM have issued guidelines regarding the necessary screening tests and timing of the screens of oocyte donors (Table 10.1). According to the FDA guidance document for eligibility for donors of human cells (www.fda.gov, section §1271.50), which USA assisted reproductive technologies programs must adhere to, required tests must be performed using FDA approved methodologies. Such methodologies are not performed in all hospitals or commercial laboratories, so investigation must

Table 10.2 Required screening for recipients

Test	< 40 year	≥ 40 year	≥ 45 year	≥ 50 year, MP or POF*
CBC	√	√	√	√
Blood type	√	√	√	√
Serum electrolytes	√	√	√	√
TSH	√	√	√	√
Pap smear	√	√	√	√
Cervical or urine DNA screen (chlamydia/gonorrhea)	√	√	√	√
HIV 1 and 2	√	√	√	√
RPR	√	√	√	√
Hepatitis B and C	√	√	√	√
Rubella antibody	√	√	√	√
Uterine cavity evaluation	√	√	√	√
ECG		√	√	√
Chest radiograph		√	√	√
Mammogram		√	√	√
Glucose tolerance test		√	√	√
Cholesterol/lipid profile		√	√	√
Exercise tolerance test			√	√
Pre-pregnancy maternal-fetal medicine consultation			√	√
Bone densitometry				√

MP menopausal, *POF* premature ovarian failure

be done prior to selecting a laboratory for donor screening. Furthermore, it is recommended that a thorough questionnaire is administered and an interview conducted regarding travel history, sexual practices, and other factors that may identify candidates who present a higher risk for transmissible disease, as determined by the FDA. An additional issue relevant to donor suitability is the presence of heritable genetic disorders. ASRM guidelines on this issue are relatively open-ended [17]:

1. Donors with a known specific personal or family history of genetic disorders should be excluded or appropriately tested.
2. Routine screening for cystic fibrosis and/or other genetic diseases should be performed in accordance with current American College of Obstetricians and Gynecologists recommendations.
3. With regard to other diseases, donor candidates belonging to "high risk groups" should be tested for diseases appropriate to their ethnicity.
4. Donors may be tested for Fragile X at the discretion of the program.
5. Routine karyotyping of all donors is optional.

Recipient Selection and Screening

ASRM endorses five categories of indications for oocyte donation:

1. Hypergonadotropic hypogonadism (i.e., ovarian failure)
2. Advanced reproductive age
3. Diminished ovarian reserve
4. Genetic disease
5. History of poor oocyte/embryo quality and/or multiple failed ART attempts

With the goal of a healthy live birth in mind, OD recipient candidates are generally screened for eligibility in a manner similar to any patient interested in pursuing ART, including a thorough medical history, physical examination with cervical cytology, transvaginal ultrasound, and routine prenatal laboratory tests (Table 10.2); the following are several considerations that demand special attention in the setting of oocyte donation.

Advanced Age and Medical Health

Common medical conditions that threaten general medical and obstetric health, including obesity, hypertension, impaired glucose tolerance, and/or diabetes all demonstrate increasing incidence as women progress through their fourth, fifth, and sixth decades of life. In particular, although no clear biological mechanism has been elucidated, the incidence of hypertensive disorders of pregnancy is significantly increased in OD recipients as compared with age-matched non-OD patients (Keegan, Le Ray). Furthermore, the risk for obstetric complications such as pre-eclampsia and gestational diabetes is further exacerbated in the setting of multiple gestation, an undesirable but not infrequent outcome in OD.

Therefore, as indicated in Table 10.2, a heightened level of vigilance is appropriate when screening a potential OD recipient for cardiovascular and metabolic fitness. This includes routine EKG, chest X-ray, glucose tolerance test, and lipid profile for women older than 40, and an exercise tolerance test for women older than 45. If the patient is menopausal and/or demonstrates premature ovarian failure of some duration, bone densitometry testing by DEXA scan is appropriate as well. If any comorbid conditions are identified, consultation with appropriate medical and/or maternal fetal medicine specialists is required to reduce the risk of avoidable and/or unexpected morbidity associated with pregnancy.

Turner Syndrome

Despite being a relatively rare condition (approximately 1 in 2,000 female births), patients with Turner syndrome have deservedly attracted a disproportionate amount of attention in the OD literature. Because this condition is frequently associated with cardiovascular malformations, Turner Syndrome patients who conceive via oocyte donation carry a 2% risk of mortality from aortic dissection or rupture during the peripartum period [21]. ASRM guidelines require preconception consultation with cardiology and with maternal fetal medicine, as well as evaluation of the aortic anatomy by trans-esophageal echocardiography in combination with cardiac MRI. An enlarged aortic size index (ASI) >2.0 cm/m^2) or any other abnormality identified on imaging should identify the patient as particularly high-risk and should be considered a strong contraindication to pregnancy.

Endometrial Response

Given the resources required to proceed with oocyte donation, and the importance of a receptive endometrium to all ART success, many programs routinely perform a "mock cycle" in which the recipient undergoes hormonal preparation in order to verify adequate uterine response prior to proceeding with OD. Endometrial response is typically evaluated either by histological evaluation on endometrial biopsy, or more commonly, by endometrial thickness on transvaginal ultrasound, with 6–7 mm being a typical minimum threshold value supported in the literature [22, 23].

The evidence in support of this practice is conflicting, and the need for universal endometrial "screening" has been questioned [24]. We advocate a selective approach to performing mock cycles. In general, the risk for inadequate response to hormonal preparation is relatively remote in the absence of specific risk factors. In the presence of these risk factors, such as a history of pelvic irradiation, severe intrauterine adhesive disease, extensive uterine surgery, or a history of multiple failed OD cycles, a mock cycle may be warranted.

Psychosocial Considerations

While many patients struggling with infertility carry a heavy emotional and psychological burden, some of these stressors are particularly amplified in the setting of OD. The emotional consequences of the loss of genetic parentage should not be underestimated. OD patients should be offered the support of social workers or other mental health professionals. Specific psychological challenges are unique to the setting of

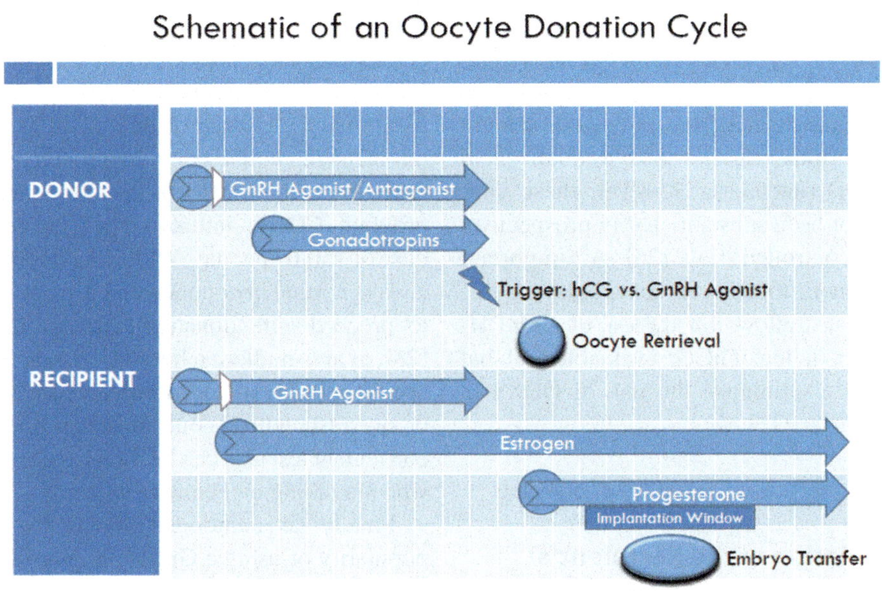

Fig. 10.2 Schematic of an oocyte donation cycle

anonymous (e.g., disclosure, worries about "unknown" genetic problems, etc.) as well as known donation (e.g., tension and/or resentment amongst the donor, recipient, partner, etc.). Finally, in cases involving more complex arrangements (e.g., surrogacy- see Chap. 11), consultation with legal counsel experienced in this specialized area of the law is mandatory.

Cycle Management/Synchronization

In order for an OD cycle to be completed successfully, several biological processes must be pharmacologically replicated in a synchronized fashion. A schematic of an OD cycle is presented in Fig. 10.2.

As a starting point, the oocyte donor, and sometimes the recipient, is typically started on a daily oral contraceptive in order to gain some leverage on the timing of their respective menses. In order to minimize the possibility of scheduling conflicts and/or non-compliance, a schedule that incorporates necessary monitoring and procedures and takes into account the specific protocol being implemented should be created and reviewed with the donor, recipient, nursing, medical, and embryology teams prior to initiating any treatment plan.

While the OD literature is replete with data regarding the relative advantages and disadvantages of various OD protocols, it is instructive to note that a recent Cochrane meta-analysis of 22 randomized trials demonstrated similar pregnancy rates for multiple different approaches to endometrial preparation and hormone replacement [25]. We review here some of the highlights and more current considerations that are important in choosing an OD protocol.

Downregulation of the Donor's Hypothalamic–Pituitary–Gonadal Axis

Donor downregulation can be accomplished in a manner similar to that of any patient undergoing non-donor IVF. While historically a GnRH-agonist (e.g., leuprolide acetate) was considered first-line option, the rising popularity and provider comfort with GnRH antagonists (e.g., ganirelix acetate), in combination with the added convenience of the shorter treatment duration using an antagonist, have led many programs to routinely use antagonist for donor downregulation. Concerns have been raised that use of the antagonist would decrease LH and that this might exert a deleterious effect on oocyte quality and ultimately OD outcomes. However, these concerns have not been substantiated in prospective, randomized controlled trials [26]. An important additional benefit to using an antagonist for this purpose is that it allows for the use of a GnRH-agonist trigger in lieu of hCG, a valuable tool that may be used to minimize the risk of OHSS in oocyte donors (see below).

Downregulation of the Recipient's Hypothalamic–Pituitary–Gonadal Axis

Strictly speaking, recipient downregulation is required only if the patient demonstrates the presence of a functional central axis to begin with; the GnRH agonist is typically considered first line for this indication. In postmenopausal women or patients with complete premature ovarian failure, endometrial preparation can be initiated without prior downregulation.

Controlled Ovarian Hyperstimulation (COH) of the Donor

The approach to COH in the oocyte donor is not fundamentally different from COH in non-donor IVF. Overall, OD outcomes have not been shown to vary significantly in association with specific gonadotropins and/or their relative LH activity. For example, in one large recent study, 1,028 donors were prospectively randomized to recombinant FSH alone (rFSH), highly purified menotropin (HP-hMG), or a mixed rFSH plus HP-hMG protocol. Other than cost, no differences were observed amongst the three groups in any clinically significant parameter, including the number of days of stimulation, number of oocytes retrieved, cancellation rate, implantation rate, pregnancy rate, and miscarriage rate [27].

The most important consideration when it comes to COH in oocyte donors is achieving stimulation that will yield a response sufficient to maximize the chance of treatment success without incurring undue risk of ovarian hyperstimulation syndrome (OHSS) in the donor. In our program, COH is initiated in a typical donor at a dose of 150 IU per day. While day 3 FSH is almost always normal in donors who have been approved to proceed with donation, antral follicle count [28], or anti-mullerian hormone levels [29] can be used to identify donors at increased risk of under- or overresponding. Anti-mullerian hormone is a convenient test as it can be drawn to screen donors who are taking oral contraceptives.

Finally, as mentioned above, the increased popularity of using a GnRH antagonist for donor downregulation has also facilitated the use of a GnRH agonist to trigger oocyte maturation prior to retrieval rather than hCG in an effort to minimize OHSS. Several clinical trials have demonstrated that GnRH trigger in OD cycles does not lead to any diminished clinical outcomes but essentially eliminates OHSS in donors (as compared with OHSS incidence of 4–17% in hCG trigger OD cycles) [30]. Hence, it seems reasonable that the use of GnRH agonist trigger in OD cycles should be considered, if not encouraged, especially in OD cycles at significant risk of OHSS.

Endometrial Preparation of the Recipient

As mentioned previously, despite the abundance of published data regarding the relative merits of various approaches to endometrial preparation and hormone replacement (specific agents, routes, and dosage), there are multiple options available that yield similarly successful outcomes.

With regard to estrogen, most programs initiate oral micronized estradiol 2–4 mg twice daily, or transdermal estrogen 0.2–0.4 mg/day, approximately 14 days prior to planned progesterone exposure. In the case of logistical complications or other reasons for delay, there are data to suggest that the duration of unopposed estrogen exposure can be extended for 5 weeks or more without impacting the chances of success [31]. Of note, monitoring serum estradiol in the recipient does not lead to improved outcomes in OD [23].

Progesterone is typically administered either transvaginally (100–600 mg/day) or intramuscularly (50–100 mg/day) in order to avoid first-pass hepatic metabolism. If tested, serum levels of progesterone will be lower when progesterone is administered transvaginally, but serum testing does not accurately reflect local/endometrial progesterone concentrations and is not clinically significant; this practice should therefore be discouraged [32].

The duration of progesterone exposure prior to embryo transfer is much more important as compared with estrogen preparation; optimal outcomes are seen when embryo transfer is performed approximately 4–5 days after progesterone exposure for cleavage stage embryos and on day 7 with blastocysts [26, 33, 34]. Our practice is to initiate 200 mg of vaginal micronized progesterone on the day prior to oocyte retrieval and continue at "full dose" (200 mg TID) thereafter, with embryo transfer occurring on Day 3, 5, or 6 of embryo culture (days 4, 6, or 7 of progesterone exposure).

Adequacy of endometrial response can be evaluated by measurement of the endometrial stripe on transvaginal ultrasound, although the literature does not consistently support this practice. While some groups report worse outcomes with an endometrium ≤6–7 mm [35], others did not observe an association between endometrial thickness and clinical outcomes [36], and pregnancies have occurred in recipients with linings as thin as 4 mm [37].

Typically, serum hCG is tested approximately 2 weeks after oocyte retrieval. When pregnancy is achieved, hormone replacement is then continued until 10–12 weeks, well past the time the luteo-placental shift is expected to occur and placental steroidogenesis is firmly established. In our program, we routinely check progesterone levels 3 days after hormone replacement is discontinued; serum progesterone >25 ng/mL is typically considered adequate and no further supplementation is needed.

Clinical Outcomes

Recipient

In terms of chances for pregnancy and live birth, at any age, the prognosis for OD recipients equals or exceeds any other subgroup of patients pursuing ART (Fig. 10.3). After four OD cycles, cumulative OD live birth rates approach 90%, regardless of indication for treatment or recipient age [11, 38].

Several clinical and demographic factors have been demonstrated to be associated with OD outcomes. Obesity, smoking, and the presence of hydrosalpinx are consistently associated with diminished OD success [36], whereas blastocyst transfer is consistently associated with increased success [11, 34]. As mentioned above, the significance of a thin endometrium (<8 mm) is unclear. Donor age, also mentioned above, is undoubtedly important [18, 19]; in contrast, the significance of recipient age is controversial. While almost no study has shown a relationship between increased recipient age and diminished OD success in younger (i.e., age <40–45) recipients, an analysis of a very large number of OD cycles reported to the SART registry did suggest the possibility of decreased success in recipients older than age 45 [39]. A more recent SART registry analysis of cumulative live birth in OD, however, failed to confirm this finding [40]. Finally, regarding male age and OD outcome, data are also mixed, but overall it seems unlikely that male age is a major determinant of OD outcomes, again reflecting the primary importance of the health of the oocyte over other factors in oocyte donation [41–43].

The risk for multiple births in OD cycles is considerable and is related to high implantation rates of embryos created resulting in high ongoing pregnancy rates. In 2009, 38% of live births resulting from OD in the USA were multiples, although it should be noted that the vast majority of these were twins, with triplets or higher-order multiples representing only 1.2% of births (2.8% of pregnancies) (CDC). Prior to initiating treatment and again at the time of embryo transfer, recipients should be thoroughly counseled

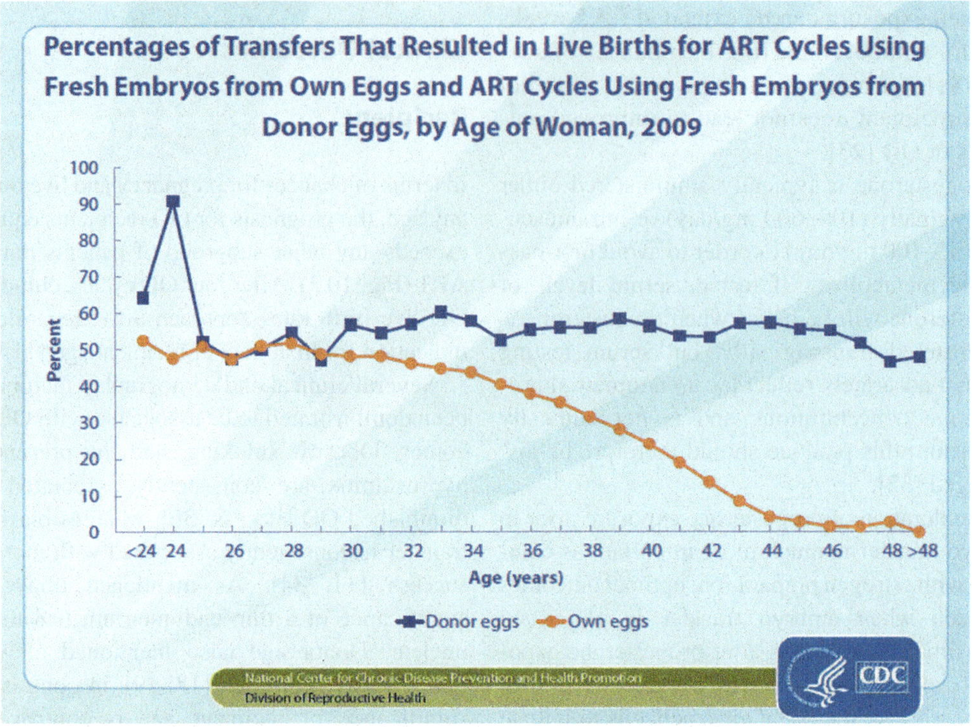

Fig. 10.3 Percentages of transfers that resulted in live births for ART cycles using fresh embryos from own eggs and ART cycles using fresh embryos from donor eggs, by age of woman, 2009

regarding the increased risk for obstetric complications in the setting of multiple gestations, further compounded in recipients of advanced reproductive age. ASRM guidelines state that donor age should be considered the primary factor in deciding on the number of embryos to transfer, in which case (assuming donor age <35 years) the number of embryos transferred in OD should never exceed two. In our opinion, elective single embryo transfer should be routinely offered and should be strongly encouraged in recipients age >40 years or with comorbid conditions (e.g., obesity, hypertension, myomatous uterus, Turner syndrome).

It should also be emphasized that overall, obstetric and pediatric outcomes in OD pregnancies are quite good. OD recipients generally demonstrate an incidence of perinatal complications similar to those of age-matched women undergoing IVF with their own oocytes. However, one prominent exception is the increased risk of hypertensive disorders of pregnancy, which has been demonstrated in multiple reports [44–46]. No abnormal pediatric complications have been reported in OD offspring; one study described follow-up of a cohort of OD offspring and their parents at 12 years without noting any significant social or emotional developmental problems [47].

Donor

As the practice of oocyte donation has matured and outcomes have continued to improve, increased attention has been devoted in the literature to issues specific to oocyte donors. Medical and surgical complications related to oocyte donation are rare, estimated at approximately 1% [48]. In one of the largest recent reviews of this subject, the rate of surgical complication in over 4,000 OD cycles was 0.4%, most commonly peri-operative bleeding issues and adnexal torsion. Surgical intervention was rarely required (0.15%); notably, organ injury, postoperative infection, and anesthesia complications did not occur in this series. The rate of moderate–severe ovarian hyperstimulation syndrome was 0.87%; all cases of moderate–severe OHSS were observed when using an hCG trigger, and no OHSS was observed when using a GnRH agonist trigger [49].

Reproductive outcomes in oocyte donors is a subject which requires further study, but data thus far have been encouraging. A common concern amongst prospective donors is premature depletion of ovarian reserve; no data currently exists to support this hypothesis. One recent study, in fact, demonstrated no decrease in response to stimulation or ovarian reserve (as measured by anti-Mullerian hormone) over the course of six OD cycles [50]. ASRM Guidelines suggest limiting ODs to six stimulated cycles, and limiting the number of offspring per donor to 25 to reduce risk of consanguinity [17]. Other recent survey-based studies of previous oocyte donors have demonstrated an incidence of subfertility of 5–10%, consistent with the general background rate of subfertility in most populations [51, 52].

Psychosocial Considerations

The complexity of oocyte donation is perhaps most deeply appreciated when its psychosocial ramifications and repercussions are considered. Numerous ethical questions and concerns have long been debated [11]; prominent amongst these are issues of compensation for donors (discussed briefly above) as well as OD in older postmenopausal recipients, a practice that the ASRM Ethics Committee (perhaps surprisingly) actually discourages due to its "unnatural" quality [53].

Another important focus of concern regarding OD is that of disclosure. While in practice many OD donors and recipients currently choose to preserve their anonymity, studies imply a growing trend toward increased disclosure of identity amongst donors and offspring for psychological, emotional, and even medical reasons [54]; indeed, some countries have enacted legislation mandating disclosure of participants involved in gamete donation.

Future Directions and Conclusion

While enormous progress has been made in the first three decades of clinical practice involving oocyte donation, numerous challenges and potential applications still lie ahead. Long-term studies of the health of oocyte donors and OD offspring are lacking and will be important to reinforce the safety of the practice and identify important risks which may currently be unknown. The ongoing challenge of access to oocyte donors may soon be eased by advances in oocyte cryopreservation technology and methodology, and the availability of commercial "egg banks" that are marketing lower cost services to ART patients and providers. In one recent study, 600 recipients were randomized to receive fresh vs. vitrified ("banked") oocytes in an oocyte donation program; outcomes were similar in both groups, demonstrating at least the feasibility of establishing cryopreserved "egg banks" for clinical use in OD [55]. Finally, advances in stem cell biology have introduced the novel field of oocyte donation for the generation of stem cells, currently for purely academic research use, but possibly for clinical application in the not-too-distant future [56].

It is fair to say that 30 years after its introduction, OD is now an established mainstream method of assisted reproduction. Despite the controversy, it has survived as an important adjunct to standard IVF. Indeed, OD has been responsible for over 200,000 births worldwide and its popularity continues to grow. Oocyte donation is truly the gift that keeps on giving, as the children of the children impact upon generations to come.

References

1. Heape W. Preliminary note on transplantation and growth of mammalian ova within a uterine foster-mother. Proc R Soc Lond. 1890;48:457–8.
2. Willett EL, Black WG, Casida LE, Stone WH, Buckner PJ. Successful transplantation of a fertilized bovine ovum. Science. 1951;113(2931):247.
3. Hasler JF. Current status and potential of embryo transfer and reproductive technology in dairy cattle. Journal of dairy science. 1992;75(10):2857–79.

4. Buster JE, Bustillo M, Thorneycroft IH, Simon JA, Boyers SP, Marshall JR, et al. Non-surgical transfer of in vivo fertilised donated ova to five infertile women: report of two pregnancies. Lancet. 1983;2(8343):223–4.
5. Bustillo M, Buster JE, Cohen SW, Hamilton F, Thorneycroft IH, Simon JA, et al. Delivery of a healthy infant following nonsurgical ovum transfer. JAMA. 1984;251(7):889.
6. Trounson A, Leeton J, Besanko M, Wood C, Conti A. Pregnancy established in an infertile patient after transfer of a donated embryo fertilised in vitro. British medical journal. 1983;286(6368):835–8.
7. Lutjen P, Trounson A, Leeton J, Findlay J, Wood C, Renou P. The establishment and maintenance of pregnancy using in vitro fertilization and embryo donation in a patient with primary ovarian failure. Nature. 1984;307(5947):174–5.
8. Sauer MV, Paulson RJ, Lobo RA. A preliminary report on oocyte donation extending reproductive potential to women over 40. The New England journal of medicine. 1990;323(17):1157–60.
9. Sauer MV, Paulson RJ, Lobo RA. Reversing the natural decline in human fertility. An extended clinical trial of oocyte donation to women of advanced reproductive age JAMA: the journal of the American Medical Association. 1992;268(10):1275–9.
10. Van Voorhis BJ, Williamson RA, Gerard JL, Hammitt DG, Syrop CH. Use of oocytes from anonymous, matched, fertile donors for prevention of heritable genetic diseases. Journal of medical genetics. 1992; 29(6):398–9.
11. Klein JU, Sauer MV. Ethics in egg donation: past, present, and future. Seminars in reproductive medicine. 2010;28(4):322–8.
12. Ethics Committee of the American Society for Reproductive Medicine. Financial compensation of oocyte donors. Fertility and sterility. 2007;88(2):305-9. http://www.asrm.org/uploadedFiles/ASRM_Content/News_and_Publications/Ethics_Committee_Reports_and_Statements/financial_incentives.pdf.
13. Covington SN. Gibbons WE; Society for Assisted Reproductive Technology. Fertil Steril. 2007;87(5):1001–4.
14. Mullin CM, Fino ME, Talebian S, Keegan D, Grifo JA, Licciardi F. Comparison of pregnancy outcomes in anonymous shared versus exclusive donor oocyte in vitro fertilization cycles. Fertility and sterility. 2010;93(2):574–8.
15. Sachs P, Covington SN, Toll C, Richter KS, Purcell M, Chang FE. Demographic variables related to successful anonymous oocyte donor recruitment. Fertility and sterility. 2010;93(1):311–3.
16. Levine BA, Klein JU, Charles A, Sauer MV. Routine toxicology screening of oocyte donors. Fertility and Sterility. 2011;96:S6.
17. Practice Committee of American Society for Reproductive Medicine, Practice Committee of Society for Assisted Reproductive Technology. 2008 Guidelines for gamete and embryo donation: a Practice Committee report. Fertility and sterility. 2008;90(5 Suppl):S30-44. http://www.asrm.org/uploadedFiles/ASRM_Content/News_and_Publications/Practice_Guidelines/Guidelines_and_Minimum_Standards/2008_Guidelines_for_gamete(1).pdf.
18. Barton SE, Missmer SA, Ashby RK, Ginsburg ES. Multivariate analysis of the association between oocyte donor characteristics, including basal follicle stimulating hormone (FSH) and age, and IVF cycle outcomes. Fertility and sterility. 2010;94(4):1292–5.
19. Cohen MA, Lindheim SR, Sauer MV. Donor age is paramount to success in oocyte donation. Human reproduction. 1999;14(11):2755–8.
20. Practice Committee of American Society for Reproductive Medicine, Practice Committee of Society for Assisted Reproductive Technology. 2012 Guideline: Mature oocyte cryopreservation. http://www.asrm.org/uploadedFiles/ASRM_Content/News_and_Publications/Practice_Guidelines/Committee_Opinions/Ovarian_tissue_and_oocyte(1).pdf.
21. Karnis MF, Zimon AE, Lalwani SI, Timmreck LS, Klipstein S, Reindollar RH. Risk of death in pregnancy achieved through oocyte donation in patients with Turner syndrome: a national survey. Fertility and sterility. 2003;80(3):498–501.
22. Hofmann GE, Thie J, Scott Jr RT, Navot D. Endometrial thickness is predictive of histologic endometrial maturation in women undergoing hormone replacement for ovum donation. Fertility and sterility. 1996;66(3):380–3.
23. Noyes N, Hampton BS, Berkeley A, Licciardi F, Grifo J, Krey L. Factors useful in predicting the success of oocyte donation: a 3-year retrospective analysis. Fertility and sterility. 2001;76(1):92–7.
24. Jun SH, Hornstein MD. Is there a role for preparatory cycle in ovum donation recipients? Current opinion in obstetrics & gynecology. 2006;18(3):333–7.
25. Glujovsky D, Pesce R, Fiszbajn G, Sueldo C, Hart RJ, Ciapponi A. Endometrial preparation for women undergoing embryo transfer with frozen embryos or embryos derived from donor oocytes. Cochrane database of systematic reviews. 2010(1):CD006359.
26. Prapas N, Prapas Y, Panagiotidis Y, Prapa S, Vanderzwalmen P, Schoysman R, et al. GnRH agonist versus GnRH antagonist in oocyte donation cycles: a prospective randomized study. Human reproduction. 2005;20(6):1516–20.
27. Melo M, Beliver J, Garrido N, Meseguer M, Pellicier A, Remohi J. A prospective, controlled randomized trial comparing three different gonadotropin regimens in oocyte donors: response, in vitro fertilization outcome and analysis of cost minimization. Fertility and Sterility. 2010;94:958–64.
28. Melo MA, Garrido N, Alvarez C, Bellver J, Meseguer M, Pellicer A, et al. Antral follicle count (AFC) can be used in the prediction of ovarian response but cannot predict the oocyte/embryo quality or the in vitro fertilization outcome in an egg donation program. Fertility and sterility. 2009;91(1):148–56.

29. Nakhuda GS, Douglas NC, Thornton MH, Guarnaccia MM, Lobo R, Sauer MV. Anti-Mullerian hormone testing is useful for individualization of stimulation protocols in oocyte donors. Reproductive biomedicine online. 2010;20(1):42–7.
30. Humaidan P, Kol S, Papanikolaou EG, Copenhagen GN. Rhatwg. GnRH agonist for triggering of final oocyte maturation: time for a change of practice? Human reproduction update. 2011;17(4):510–24.
31. Yaron Y, Amit A, Mani A, Yovel I, Kogosowski A, Peyser MR, et al. Uterine preparation with estrogen for oocyte donation: assessing the effect of treatment duration on pregnancy rates. Fertility and sterility. 1995;63(6):1284–6.
32. Miles RA, Paulson RJ, Lobo RA, Press MF, Dahmoush L, Sauer MV. Pharmacokinetics and endometrial tissue levels of progesterone after administration by intramuscular and vaginal routes: a comparative study. Fertility and sterility. 1994;62(3):485–90.
33. Navot D, Scott RT, Droesch K, Veeck LL, Liu HC, Rosenwaks Z. The window of embryo transfer and the efficiency of human conception in vitro. Fertility and sterility. 1991;55(1):114–8.
34. Schoolcraft WB, Gardner DK. Blastocyst culture and transfer increases the efficiency of oocyte donation. Fertility and sterility. 2000;74(3):482–6.
35. Dessolle L, Darai E, Cornet D, Rouzier R, Coutant C, Mandelbaum J, et al. Determinants of pregnancy rate in the donor oocyte model: a multivariate analysis of 450 frozen-thawed embryo transfers. Human reproduction. 2009;24(12):3082–9.
36. Soares SR, Velasco JA, Fernandez M, Bosch E, Remohi J, Pellicer A, et al. Clinical factors affecting endometrial receptiveness in oocyte donation cycles. Fertility and sterility. 2008;89(3):491–501.
37. Sauer MV, Kavic SM. Oocyte and embryo donation 2006: reviewing two decades of innovation and controversy. Reproductive biomedicine online. 2006; 12(2):153–62.
38. Paulson RJ, Hatch IE, Lobo RA, Sauer MV. Cumulative conception and live birth rates after oocyte donation: implications regarding endometrial receptivity. Human reproduction. 1997;12(4):835–9.
39. Toner JP, Grainger DA, Frazier LM. Clinical outcomes amongst recipients of donated eggs: an analysis of the US national experience, 1996–1998. Fertility and sterility. 2002;78(5):1038–45.
40. Stern JE, Brown MB, Luke B, Wantman E, Lederman A, Missmer SA, et al. Calculating cumulative live-birth rates from linked cycles of assisted reproductive technology (ART): data from the Massachusetts SART CORS. Fertility and sterility. 2010;94(4): 1334–40.
41. Gu L, Zhang H, Yin L, Bu Z, Zhu G. Effect of male age on the outcome of in vitro fertilization: oocyte donation as a model. Journal of assisted reproduction and genetics. 2012;29(4):331–4.
42. Luna M, Finkler E, Barritt J, Bar-Chama N, Sandler B, Copperman AB, et al. Paternal age and assisted reproductive technology outcome in ovum recipients. Fertility and sterility. 2009;92(5):1772–5.
43. Whitcomb BW, Turzanski-Fortner R, Richter KS, Kipersztok S, Stillman RJ, Levy MJ, et al. Contribution of male age to outcomes in assisted reproductive technologies. Fertility and sterility. 2011;95(1):147–51.
44. Keegan DA, Krey LC, Chang HC, Noyes N. Increased risk of pregnancy-induced hypertension in young recipients of donated oocytes. Fertility and sterility. 2007;87(4):776–81.
45. Krieg SA, Henne MB, Westphal LM. Obstetric outcomes in donor oocyte pregnancies compared with advanced maternal age in in vitro fertilization pregnancies. Fertility and sterility. 2008;90(1):65–70.
46. Le Ray C, Scherier S, Anselem O, Marszalek A, Tsatsaris V, Cabrol D, et al. Association between oocyte donation and maternal and perinatal outcomes in women aged 43 years or older. Human reproduction. 2012;27(3):896–901.
47. Murray C, MacCallum F, Golombok S. Egg donation parents and their children: follow-up at age 12 years. Fertility and sterility. 2006;85(3):610–8.
48. Sauer MV. Defining the incidence of serious complications experienced by oocyte donors: a review of 1000 cases. American journal of obstetrics and gynecology. 2001;184(3):277–8.
49. Bodri D, Guillen JJ, Polo A, Trullenque M, Esteve C, Coll O. Complications related to ovarian stimulation and oocyte retrieval in 4052 oocyte donor cycles. Reproductive biomedicine online. 2008;17(2): 237–43.
50. Bukulmez O, Li Q, Carr BR, Leader B, Doody KM, Doody KJ. Repetitive oocyte donation does not decrease serum anti-Mullerian hormone levels. Fertility and sterility. 2010;94(3):905–12.
51. Kramer W, Schneider J, Schultz N. US oocyte donors: a retrospective study of medical and psychosocial issues. Human reproduction. 2009;24(12):3144–9.
52. Stoop D, Vercammen L, Polyzos NP, de Vos M, Nekkebroeck J, Devroey P. Effect of ovarian stimulation and oocyte retrieval on reproductive outcome in oocyte donors. Fertility and sterility. 2012;97(6): 1328–30.
53. Ethics Committee of the American Society for Reproductive Medicine. Oocyte Donation to Postmenopausal Women. Fertil Steril 2004. http://www.asrm.org/uploadedFiles/ASRM_Content/News_and_Publications/Ethics_Committee_Reports_and_Statements/postmeno.pdf.
54. Soderstrom-Anttila V, Salevaara M, Suikkari AM. Increasing openness in oocyte donation families regarding disclosure over 15 years. Human reproduction. 2010;25(10):2535–42.
55. Cobo A, Meseguer M, Remohi J, Pellicer A. Use of cryo-banked oocytes in an ovum donation programme: a prospective, randomized, controlled, clinical trial. Human reproduction. 2010;25(9):2239–46.
56. Noggle S, Fung HL, Gore A, Martinez H, Satriani KC, Prosser R, et al. Human oocytes reprogram somatic cells to a pluripotent state. Nature. 2011; 478(7367):70–5.

11 Gestational Carrier

Pravin Patel and Manish Banker

Introduction

Gestational carrier is defined as a treatment in which embryos generated from the gametes of a "commissioning couple" or "intended parents" or "genetic parents" are transferred into the uterus of a woman who is contracted to act as a host for these embryos. The host or "carrier" does not contribute any genetic material to the child born through this process. In India, the term surrogate is used in lieu of carrier, and therefore also pertains to situations in which a woman is carrying a pregnancy for another, with no genetic connection to the child herself.

In contrast to gestational carrier, in traditional surrogacy, also called "Natural Surrogacy" or "Partial Surrogacy," the surrogate is inseminated with semen of the husband of the "commissioning couple." The child born through this will therefore be the biological offspring of the surrogate. Examples of surrogacy date back to the time of the Old Testament and are also mentioned in Hindu mythology. The Bible describes the story of Abraham, who fathered a child through his maid Hagar, on his wife Sarah's request [1]. There is also the story of Jacob and one of his two wives, Rachel, who was unable to bear a child, and thus had her maid Bilhah act as a surrogate for her. The maid gave birth to two sons: Dan and Naphtali [2]. According to Hindu Mythology, the Bhagwad Purana mentions the transfer of the fetus from the womb of Devaki to Rohini (Vasudev's second wife) to prevent the child from being killed by Kans.

These early examples of surrogacy illustrate the need even many hundreds of years ago to assist infertile couples to have children. Today, however, use of a woman's own eggs (typically the intended mother) to create an embryo(s) that is then transferred to the uterus of a gestational carrier is more common. Aside from enabling such couples to have their own biological children, contracting a woman as a traditional surrogate (i.e., to be both the genetic and gestational mother), is tricky legally as in many countries and, indeed, in some states in the USA, she may retain custody of a child if she wishes. Such treatment does not require in vitro fertilization and is therefore outside the scope of this book.

Gestational carrier (GC) is associated with complex medical, social, ethical, and legal issues, particularly regarding the following circumstances.

1. Cross Border reproductive care, in which case the laws of both countries need to be taken into account, especially with respect to ensuring that the child is able to get back into the parent's home country. This can get further complicated when both partners of the commissioning couple have different nationalities.

P. Patel, M.D. • M. Banker, M.D. (✉)
Department of Endoscopy, Nova IVI Fertility and Pulse Women's Hospital, 108, Swastik Society, Navrangpura, Ahmedabad, Gujarat 380009, India
e-mail: drpravinpatel@pulse-hospital.com; drbanker@pulse-hospital.com

E.S. Ginsburg and C. Racowsky (eds.), *In Vitro Fertilization: A Comprehensive Guide*,
DOI 10.1007/978-1-4419-9848-4_11, © Springer Science+Business Media New York 2012

2. Use of donor gametes along with a GC as this leads to separation of the "parent" into three separate entities—the genetic parent, the gestational parent/mother, and the social parent [3].
3. Use of a GC by single parents and same sex couples.

This chapter will discuss these issues in the context of using a woman commissioned to carry the pregnancy and who has no genetic relationship to the child. That is, the focus will be exclusively on GC cycles.

Indications for Gestational Carrier

GC for Women with an Absent or Abnormal Uterus, or Medical Contraindications for Pregnancy

A GC option is offered to women who either cannot or are not medically fit to carry a pregnancy. In practice, GC cycles account for less than 1% of IVF cases internationally [4]. Table 11.1 lists indications for using a GC. The majority of GC cycles occur when the intended female parent has ovaries and is a genetic parent. Specific medical indications for use of either both an egg donor and a GC are much less common. For example, women undergoing pelvic irradiation as part of cancer treatment often have neither a functional uterus nor ovarian function. Another increasingly common scenario is that of a woman of advanced reproductive age who has both decreased ovarian reserve and a higher risk of medical complications of pregnancy; in this case, she contracts with both an oocyte donor and a GC. It can be difficult to know when to recommend use of a GC to women with a uterine factor for infertility, such as recurrent fibroids or partially treated Asherman's syndrome.

Table 11.1 Indications for use of gestational carrier

Indication
Women with ovaries
Congenital absence of uterus • i.e., Mayer Rokitansky Kuster Hauser Syndrome
Surgical absence of uterus • Hysterectomy, e.g., fibroids, cancer, postpartum hemorrhage
Recurrent pregnancy loss
Repeated IVF failure with good embryo quality • ≥6 cycles
Medical contraindication for pregnancy • e.g., Renal insufficiency, significant heart disease
Single sex couples
Male couples • May chose to use an egg donor and gestational carrier
Female couples • May chose to share pregnancy by having embryos created from the eggs of one partner carried by the other
Single men
• May chose traditional surrogacy, or hire both an egg donor and a gestational carrier
Social indications (controversial)
• Concern about disruption of lifestyle by pregnancy
Poor endometrial development
Intrauterine pathology • Adhesions, Asherman's syndrome Infections • Tuberculosis

GC for Single Parents or Same Sex Couples

One of the issues concerning surrogacy is whether it is acceptable only for heterosexual couples or whether it can be provided to gay couples as well. The Ethics Committee Report of ASRM in 2009 [5] carefully considered "the changing nature of reproduction and the family." This committee concluded that there is no sound basis for denying to single persons and gay couples the same rights to reproduce shared by other individuals. The committee further concluded that it is a matter of ethical duty to treat every person with equal respect, and that this requires fertility programs to treat single persons and gay couples equally with married couples in determining which services to provide. Indeed, in some countries, including the USA, the law allows for use of a GC by same sex couples or single parents using anonymous gamete donors.

GC with Embryo Donation

Use of a GC with embryo donation is analogous to adoption, as the commissioning couple neither contributes any genetic material nor carries the pregnancy [6]. Theoretically, a rare possibility for embryo donation with GC is in case of severe genetic defects in both parents. However, there is no legal precedence for this in India yet, and legal advice is recommended prior to undertaking this in the USA as well, as legal parentage of the future child must be established prior to undertaking the embryo donation and surrogacy.

The Gestational Surrogacy Process

There are several critical steps involved in undertaking pregnancy with a GC; these steps are outlined in the following sections.

Legal Compliance

Ensuring that proper legal advice is obtained prior to embarking on the GC arrangement is of utmost importance as GC, while legal in some countries, or regions of some countries, is illegal in others. In the USA, the state in which the GC delivers is critical, as the laws of that state determine the legal parentage of the child born.

When a couple wishes to use an international GC, the nationality of both partners (the husband and wife can be of different nationalities), as well as the nationality of the carrier, need to be taken into account. Proper legal advice should be sought and if required, advice from the appropriate government agency obtained. Some countries require the commissioning couple to sign a declaration/undertaking to this effect (Appendix 1). This is to ensure that no legal problem arises after a child is born from a GC and that the child is issued a passport and citizenship by the country of the commissioning couple.

According to International Federation of Fertility Societies (IFFS) surveillance, of the total 105 countries to which the questionnaires on GC were sent, only 71 (68%) responded. Of those countries which did not respond, most do not perform GC cycles for religious reasons. Out of the 71 responding countries, 15 (21%) allow GC by statute, 13 (23%) countries have guidelines, 30 (42%) do not allow it, and 10 countries (14%) had no comment on GC at all. In 17 of the 71 countries (24%), GC is practiced, but 9 of these countries have no statutes or guidelines [4]. Most countries that follow Islam do not allow use of GCs.

In India, each center where GC cycles are performed must be registered and must follow guidelines laid out by the Indian Council for Medical Research [ICMR]. General considerations include the following [7].

- GC by assisted conception should normally be considered only for patients for whom it would be physically or medically impossible to carry a baby to term.
- Payments to carriers should cover all genuine expenses associated with the pregnancy. Documentary evidence of the financial arrangement for the GC cycle must be available. An "ART Bank," a separate legal entity operating independently of the ART clinic, should handle the monetary aspects; the ART center should not be involved in this. [In the USA, this is often managed by GC agencies]. The reason for this is to avoid any conflict of interest, so that the ART center does not have a vested interest regarding which carrier the intended parents employ.
- In India, advertisements regarding gestational carrier as an option should not be made by the ART clinic. The responsibility of finding a GC, through advertisement or otherwise, should rest with the couple, or an ART bank.

Legal Steps of Gestational Carrier

The Agreement

The contract, which must be vetted by the intended parent's attorney as well as the attorney representing the GC must outline the rights and duties of the GC. Typically, all expenses incurred for care and treatment by the carrier are to be borne by the commissioning couple. The carrier has a right to receive monetary compensation for agreeing to act as a carrier, apart from the financial

Table 11.2 Logistics of gestational carrier cycle in India

Agreements	Brief description of the document
Financial contract between patient and GC	Financial contract between the commissioning couple and the GC; payment schedule, total reimbursement, and prorating
Agreement between commissioning couple and GC	Details about the purpose, methods, medical risks, maintenance of pregnancy, abortion/death, custody, legal processes, termination and breach of agreement, confidentiality
Appointment of local guardian	Explanation regarding the local guardian's responsibilities
Agreement of surrogacy between GC and the IVF clinic	Medical and social information regarding intended parent(s), hospital of delivery, IVF process, process of handing over of child at birth, right to amniocentesis, selective reduction, pregnancy termination, testing for STDs, and nondisclosure of identity

agreement. She should be assured that confidentiality about specifics of the procedure will be maintained. She understands that it is her duty to relinquish all parental rights of the child; she must register in a hospital under her own name; and she must declare that she is a GC. She must undergo standard prenatal care, and she cannot engage in any act that would cause harm to the child during pregnancy. In case of use of donor eggs, the GC cannot act as a donor for the same couple.

If the surrogate is married, consent of her spouse is required. This latter requirement is important, because if the pregnancy requires bed rest, her husband will have to be the primary caregiver for their children.

Issues related to medical management of the pregnancy must be outlined in detail in the legal agreement. For example, in the USA, performance of amniocentesis if indicated, pregnancy termination, selective reduction, and other details about possible occurrences that would require decision making during pregnancy are discussed by the commissioning couple and the GC and agreed to prior to beginning treatment.

The rights of a child born from a GC are controversial and not well defined. In India, a child born through ART has a right to seek information about his/her GC on reaching 18 years, excluding her personal identity. The identity of the GC can only be released in cases of life threatening medical conditions which may require physical testing [8].

Signing Consent Forms

The legal documents that need to be signed depend on the country where the procedure is to be carried out. Some of these may have to be signed in the presence of a Legal Representative of the government or a notary public (Table 11.2).

Financial Arrangements

Payment of the GC continues to be a debatable issue [9, 10]. Many countries, such as the UK, ban paying a GC, which has crippled the ability of women to employ a GC because there are not enough women willing to become uncompensated GCs. In these countries, carriers tend to be relatives or friends of the commissioning couple, willing to go through treatment for their family member or friend and are only allowed to receive "reasonable expenses." Other countries do allow payment to GCs, as in India, which allows easy availability of women as GCs. In India, such a treatment option is often described as "commercial surrogacy." Laws vary tremendously in other countries with state by state variation common in the USA.

The contract with a GC prorates the reimbursement schedule. For example, in case of a miscarriage, payment is to be made until the stage of the pregnancy at which the GC miscarried. If, however, the GC chooses to terminate the pregnancy, she forfeits all further payment, and returns the amount she has already received. Reimbursement is typically also prorated for effort and risk, with payments higher for twin pregnancies or deliveries by cesarian section.

Record Keeping

Records related to the entire GC process must be kept, including those created at the initial screenings and blood testing, as well as those documenting all results, financial and other contracts, counseling, IVF treatment details, number of embryo transfers the GC has undergone along with their outcomes. The duration of time for which the records need to be maintained and the place where they should be maintained (i.e., whether at the ART clinic or a regulatory data base) are dictated by the law/guidelines of the country.

Selection of the Gestational Carrier

As there are general medical and psychological criteria which make a woman a desirable GC, both medical screening and counseling are mandatory [7].

Medical Screening

All information should be collected on a standard screening form such as that in Appendix 2.

- A surrogate mother should ideally not be less than 21 or more than 35 years of age, although in the USA an age cutoff of 40 is common.
- Her obstetric history should have no more than 4 prior births including those of her own children, though in India 5 prior births is the standard cutoff. (The reason for the limitation in the number of prior births is to avoid risks of grand multiparity such as postpartum hemorrhage). The GC may be a relative or friend or recruited person, but must meet the same eligibility criteria regardless.
- It is likely wise to have a body mass index cut off as well; overweight and underweight women are known to have higher miscarriage rates and lower pregnancy rates in the context of IVF. At Brigham & Women's Hospital in Boston, for example, the GC must have a BMI less than 35.

Counseling

Initially, of course the potential GC must be educated about the medical interventions required to carry a pregnancy, including use of medications such as oral contraceptives, GnRH agonists, estrogen, and progesterone, and the route of delivery of each, as well as the likely number of visits and how long a treatment cycle is likely to take.

Assessment of the GC also includes evaluation by a skilled social worker or psychologist of the GC's motives for wanting to become a carrier and to ensure that no coercion exists, particularly if she is a friend or family member. A formal assessment of mental health to exclude psychiatric illness and to determine suitability is important. In addition, determination of family support during the pregnancy, including any societal and religious implications, is critical. The possible need for interventions such as D&E, amniocentesis, fetal reduction, bed rest, hospitalization, abstinence from intercourse during the cycle, need for leave from work are all critical. Discussion about whether the GC plans to remain in touch with the commissioning couple and the child is also important before the process begins.

Many programs have the GC (and husband, if she is married) meet the intended parent(s) to ensure that expectations are understood for all those concerned.

Screening of the Intended Parents

Medical Screening

In the USA, FDA regulations have been established to protect the GC against transmission of potentially sexually or blood transmitted diseases

Table 11.3 Required screening for genetic parents in gestational carrier cycles in the USA

Required tests	Oocyte donor (within 30 days of oocyte retrieval)	Sperm donor (within 7 days of oocyte retrieval)
Physical exam	Yes	Yes
HIV	Yes	Yes
Hepatitis B core antibody	Yes	Yes
Hepatitis B surface antigen	Yes	Yes
Hepatitis B surface antibody	Yes	Yes
Hepatitis C antibody	Yes	Yes
Rapid Plasma Reagin (syphilis)	Yes	Yes
CMV IgG and IgM	Yes	Yes
Rubella Virus IgG	Yes	No
HTLV I and II	No	Yes
Recommended tests		
Blood Type and Antibody screen	Yes	Yes

from the intended parents, similar to the screening required for ovum donors (Table 11.3). As is the case with use of fresh donor oocytes, the genetic oocyte donor must be screened within 30 days of the oocyte retrieval, and the male partner within 7 days; screening must include a physical exam which includes documentation of piercings, tattoos, and any signs of potentially sexually transmitted diseases.

If one of the intended parents tests positive, but the test is likely a false positive, or unlikely to cause infection in the carrier (e.g., positive hepatitis core antibody screen with negative hepatitis surface antigen, and no detectable virus on RNA screening) it is allowable for the GC to sign a waiver and agree to undergo embryo transfer. ASRM guidelines also suggest freezing and quarantine of embryos for 6 months prior to embryo transfer, though this is rarely done in practice due to the currently lower pregnancy rates associated with the use of cryopreserved embryos [11]. Performance of the tests is, however, required and programs performing donor oocytes or GC cycles in the USA are audited to ensure compliance. Extensive information on regulations is available online and US providers must be familiar with and adhere to them. The website, http://www.fda.gov/biologicsbloodvaccines/guidancecomplianceregulatoryinformation/guidances/tissue/ucm073964.htm, includes a downloadable PDF file.

Counseling

Counseling for the intended parent(s) must cover many factors [12, 13] including a discussion of the reasons for requiring surrogacy, and exploration of alternative treatments, such as adoption. As with other ART treatments, using a GC neither guarantees a live birth nor a medically healthy child. Discussion of the possibility of failed cycles or pregnancy losses is important. Parental expectations must therefore be explored. A mental health assessment by a trained social worker or psychologist is critical in this discussion. Religious and societal implications of undergoing this procedure for the couple or individual, a discussion on how to reveal the news to family members and later to the child, and a discussion of expectations as to the future relationship with the GC are critical. In this area, striking a balance between the patient's need to oversee every aspect of the pregnancy and the carrier's right to privacy is critical to a good experience, with expectations set in advance as much as possible.

Treatment Procedure

Paradigms

There are several ways in which a gestational carrier cycle may be accomplished, as the commissioning couple and/or the carrier may be living in different

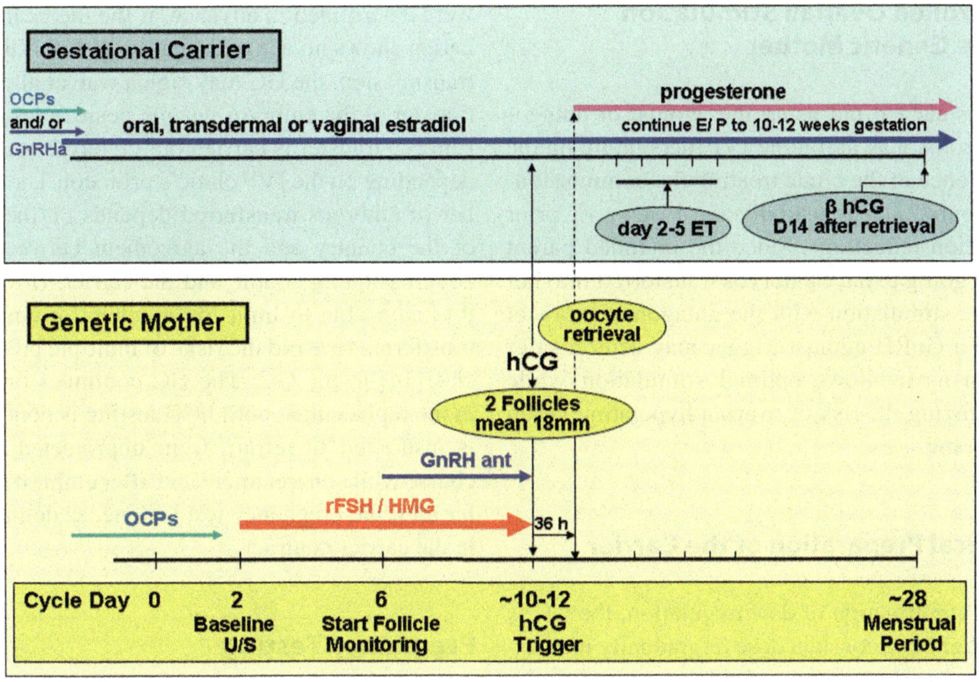

Fig. 11.1 Schematic diagram of synchronization and medical treatment in gestational carrier cycle

cities or countries than where the IVF clinic is located. These paradigms include the following.

1. The genetic/commissioning parent (s) can start stimulation with her own gynecologist and only come for egg retrieval to the ART clinic. This reduces the amount of time and number of visits, but control over the ovarian stimulation may not be optimal.
2. Shipping of frozen embryos: the patient can undergo the entire procedure at her own ART clinic with embryos cryopreserved and the frozen embryos then shipped to the ART clinic where the GC is to undergo embryo transfer. This is especially useful in cases of cross border treatments, so that the intended parent does not require extended stay in a foreign city/country and can have the entire procedure in familiar environment. In such cross border cases the intended parent may only be present in the GC's country for a few days. Utilization of frozen embryos allows for flexibility for timing the transfer so that they can be present at the time of transfer.
3. The entire treatment can occur at the ART clinic which manages both the ovulation induction of the genetic mother, preparation of the GC, and embryo transfer.

Synchronization of Cycles

After the GC has been selected and contracts signed, her cycle is synchronized with that of the genetic mother (who can be the intended parent or an egg donor). This is done using oral contraceptive pills with or without GnRH analogues. Depending on the date of their expected menses either one or both are started on oral contraceptive pills. This helps to regulate the cycle and hence program the cycles to match each other. Downregulation of the GC is then done with a GnRH analogue. The cycles are programmed in such a way that the surrogate is ready for endometrial preparation before stimulation of the genetic mother is started; this is the same process that is performed in ovum donation cycles (Fig. 11.1).

Controlled Ovarian Stimulation of the Genetic Mother

This is carried out using the agonist or antagonist protocol as in routine IVF, depending on the preference of the clinic treating the commissioning couple and potentially the history of prior ovulation inductions. Since the intended parent is not going to have embryos transferred into her uterus, stimulation with the antagonist protocol using a GnRH-agonist trigger may offer a safer option as it allows optimal stimulation while minimizing the risk of ovarian hyperstimulation syndrome.

Medical Preparation of the Carrier

After confirmation of downregulation, the GC is put on either a constant dose or gradually increasing doses of estradiol valerate or estradiol for endometrial preparation to achieve optimal endometrial thickness at the time of egg retrieval. This can be administered orally, vaginally, or by transdermal patches. Progesterone is begun the day of egg retrieval of the genetic mother. Programs typically use the same uterine preparation for the GC as they do for women undergoing cryopreservation embryo transfer.

Oocyte Retrieval and Embryo Transfer

Egg retrieval is done transvaginally and the eggs inseminated with the intended male parent's prepared semen sample, or with ICSI if indicated by semen parameters. In some countries, it is mandatory to freeze the embryos for a quarantine period of 6 months and during this period the couple is again tested for HIV virus and embryos transferred to the carrier if they are seronegative [14]. In other countries, a fresh transfer is allowed. In the USA, if a fresh embryo transfer is performed, the genetic mother must have STD testing performed within 30 days of embryo transfer by FDA approved testing, and the genetic father must have such testing performed within 7 days, as noted previously. In cases of positive tests that were determined in advance, if the medical evaluation shows no active disease or risk for disease transmission, the GC may sign a waiver allowing transfer of the embryos despite positive testing. Embryo transfer is carried out on day 2 or 3 or 5 depending on the IVF clinic's protocol. The number of embryos transferred depends on the laws of the country and the agreement between the commissioning couple and the carrier. However, it is advisable to limit the numbers of embryos transferred to avoid the risks of multiple pregnancies [14] to the GC. The GC continues on hormone replacement until hCG testing is done. She is instructed to refrain from unprotected intercourse while on treatment and after embryo transfer until the pregnancy test is done, as delineated in the carrier contract.

Pregnancy Testing

Serum beta hCG is typically measured 13–15 days after embryo transfer and often repeated in 48 h to document a normal rise. The GC is then scheduled for ultrasonic confirmation of intrauterine pregnancy between 5 and 6 weeks gestation, with dating determined by the oocyte retrieval equivalent to a date of ovulation. Ultrasound for cardiac activity confirmation follows 1–2 weeks days after the first scan.

Care During Pregnancy

Care of the Carrier

If the IVF clinic has an obstetric unit, the GC can obtain prenatal care with the clinic itself. If not, she can obtain care from the obstetrician of her choice, provided she registers in her own name, and informs the treating obstetrician of having undergone surrogacy.

The GC prenatal care is covered by the commissioning couple or health insurance in some states in the USA. However the intended parent(s) must be prepared to cover all the expenses related to the pregnancy and its management. The carrier contract should make it clear that the carrier must attend regular obstetrical check ups and must follow the obstetrician's advice.

If the commissioning couple does not live in the same country as the carrier, at least in some countries, they must appoint a local guardian in the same city who will take responsibility of the carrier and the unborn child in their absence. The local guardian is especially required in cases of premature delivery occurring in the absence of the commissioning couple, a complication such as miscarriage or ectopic pregnancy requiring surgical intervention, a medical condition requiring hospitalization of the surrogate, or in event of death of the genetic parents before delivery.

In cases of patients with no local contacts, in some countries, e.g., India, the hospital can appoint a guardian for them.

In a few countries, GCs live in carrier houses where their health and nutrition can be closely monitored. Most prefer to allow the carriers to stay in their own homes with their own children and families to avoid homesickness and to avoid disturbing their domestic environment. Medical care is standard for GCs pregnant after transfer. Luteal support with estradiol and progesterone, started before embryo transfer, are continued till 10–12 weeks of pregnancy. The GC is expected to undergo screening for genetic abnormalities as indicated, and tests are performed keeping in mind the age of the genetic mother and not the carrier. Regular updates are given to the genetic parents, typically by the GC or the obstetrician or IVF clinic if it is providing prenatal care. The genetic parents can be present at each hospital visit if they wish. Many intended parents also are present inside the delivery room at the time of the birth of the baby.

The timing and mode of delivery is essentially an obstetric decision, but many commissioning couples request a planned cesarean section at term. This is often due to the feeling that it will avoid emergency child birth and also allows the genetic parents to be present at the time of birth. However, this is a highly controversial and debatable issue.

After delivery it should be made clear that the child will be handed over immediately to the intended parents, and this is included in the legal agreement. In case of absence of the commissioning parents at the time of the birth, the baby is handed to the local guardian. Breast feeding by the GC is not recommended to avoid bonding of the carrier with the baby. After delivery, the GC undergoes standard postnatal follow-up until 6 weeks postdelivery; lactation suppression is advised.

In the case of fetal anomalies, the GC may have the right to terminate the pregnancy if she is unwilling to carry an anomalous baby. It is critical that this be detailed in the GC contract. The commissioning couple can also request for termination of pregnancy on the obstetrician's advice.

Obstetric complications can arise as in any pregnancy. If more than one embryo is transferred into the GC multiple pregnancy may occur, along with an increased risk of complications. These include pregnancy induced hypertension, preterm delivery, postpartum hemorrhage, etc. In case of any medical complications that pose a risk to the health of the GC, pregnancy can be terminated on the advice of the obstetrician, irrespective of the consent of the genetic parents.

Social Complexities

These include occurrences such as the GC changing her mind and requesting pregnancy termination, the GC refusing to give up the child, or the commissioning couples refusing to accept an abnormal child. Proper counseling of the carrier and the commissioning couple before and during the treatment and a detailed contract helps reduce these risks. Psychological effects [15, 16] in the GC that can also complicate the situation include the GC bonding with the child, or having discomfort and feelings of stigma if others find out about the carrier arrangement. In the intended parent, concerns include lack of emotional attachment to the child, guilt about not being able to carry the child herself, and strain in the husband–wife or partner–partner relationship. Proper counseling before and during treatment can minimize all these issues.

The status of the child is determined by the law of the country where surrogacy is carried out

[8, 14]. The goal is that the child born through the process of GC, whether to a married couple, unmarried couple, or single person, be considered by law to be the legitimate child of the commissioning individuals, with the same legal rights as a child born through intercourse. As stated previously, it is critical that careful legal documentation and contracts are written to ensure no confusion about parentage when the child is born.

The law of the country where the delivery occurs governs the process for issuance of the birth certificate. The names of both the genetic parents and the carrier may be mentioned, though anonymous egg donor names are not included [8]. In India after the birth of the child, the hospital issues a certificate to the Birth and Deaths Registry office. This will only have the names of the genetic parents without mention of the GC process or name of the GC indicated, although it will state "anonymous donor eggs/sperm" in cases of donor gamete. In the USA, the law of the state in which the GC delivers dictates the names present on the birth certificate.

Other Important Issues

DNA Fingerprinting

DNA fingerprinting may be used to remove any doubt that the genetic parents may have about the child being genetically their own, and not the carrier's or her husband's. This is also mandatory in some countries, especially when the GC resides and delivers in a foreign country.

Payment to the Carrier

Payment to be made to the carrier is agreed upon in the contract between the commissioning couple and the carrier. The manner in which this is to be paid varies from country to country. The amount may have to be paid in one or multiple installments. In any case, the entire amount has to be paid before or at the time of handing over the child.

Insurance

Some countries, including the USA, have a provision for insurance for the carriers to protect them in case of any adverse events. Part of the payment that is made for antenatal care of the carrier is used as premium for additional medical and life insurance of the carrier, in case of a medical emergency requiring hospitalization, or in case of death of the surrogate during pregnancy or delivery.

Right to Terminate the Pregnancy

This is a controversial issue and is also governed by the laws of the country in relation to abortion [6, 17]. Where abortion is legal, the carrier has the right to terminate the pregnancy at any time (within the legal limit). If the termination is done with the understanding and consent of all parties, the carrier is entitled to the payment corresponding to her period of gestation at the time of termination. If however, she chooses to terminate at her own will, she is obligated to return all payments and expenses incurred by the genetic parents. Although termination is acceptable in the legal sense, it has to be impressed upon the carrier that the psychological effects of the loss of this much-awaited pregnancy could be disastrous for the genetic parents. To avoid such situations, psychological counseling of the carrier is essential. If there is indication that she is unwilling or uncertain about carrying the pregnancy, she should not be recruited as a carrier.

Selective Termination

In case of a triplet or higher order pregnancy, the genetic parents have a right to ask for selective reduction of one or more fetuses, subject to the provisions of the law. In India, the carrier is obligated to undergo the procedure regardless of her wishes as long as it is agreed upon by the obstetrician and does not endanger the life of the remaining fetuses. In the USA, the GC has the right to refuse procedures, however standard

GC contracts include selective termination in the list of eventualities that must be agreed on prior to the GC cycle taking place. Clearly transfer of fewer embryos will reduce the need for reduction.

Expected Pregnancy Rates and Outcomes

The earliest reports of GC outcomes were reported in the mid to late 1980s [18, 19]. These early reports indicated clinical pregnancy rates of 18%, in cycles utilizing GCs. Although there were increasing numbers of published series in the 1990s and 2000s (see below), the data on the delivery rates, course of pregnancy, and the impact of pregnancy on the GC herself remain scanty.

The first GC pregnancy and delivery was undertaken by Edwards and Steptoe [20] in 1989, at Bourne hall. Since then, other case series have been reported with varying delivery rates per cycle. For example, a case series published in 2000 listed outcomes of 11 GC cycles in 6 patients with Rokitansky syndrome; the median age was 33 year, mean oocytes retrieved 14.6, mean fertilization rate 69%, and a mean of 6 embryos were frozen per patient. The pregnancy rate was 42.9% per embryo transfer, with the live birth rate per cycle and per transfer 21.4 and 27.3%, respectively. Half of the patients had at least one live birth [21]. A series of 75 couples undergoing 117 GC cycles performed from 1988 to 1999 found that no pregnancies occurred in 26 cycles in women over age 40, but reported a delivery rate of 29% per cycle for the population overall, with approximately 50% of women less than 40 having a delivery [22]. A series of GC cycles from Bourne Hall in Cambridge from 1990 to 1998 included 49 patients (see Table 11.4). Of note, 61 were referred but only 49 were accepted for treatment. On average 10 oocytes were obtained per retrieval, 5.4 embryos frozen and on average 2 embryos were transferred to each carrier. Indications included hysterectomy for cancer or postpartum hemorrhage or menorrhagia, congenital uterine absence, repeated IVF failures, recurrent pregnancy loss, or severe medical illness precluding pregnancy [23]. In another series, a mean pregnancy rate of 17% per cycle was reported for 19 couples (from 60 cycles), reflecting the need for 3 cycles to obtain a delivery [24]. A series of 16 patients with a median age of 40 undergoing GC due to hysterectomy reported that of 22 cycles there were 4 deliveries. Not surprisingly, the likelihood of pregnancy and delivery was higher at younger ages (<37) [25].

Table 11.4 Gestational Surrogate Treatment Outcomes at Bourne Hall 1990–1998

Variable	Outcome
Genetic couples	
No. patients (intended parents)	49
Mean (range) age	32.9 (22–40)
No. total stimulated cycles (range)	80 (1–5)
Gestational surrogates	
No. GS starting treatment	53
No. cycles having embryo transfer	87
No. embryo transfers per GS (mean)	1.6
Pregnancy rates	
No. (%) clinical pregnancies per GS	31/53 (59)
No. (%) delivered/ongoing pregnancies per GS transfer	18/87 (21)
No. (%) delivered/ongoing pregnancies per GS	18/53 (34)
No. (%) clinical pregnancies per genetic couple	31/49 (63)
No (%) delivered/ongoing pregnancies per genetic couple	18/49 (37)

Adapted from Brinsden PR et al. BMJ 2000

In 2011, Gibbons et al. published outcomes on birth weights in GC deliveries compared to those of donor egg and IVF. The mean (±SD) birth weight associated with standard IVF was 3,265±611 g, which was statistically greater ($P<0.002$) than that associated with donor oocyte cycles (3,236±652.7 g) and statistically less ($P<0.009$) than that with GC (3,309±635.4 g) (Fig. 11.2) [26]. The reason for these disparities in birth weight is unknown, but it was postulated that the uterine environment may be the most important determinant of birth weight; this was thought to explain the lower birth weights when infertile women utilizing donor oocytes delivered. An older report from 1992 of GC outcomes highlighted that premature delivery rates are high

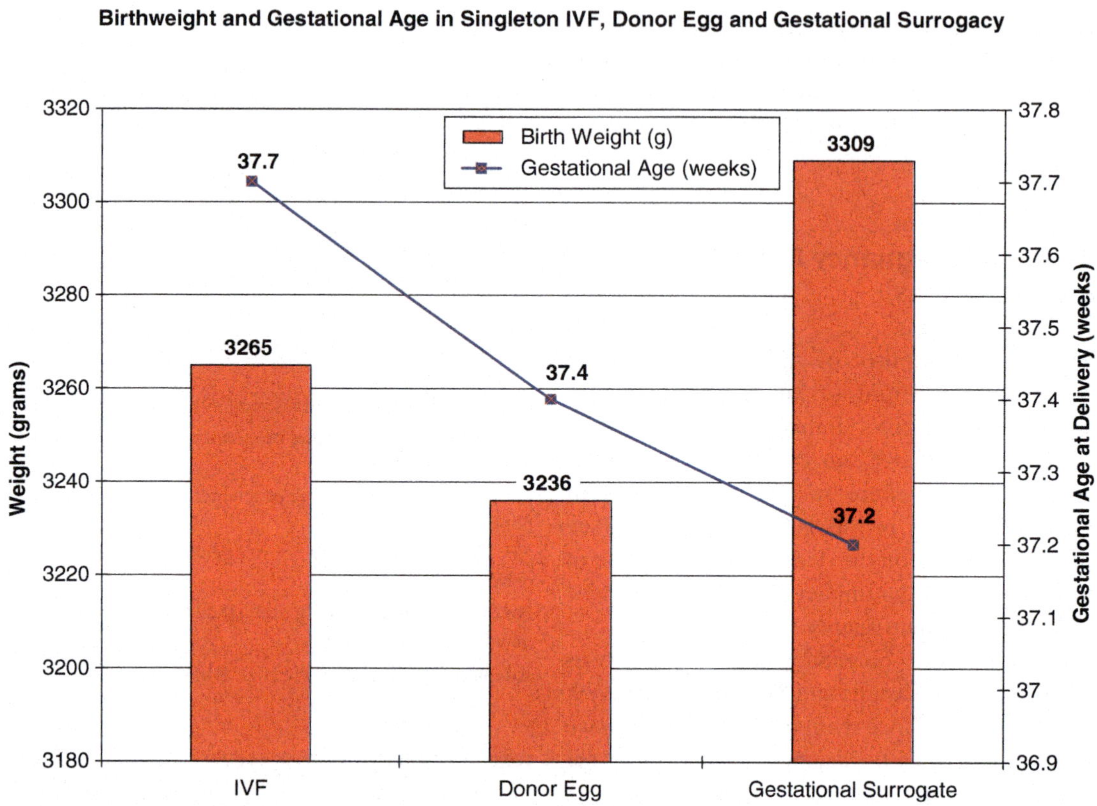

Fig. 11.2 Birth outcomes in gestational carrier, IVF, and oocyte donation cycles

if twins (43%) or triplets (100%) occur, so that controlling the number of embryos transferred is vitally important and should be related to the oocyte age [27].

One of the largest GC series reported on 180 GS cycles in 112 couples performed from 1984 to 1999 [28]. The mean age was 34, mean oocyte number was 11, mean number of embryos 7, and delivery rate per cycle was 15.8%, comparable to the overall pregnancy rate in their program. Couples utilized GCs for a variety of indications. Sixteen cycles were canceled. Of note, 51 patients had hysterectomies and 15 had congenital uterine absence (Mayer-Rokitansky-Kuster-Hauser Syndrome, [MRKH]). Patients in these groups were of similar ages (32 vs. 33), however the MRKH patients had more oocytes (15 vs. 9) as well as more embryos and more embryos cryopreserved. This may suggest that there was vascular compromise to the ovaries though ovarian reserve testing was not available. Not surprisingly, delivery rate per cycle was related to oocyte age: 26–30: 36.7%, 31–35: 11.1%, 36–40: 6%, 41–45: 10.5% [28].

In 2010, the US national summary data reported that the live birth rate per cycle of IVF/ICSI initiated and per transfer for women <35 with uterine factor infertility was 35.3 and 40.6% respectively, compared to 48.7 and 55.9% when a gestational surrogate was used in that age group [29]. These data, however, do not separate causes of uterine factor, so which infertile patients would most benefit from use of a GC is not entirely clear. Overall, it is clear that delivery rates from use of GC vary among programs and are affected by multiple factors, the most important of which is likely the age of the genetic egg donor.

Conclusions

Gestational carrier provides the opportunity for couples to have children in circumstances that would make childbirth impossible or medically dangerous for the mother. However, the process is highly complex, involving many medical, legal, and social issues. It is critical that screening and counseling processes are undertaken in a rigorous manner in order to provide a successful and rewarding experience to all parties involved. Gestational carrier cycles should be undertaken in programs with all the resources necessary to maximize the likelihood of good outcomes.

Appendix 1

APPENDIX 1

SAMPLE UNDERTAKING AS PER INDIAN GUIDELINES

This letter of undertaking is executed by

(1) Name: Mrs.
Address:

(2) Name: Mr.
Address:

In favour of (hospital name and address)

We say that we are the nationals of the.......................("Country") having the nationality of the country. The proof of the same i.e. attested copy of the Passport is attached. Our Nationality ID is .... and .... Hereinafter, in this undertaking, we will be referred to as "Intending Parent(s)"

1. We say that we desire to have a child through Surrogacy Process in India as explained to us by the Doctors at (Hospital name).
2. We say that we want to undergo IVF with Mrs.________________ 's eggs and Mr.________________'s sperm at (Hospital name).
3. We undertake that Surrogacy process is legal and recognized by the government of our Country.
4. We also undertake that the child born out of Surrogacy process on birth will get the nationality of the Country & will be issued a valid passport by the Government of our Country
5. We also have attached a copy of the letter furnished to us by our Consulate/ Government accepting Surrogacy as Legal & Valid under the laws of the country.
6. We are aware that at the time of getting passport for the child(ren) born out of surrogacy, we as the "Intending Parent(s)" may have to prove the genetic relationship with the child(ren) by the DNA fingerprinting or as required by the passport issuing authorities.
7. We undertake to appoint a local guardian in India for the child(ren) born out of surrogacy. We assure that the local guardian will take possession of the child(ren) delivered out of surrogacy in an event of we not able to take possession of the child(ren). The attested identity proof of the guardian along with the undertaking duly signed by us and the guardian shall be submitted to (Hospital name) before the commencement of the treatment.
8. We undertake to purchase medical insurance for the surrogate for the insurance value of (amount) for the entire duration of surrogacy treatment. The insurance policy will expire on the date of handover of the child(ren) to the "Intending Parent(s)"
9. We undertake that the information furnished by us in the declaration is true, correct, valid & unambiguous. We undertake the responsibility of everything we have mentioned in the declaration and the consequences of the same.

Signature of the "Intending Parent(s)"

____
Name of female Parent 1:
Passport Number:

____
Name of Male Parent 2:
Passport Number:

<u>Witness</u>
Name: Date :
Signature: Place:
Address:

Appendix 2

Date of filling the form (except items 20–31)		
Date of filling items 20–31		
Basic information:	History:	Investigations
1. Identification number	12. Obstetric history :	20. Blood group and Rh status
2. Name	a. Number of deliveries	21. Complete blood picture
3. Age/Date of birth	b. Number of abortions	a. Hb
4. Address	c. Other points of note	b. Total RBC count
5. Photograph	13. Menstrual history	c. Total WBC count
6. Tel no.	14. History of use of contraceptives	d. Differential WBC count
7. Marital status	15. Medical history	e. Platelet count
8. Education :	16. Family history	f. Peripheral smear
a. Surrogate	17. Has she acted as surrogate earlier : Yes No	22. Random blood sugar
b. Spouse	If so, how many times did it lead to a successful pregnancy?	23. Blood urea/Serum creatinine
9. Occupation :	18. History of blood transfusion	24. SGPT
a. Surrogate	19. History of substance abuse	25. Routine urine examination
b. Spouse		26. HBsAg status
10. Monthly Income		27. Hepatitis C status
11. Religion		28. HIV status
		29. Hemoglobin A2 (for thallasemia) status
		30. HIV PCR
		a. Surrogate
		b. Spouse
		31. Any other specific test
Footnotes		FEATURES:
(1) To be carried out within 15 days prior to embryo transfer. Test no.30 to be done only if test 28 is negative		32. Height
		33. Weight
(2) Any additional test carried out on the basis of the history and examination of the surrogate OR any test requested by the recipient who shall pay for the additional requested test		Detailed physical examination:
		34. Pulse
		35. Blood pressure
		36. Temperature
To the patient, a copy of this form without items 20–31 filled in, may be provided when asked for. The investigations in items 20–31 may be done when the patient has chosen the surrogate provisionally, subject to the results of tests in items 20–31 being satisfactory		37. Respiratory system
		38. Cardiovascular system
		39. Per abdominal examination
		40. Per speculum examination
		41. Per vaginal examination
Name(s) and signature(s) with date(s) of person(s) filling the form:		42. Trans-vaginal sonography
		43. Other systems

References

1. Old Testament, Book of Genesis *16:2*, KJV.
2. Old Testament, Book of Genesis *30:3*, KJV.
3. Ber R. Theoretical Medicine and Bioethics. Ethical Issues in Gestational Surrogacy. Theor Med Bioeth. 2000;21:153–69.
4. Jones HW, Cooke I, Kempers R, Brinsden P, Saunders D. International Federation of Fertility Societies Surveillance 2010: preface. Fertil Steril. 2010;95: 491–6.
5. Ethics Committee of the American Society for Reproductive Medicine. Access to fertility treatment by gays, lesbians, and unmarried persons. Fertil Steril. 2009;92:1190–3.
6. Shenfield G, Pennings G, Cohen J, Devroey P, de Wert G, Tarlatzis B. ESHRE Task Force on Ethics and Law. Hum Reprod. 2005;20:2705–7.
7. Indian Council of Medical Research. National Guidelines for Accreditation, Supervision and Regulation of ART Clinics in India. Code of practice and ethical considerations and legal issues. New Delhi, India. National Academy of Medical Sciences (India). 2005, 68-69.
8. Indian Council of Medical Research. The Assisted Reproductive Technologies (Regulation) Bill. 2010; 25–29.
9. Cotton K. Surrogacy should pay Br Med J. 2000;320: 928–9.
10. Tieu MM. Altruistic surrogacy: the necessary objectification of surrogate mothers. J Med Ethics. 2009;35:171–5.
11. Practice Guideline, Recommendations for practices using gestational carriers. (https://www.asrm.org/uploadedFiles/ASRM_Content/News_and_Publications/Practice_Guidelines/Committee_Opinions/recommendations_for_practices_utilizing_gestational_carriers_nonmembers.pdf.
12. Boivin J, Appleton TC, Baetens P, Baron J, Bitzer J, Corrigan E, et al. Guidelines for counseling in infertility: outline version. Hum Reprod. 2001;16:1301–4.
13. Van Den Ekker OB. Psychosocial aspects of surrogate motherhood. Hum Reprod Update. 2007;13:53–62.
14. Parliament by the Secretary of State for Health. Donor recruitment, assessment and screening; Surrogacy. Code of Practice for clinics licensed by the Human Fertilisation and Embryology Authority, 8th Edition. London 2011.
15. Jadva V, Murray C, Lycett E, MacCallum F, Golombok S. Surrogacy: the experiences of surrogate mothers. Hum Reprod. 2003;18:2196–204.
16. MacCallum F, Lycett E, Murray C, Jadva V, Golombok S. Surrogacy: the experience of commissioning couples. Hum Reprod. 2003;18:1334–42.
17. Schenker JG. Assisted reproduction practice in Europe: legal and ethical aspects. Hum Reprod. 1997; 3:173–84.
18. Utian WH, Sheean L, Goldfarb JM, Kiwi R. Successful pregnancy after in vitro fertilization and embryo transfer from an infertile woman to a surrogate. N Engl J Med. 1985;313:1351.
19. Utian WH, Goldfarb JM, Kiwi R, et al. Preliminary experience with in vitro fertilization-surrogate gestational pregnancy. Fertil Steril. 1989;52:633.
20. Steptoe P. Surrogacy. Br Med J (Clin Res Edn). 1987;294:1688–9.
21. Beski S, Gorgy A, Venkat G, et al. Gestational surrogacy: a feasible option for patients with Rokitansky syndrome. Hum Reprod. 2000;15:2326.
22. Corson SL, Kelly M, Braverman AM, English ME. Gestational carrier pregnancy. Fertil Steril. 1998;69:670–4.
23. Brinsden PR, Appleton TC, Murray E, et al. Treatment by in vitro fertilisation with surrogacy: experience of one British centre. BMJ. 2000;320:924.
24. Raziel A, Schachter M, Strassburger D, et al. Eight years' experience with an IVF surrogate gestational pregnancy programme. Reprod Biomed Online. 2005;11:254.
25. Meniru GI, Craft I. Assisted conception options for patients with good-prognosis cervical cancer. Lancet. 1997;349:542.
26. Gibbons WE, Cedars M, Ness RB. Society for Assisted Reproductive Technologies Writing Group. Toward understanding obstetrical outcome in advanced assisted reproduction: varying sperm, oocyte, and uterine source and diagnosis. Fertil Steril. 2011;95:1645.
27. Parkinson J, Tran C, Tan T, Nelson J, Batzofin J, Serafini P. Perinatal outcome after in-vitro fertilization-surrogacy. Hum Reprod. 1999;14(3):671–6.
28. Goldfarb JM, Austin C, Peskin B, et al. Fifteen years experience with an in-vitro fertilization surrogate gestational pregnancy programme. Hum Reprod. 2000;15:1075.
29. https://www.sartcorsonline.com/rptCSR_PublicMultYear.aspx?ClinicPKID=0.

12 Adjunctive Treatments in ART

Eric Surrey

Beyond the critical issues of ovarian hyperstimulation, oocyte retrieval, in vitro fertilization, and embryo transfer, a variety of approaches have been proposed to enhance outcomes from the assisted reproductive technologies. Many have become routine components in the practices of many centers. However, adequate data supporting their use have often been sparse at best. In this chapter, we shall investigate four commonly employed adjunctive treatments and critically assess both the logic behind and the evidence supporting their use. Two have been theoretically employed to aid the poor responder: dehydroepiandrosterone (DHEA) and growth hormone. Two have been theoretically employed to enhance implantation: low dose aspirin and acupuncture (Table 12.1).

Table 12.1 Adjunctive treatments in ART

Enhance ovarian response?
• DHEA (dehydroepiandrosterone)
• Growth hormone
Enhance implantation?
• Low dose aspirin
• Acupuncture

E. Surrey, M.D. (✉)
Colorado Center for Reproductive Medicine,
Lone Tree, CO 80124, USA
e-mail: esurrey@colocrm.com

Growth Hormone and the Poor Responder

Management of the poor responder represents one of the great challenges of the assisted reproductive technologies. A review of protocols designed for these individuals is presented elsewhere in this text. One of the problems in evaluating the literature in this field is the lack of a standardized definition of the "poor responder" with a host of criteria employed by prior investigators [1]. As a result, it is extremely challenging, if not impossible, to compare outcomes from various investigators given the extreme heterogeneity of the populations studied.

Growth hormone (GH) has been investigated as a means of amplifying the action of gonadotropins to improve ovarian response. The logic behind this approach lies in evidence suggesting that GH may act directly to enhance folliculogenesis and inhibit follicular atresia [2]. In addition, GH acts via insulin like growth factor-1 (IGF-1) to potentiate the action of FSH and LH on granulosa cells [2–4].

The coadministration of GH with gonadotropins to anovulatory hypogonadotropic women has been shown to reduce the gonadotropin dose required to achieve an ovulatory response and may result in a degree of follicular development which could not be achieved with gonadotropins alone [2, 5].

The outcomes are less clear when this approach is applied to the ovulatory patient and/or poor responder. A Cochrane review of nine

E.S. Ginsburg and C. Racowsky (eds.), *In Vitro Fertilization: A Comprehensive Guide*,
DOI 10.1007/978-1-4419-9848-4_12, © Springer Science+Business Media New York 2012

Table 12.2 GH and poor responders: meta-analysis[a]

Parameter	Impact (%)	95% CI[b]	NNT[c] (95% CI)
Patients reaching ET[d]	↑ 22	7–30	–
Clinical pregnancy rate	↑ 16	4–21	6 (4–21)
Live birth rate	↑ 17	5–30	6 (3–20)

[a] Adapted from Kolibianakis et al. [9]
[b] CI = Confidence interval
[c] NNT = Number needed to treat
[d] ET = Embryo transfer

prospective randomized trials including 401 IVF patients using varying doses of GH as well as growth hormone releasing hormone (GHRH) provides some insight [6]. No improvement in live birth rates was noted in the three trials in which women without a history of poor response were administered GH (OR 1.17; 95% confidence interval [CI]: 0.38–3.5). However, live birth rates were significantly improved in the three trials investigating prior poor responders as defined in a variety of ways (OR 4.37; 95% CI: 1.05–18.01). GHRH was not helpful.

Two more recent randomized trials bear attention. Kucuk et al. evaluated 61 prior poor responders receiving a long GnRH agonist protocol [7]. Patients in the study group received GH 4 mg daily from mid-luteal initiation of the agonist until the day of human chorionic gonadotropin (hCG) trigger. A significant increase in the number of fertilized oocytes with a trend towards an increase in clinical pregnancy rate was reported in the GH group.

In a larger trial of 100 women over 40 years of age who were not necessarily poor responders, Tesarik and colleagues administered GH 8 IU daily from day 7 of gonadotropin stimulation until the day of hCG administration [8]. There were no differences in the number of oocytes or embryos in either group. However, a significant increase in peak estradiol levels (1,523 ± 203 pg/mL vs. 912 ± 129 pg/mL, $P < 0.05$), implantation rates (6.2% vs. 1.7%; $P < 0.05$), and live birth rates (22% vs. 4%; $P < 0.05$) was achieved after GH coadministration.

A more recent meta-analysis evaluated six randomized trials including 169 women defined as "poor responders." Significant increases in clinical pregnancy rates and decreases in cycle cancellation rates were achieved with the coadministration of growth hormone, although the authors calculated that six patients would need to be treated in this fashion to achieve one extra birth [9] (Table 12.2). This investigation suffers from the same weaknesses as the earlier meta-analysis: a high degree of heterogeneity regarding the definition of the poor responder, growth hormone dose and duration, and ovarian stimulation protocol employed.

Thus, although it is not possible to arrive at definitive conclusions, it does appear that an as yet undefined subgroup of poor responders will benefit from GH coadministration.

Dehydroepiandrosterone (DHEA) and the Poor Responder

DHEA has recently received interest as potentially playing a role in enhancing ovarian response. The logic behind this approach is that androgens may serve as positive regulators for follicular development. Frattarelli and colleagues had previously reported a significant increase in IVF pregnancy rates in patients with basal testosterone levels >20 ng/dL [10]. Haning et al. had demonstrated that, as a precursor hormone, DHEA increases the pool of substrate for estradiol and testosterone [11]. In addition, DHEA may act by increasing ovarian IGF-1 expression and induce FSH receptor upregulation to amplify the action of gonadotropins [12, 13].

The largest clinical trial published to date is a case control study of 190 women with diminished ovarian reserve defined as follicular phase FSH level ≥12 mIU/mL or estradiol level >75 pg/mL who were not necessarily prior poor responders

Table 12.3 Low dose aspirin and IVF Outcome[a]

	Aspirin 100 mg daily	Placebo
Patients	149	140
Oocytes retrieved	16.2 ± 6.7	8.6 ± 4.6*
Peak E_2 (pg/mL)	2,924 ± 1,023	1,614 ± 792*
Cancellation (%)	11.4	23.1
Implantation (%)	17.8	9.2
Clinical pregnancy (%)	45	28
Uterine artery PI[b]	1.22 ± 0.34	1.9 ± 0.58
Ovarian artery PI[b]	1.18 ± 0.31	1.9 ± 0.57

[a]Adapted from Rubinstein et al. [18]
[b]PI = Pulsatility index on day of hCG administration
*$P<0.05$

[14]. Eighty-nine women were administered DHEA 75 mg daily for variable time periods up to 4 months before initiation of the IVF cycle. There were no differences in cancellation or implantation rates in comparison to controls. Total pregnancy rates, which included pregnancies occurring prior to IVF cycle initiation, were higher in patients administered DHEA (28.1% vs. 10.9%; $P<0.01$). However, differences in IVF pregnancy rates were not significantly different between the groups (20.6% vs. 11.9%). Surprisingly, oocyte and cleavage stage embryo quality was enhanced in the control group. The lack of uniformity in the length of treatment and inclusion of pregnancies occurring prior to the IVF cycle represent confounding variables.

It is interesting to note that despite the widespread popularity of DHEA supplementation among patients and clinicians, only a single small prospective randomized trial has to this point been published which addressed its use in the poor responder. Wiser and colleagues studied a cohort of 33 women with diminished ovarian reserve and a prior failed IVF cycle who were randomized to receive DHEA 75 mg or placebo daily before and during a similar stimulation protocol as that employed in the prior failed cycle [15]. Patients in the DHEA group were noted to have a nonsignificant increase in serum estradiol levels on the day of hCG administration ($P=0.09$). However, day 3 embryo quality was significantly improved and live birth rates were significantly increased (23.1% vs. 4.0%; $P=0.006$) after DHEA administration. Clearly, there is a need for larger scale trials addressing dose and duration of therapy before this agent should be routinely recommended.

Low Dose Aspirin

The role of low dose aspirin in enhancing implantation after embryo transfer has been investigated by a variety of groups over the last 13 years. The logic behind this approach lies in the fact that low dose aspirin has been shown to exert antithrombotic and vasodilatory effects. This is felt to be due to activation of cyclooxygenase leading to inhibition of thromboxane A2 synthesis (a vasoconstrictor and platelet aggregation promoter) and enhanced production of prostacyclin (a vasodilator) [16, 17]. The benefits of this agent for prevention of thrombotic cardiovascular disease have been well established. Its role in enhancing uterine and ovarian blood flow and likelihood of implantation after IVF is less clear.

Rubinstein et al. performed one of the first prospective randomized double blind clinical trials addressing this issue [18]. This study included 289 IVF patients of whom 149 were treated with aspirin 100 mg daily during ovarian stimulation. A significant improvement in virtually all parameters measured was described, although a trend towards a higher clinical pregnancy rate was not statistically significant (Table 12.3).

Unfortunately, a subsequent meta-analysis of seven randomized clinical trials including 1,241

Table 12.4 Low dose aspirin and IVF outcome: a meta-analysis[a]

Parameter	RR[b]	95% CI[c]	*P*
Clinical pregnancy rate	1.11	0.95–1.3	NS[d]
Live birth rate[e]	0.94	0.64–1.39	NS
Pregnancy loss rate	1.06	0.53–2.11	NS

[a]Adapted from Khairy et al. [19]
[b]RR = Relative risk
[c]CI = Confidence interval
[d]NS = Not significant
[e]Two studies only

women treated with aspirin in doses ranging from 80 to 100 mg daily as part of an IVF cycle did not confirm these largely encouraging results [19]. No treatment effects on clinical pregnancy, live birth, or pregnancy loss rates were noted (Table 12.4).

Since the publication of the aforementioned meta-analysis, three more recent randomized trials have been confirmatory, demonstrating no impact on clinical pregnancy or live birth rates after low dose aspirin use [20–22]. Although Haapsamo et al. reported a decreased incidence of abnormal uterine artery pulsatility indices in the aspirin group, others showed no effect [21, 22].

An expanded meta-analysis conducted by Ruopp and coworkers analyzed ten randomized clinical trials including 2,001 IVF cycles [23]. Although an increase in clinical pregnancy rate was noted in the aspirin groups (RR 1.15; 95% CI: 1.08–1.27), there was no effect on either implantation or pregnancy loss rates. Of note is the fact that live birth was not assessed. Thus, the impact of low dose aspirin on implantation, if any, remains undetermined in the typical IVF patient.

Acupuncture

Acupuncture has been an integral component of traditional Chinese medicine for several thousand years. More recently, this modality has been employed as an adjunct in the management of infertility. Its effectiveness remains controversial due to significant variations in study design, technique, patient populations, and description of controls [24].

The rationale behind acupuncture is that energy (Qi) flows along various pathways (meridians) in the body. Specific areas along these meridians (acupoints) can be stimulated to alter the flow of Qi and affect disease states. It has been proposed that, by stimulation of specific acupoints, particularly in the auricular region, uterine and ovarian blood flow can be enhanced, along with a decrease in anxiety and stress along with modulation of the neuroendocrine system [24].

IVF studies have employed either manual or low voltage electrical stimulation of the needle. Several of the difficulties in evaluating the impact of acupuncture on IVF outcomes center around a host of significant confounding variables: treatments are individualized based on evaluation of patient energy imbalances or deficiencies and may be administered for a variety of time periods employing different techniques. Perhaps the greatest controversy surrounds the disparate types of control groups employed in published trials. These have included matched patients undergoing similar care without acupuncture, true acupuncture performed on sites which are not acupoints for the treatment of infertility, and "sham" acupuncture in which either sham needles are attached to the skin but do not penetrate or regular needles are introduced but not placed at an appropriate depth [24, 25]. Clearly, it is impossible to compare outcomes from studies employing these different approaches.

Using a control group of patients undergoing routine care without acupuncture, Paulus et al. randomized 160 patients with good embryo quality to 25 min of therapy including needle rotation starting 25 min before and 25 min after embryo transfer in age matched controls using several therapists [26]. No differences in uterine artery pulsatility indices were reported, but a significantly

Table 12.5 Acupuncture pre- and post-embryo transfer[a]

	"Real"	"Sham"	*P* value
Overall pregnancy (%)	43.8	55.1	0.038
Ongoing pregnancy (%)	31.9	40.5	0.105
Live birth (%)	29.7	38.4	0.100
Implantation (%)	28.0	32.8	0.189
Miscarriage (%)	32.1	30.4	0.931
Ectopic (%)	2.5	1.0	0.585

[a]Adapted from So et al. [28]

higher clinical pregnancy rate was noted in the acupuncture group (42.5% vs. 26.3%; $P=0.03$). In contrast, Domar and colleagues employed a similar design but with the use of a single acupuncturist [27]. Controls were allowed to lie quietly for an equal time period. There were no differences in pregnancy rates including the subgroups of patients with only good embryos.

Smith and coworkers used a different design in a single blind randomized trial of 228 IVF patients [28]. Acupuncture was performed using variable acupoints determined by the acupuncturist on day 9 of stimulation as well as immediately before and after embryo transfer. Controls underwent needle placement at sham points near but not at the true acupoints. Embryo scores, age, and body mass index were matched between the groups. Ongoing pregnancy rates were not significantly different between groups (30.9% vs. 22%; $P=0.08$).

A more recent well-designed study attempted to address many of these variables [29]. So and colleagues performed a prospective randomized trial of 370 patients undergoing 25 min of therapy before and after embryo transfer. The placebo group was treated with retractable needles at the same acupoints. Patients were treated with similar stimulation protocols, and were matched based on age, ovarian reserve testing, duration of infertility, as well as day and number of embryos transferred. All acupuncture was performed by one experienced clinician. In this study, overall pregnancy rates were higher in the sham group, although all other outcomes were similar between the groups (Table 12.5). This would either suggest that either there is no overall benefit of acupuncture or that the placebo may not be truly inert. Given the findings of prior studies which compared acupuncture to no treatment, it is unlikely that the sham acupuncture had no effect and pregnancy rates were lowered by true acupuncture. These findings were confirmed by Andersen et al. in a similarly designed prospective randomized trial of 635 patients with a control group undergoing placebo acupuncture using a "validated" placebo needle [30]. There were no differences in clinical pregnancy, implantation, or live birth rates between the groups.

Zhang and coworkers recently reported encouraging outcomes employing transcutaneous electrical stimulation of acupoints [31]. Three hundred nine patients less than 45 years of age undergoing fresh or frozen embryo transfer were placed in one of three groups: mock treatment at the appropriate acupoints but with "weak" stimulation 30 min after transfer, a single stimulation treatment 30 min after embryo transfer and two treatments 24 h before and 30 min after the transfer. Implantation (15.6% vs. 20.7% vs. 25.9%) and live birth rates (21.2% vs. 37.8% vs. 42%) were significantly lower in the "mock" treatment group than in either of the study groups. There were no significant differences between the two treatment groups.

Three meta-analyses have attempted to pool and analyze the available data despite the heterogeneity in techniques and controls [32–34]. Manheimer et al. evaluated seven trials of 1,366 women randomized to needle acupuncture within 1 day of embryo transfer or to either no treatment or sham acupuncture [32]. Acupuncture resulted in a significant improvement in ongoing pregnancy rates in five trials (RR 1.87; 95% CI: 1.40–2.49) and live birth rates in the four trials in which this was reported (RR 1.91; 95% CI: 1.39–2.64). Based on this analysis, the number of patients

Table 12.6 Acupuncture and IVF: a meta-analysis[a]

Group	Parameter	Trials	Outcome	OR[b]	95% CI[c]
All acupuncture	LBR[d]	7	32% vs. 29%	1.31	0.88–1.95
	CPR[e]	14	38% vs. 35%	1.21	0.90–1.63
Acupuncture at retrieval	LBR	2	33% vs. 36%	0.87	0.59–1.29
	CPR	5	37% vs. 35%	1.08	0.82–1.44
Acupuncture day of transfer	LBR	4	33% vs. 29%	1.43	0.77–2.65
	CPR	8	39% vs. 37%	1.14	0.76–1.69
(Sham vs. No sham)	LBR	5	Not reported	1.35	1.04–1.75
Repeated acupuncture	LBR	2	28% vs. 17%	1.83	1.00–3.35
	CPR	2	35% vs. 19%	2.23	1.41–3.51

[a] Adapted from Cheong et al. [34]
[b] OR = Odds ratio
[c] CI = Confidence interval
[d] LBR = Live birth rate
[e] CPR = Clinical pregnancy rate

who would need to undergo acupuncture in order to achieve an additional live birth was nine (95% CI: 6–17).

El-Toukhy and coworkers identified 13 relevant trials of similar design involving 2,500 women [33]. Five trials including 877 patients evaluated acupuncture performed around the time of oocyte retrieval, analysis of which showed no impact on clinical pregnancy rates (RR = 1.06; 95% CI: 0.82–1.37, $P = 0.65$). A similar lack of benefit was noted after analysis of trials including 1,623 patients for whom acupuncture was performed around the time of embryo transfer (RR = 1.23; 95% CI: 0.97–1.58; $P = 0.1$).

A more recent and extensive meta-analysis was performed by Cheong et al. [34]. Fourteen randomized trials involving 2,670 subjects were included. The studies were divided into three groups based on the timing of acupuncture: near the time of aspiration, the day of embryo transfer, and repeated acupuncture performed on and after the day of embryo transfer. Only six of these trials included data on live birth. The authors emphasized the difficulty in merging outcomes from studies that were so heterogeneous in design. The authors concluded that acupuncture around the time of oocyte retrieval had no impact on IVF pregnancy rates and that acupuncture on the day of embryo transfer was beneficial only when therapy was repeated subsequently (Table 12.6). It is interesting to note that outcomes were enhanced in those control groups in which sham acupuncture as opposed to no treatment was employed. This may suggest that "sham" acupuncture is likely not inert.

Clearly the ideal acupuncture trial has not yet been performed. Patients must be matched based on history, protocol, and embryo quality. Acupuncture technique must be standardized and performed by a small number of experienced acupuncturists for aggregate results to be interpretable. Ideally, two control groups should be considered: "sham acupuncture" and "no treatment." The study must be of adequate power to evaluate the two most important outcomes: implantation and live birth.

Summary and Conclusions

The current state of knowledge of the four adjunctive therapies discussed in this chapter remains incomplete. Meta-analyses cannot compensate for heterogeneous patient populations, treatment regimens, indications for therapy and outcome parameters. However, based on this review of currently available evidence, the following comments can be made.

1. *Growth hormone*: The administration of growth hormone as adjunctive therapy for controlled ovarian stimulation regimes has been evaluated in a variety of randomized clinical trials. This approach does not appear to be beneficial for the average patient. There

is suggestive evidence that live birth rates and ovarian response may be improved in a subset of prior poor responders. Given the heterogeneity of regimens assessed, the ideal dose or duration has not been determined, therefore there are inadequate data on which to base a recommendation for treatment.

2. *DHEA*: Currently, the only prospective randomized trial which has been published demonstrated enhanced pregnancy rates and embryo quality after pre-cycle DHEA administration in a small group of poor responders who had previously failed IVF. Case–control studies do not consistently confirm enhanced IVF pregnancy rates, although oocyte yields may be increased and cancellation rates decreased. The appropriate dose and duration of therapy has not been defined.
3. *Low dose aspirin*: An earlier meta-analysis showed slight increases in IVF clinical pregnancy rates with no evidence of any impact on implantation or live birth rates. Recent randomized clinical trials demonstrate no benefit when administered routinely prior to IVF. Whether this approach may improve IVF outcomes, in specific patient subsets such as those with antiphospholipid syndromes, recurrent pregnancy loss, or a history of prior failed cycles despite adequate embryo quality requires further evaluation, so that there is little basis for routine treatment.
4. *Acupuncture*: Analysis of data from published trials investigating the effect of acupuncture on IVF cycle outcomes is confounded by a host of variables including variations in technique, patient populations, timing, and control groups, and the fact that sham acupuncture may have an effect. The aggregate of randomized controlled trials show no clearly defined benefit of acupuncture on IVF pregnancy and delivery rates, although the ideal study has not been performed. If there is a benefit of acupuncture, it may be when performed on the day of embryo transfer and possibly thereafter as well. The ideal candidate or technique has not been defined, and patients should be educated about this if acupuncture is discussed.

In our quest to maximize pregnancy rates associated with the assisted reproductive technologies, it is vital that new techniques, technologies, and adjunctive therapies be critically evaluated in appropriately designed trials before they are generally accepted and introduced into widespread use. It is vital that clinicians evaluate the literature themselves as well as their own outcome data so that patients can be appropriately informed and educated decisions made.

References

1. Surrey E, Schoolcraft W. Evaluating strategies for improving ovarian response of the poor responder undergoing assisted reproductive technologies. Fertil Steril. 2000;73:667–76.
2. Hull K, Harvey S. Growth hormone: roles in female reproduction. J Endocrinol. 2001;168:1–23.
3. Adashi E, Resnick C, Hernandez E, Hurwitz A, Roberts C, Leroth D, et al. Insulin-like growth factor as an intraovarian regulator: basic and clinical implications. Ann N Y Acad Sci. 1992;626:161–8.
4. Mason H, Martikainen H, Beard R, Anyaolou U, Fraiks S. Direct gonadotropin effect of growth hormone on oestradiol production by human granulosa cells on-vitro. J Endocrinol. 1990;126:1–4.
5. European and Australian Multicenter Study. Cotreatment with growth hormone and gonadotropin for ovulation induction in hypogonadotropic patients: a prospective, randomized, placebo-controlled, dose-response study. Fertil Steril. 1995;64:917–23.
6. Harper K, Proctor M, Hughes E. Growth hormone for in vitro fertilization. Cochrane Database Syst Rev. 2003(3);CD000099.
7. Kucuk T, Kozinoglu H, Kaba A. Growth hormone co-treatment within a GnRH agonist long protocol in patients with poor ovarian response: a prospective randomized clinical trial. J Assist Reprod Genet. 2008;25:123–7.
8. Tesarik J, Hazout A, Mendoza C. Improvement of delivery and live birth rates after ICSI in women aged >40 years by ovarian co-stimulation with growth hormone. Hum Reprod. 2005;20:2536–41.
9. Kolibianakis E, Venetis C, Diedrich K, Tarlatzis B, Griesinger G. Addition of growth hormone to gonadotropins in ovarian stimulation of poor responders treated by in-vitro fertilization: a systematic review and meta-analysis. Hum Reprod Update. 2009;15:613–22.
10. Frattarelli J, Peterson E. Effect of androgen levels on in vitro fertilization cycles. Fertil Steril. 2004;81: 1713–4.
11. Haning Jr R, Hackett R, Flood C, Loughlin J, Zhao Q, Longcope C. Plasma dehydroepiandrosterone sulfate serves as a prehormone for 48% of follicular

fluid testosterone during treatment with menotropins. J Clin Endocrinol Metab. 1993;76:1301–7.
12. Casson P, Santoro N, Elkind-Hirsch K, Carson S, Hornsby P, Abraham G, et al. Postmenopausal dehydroepiandrosterone administration increases free insulin-like growth factor-I and decreases high density lipoprotein: a six-month trial. Fertil Steril. 1998;70:107–10.
13. Weil S, Vendola K, Zhou J, Adesanya O, Wang J, Okafor J, et al. Androgen receptor gene expression in the primate ovary: cellular localization, regulation and functional correlations. J Clin Endocrinol Metab. 1998;83:2470–8.
14. Barad D, Brill H, Gleicher N. Update on the use of dehydroepiandrosterone supplementation among women with diminished ovarian function. J Assist Reprod Genet. 2007;24:629–34.
15. Wiser A, Gonen O, Ghetler Y, Shavit T, Berkovitz A, Shulman A. Addition of dehydroepiandrosterone (DHEA) for poor responder patients before and during IVF treatment improves the pregnancy rate: A randomized prospective study. Hum Reprod. 2010;25:2496–500.
16. Ozturk O, Greaves M, Templeton A. Aspirin dilemma: remodeling the hypothesis from a fertility perspective. Hum Reprod. 2002;17:1146–8.
17. Catella-Lawson F. Vascular biology of thrombosis: platelet vessel wall interactions and aspirin effects. Neurology. 2001;57(5 Suppl 2):5–7.
18. Rubinstein M, Marazzi A, Polak de Fried E. Low-dose aspirin treatment improves ovarian responsiveness, uterine and ovarian blood flow velocity, implantation and pregnancy rates in patients undergoing in vitro fertilization: a prospective randomized, double-blind placebo-controlled assay. Fertil Steril. 1999;71:825–9.
19. Khairy M, Banerjee K, El-Toukhy T, Coomarasamy A, Khalaf Y. Aspirin in women undergoing in vitro fertilization treatment: a systematic review and meta-analysis. Fertil Steril. 2007;88:822–31.
20. Dirckx K, Cabri P, Merien A, Galajdova L, Gerris J, Dhont M, et al. Does low-dose aspirin improve pregnancy rate in IVF/ICSI? A randomized double-blind placebo controlled trial. Hum Reprod. 2009;24:856–60.
21. Haapsamo M, Martikainen H, Räsänen J. Low-dose aspirin and uterine haemodynamics on the day of embryo transfer in women undergoing IVF/ICSI: a randomized, placebo-controlled, double-blind study. Hum Reprod. 2009;24:861–6.
22. Lambers M, Hoozemans D, Schats R, Homburg R, Lambalk C, Hompes P. Low-dose aspirin in non-tubal IVF patients with previous failed conception: a prospective randomized double-blind placebo-controlled trial. Fertil Steril. 2009;92:923–9.
23. Ruopp M, Collins T, Whitcomb B, Schisterman E. Evidence of absence or absence of evidence? A reanalysis of the effects low-dose aspirin in in vitro fertilization. Fertil Steril. 2008;90:71–6.
24. Ng Y, So W, Gao J, Wong Y, Ho P. The role of acupuncture in the management of subfertility. Fertil Steril. 2008;90:1–13.
25. Dieterle S, Ying G, Hatzmann W, Neurer A. Effect of acupuncture on the outcome of in vitro fertilization and intracytoplasmic sperm injection: a randomized, prospective, controlled clinical study. Fertil Steril. 2006;85:1347–51.
26. Paulus W, Zhang M, Strehler E, El-Danasouri I, Sterzik K. Influence of acupuncture on the pregnancy rate in patients who undergo assisted reproductive therapy. Fertil Steril. 2002;77:721–4.
27. Domar A, Meshay I, Kelliher J, Alper M, Powers R. The impact of acupuncture on in vitro fertilization outcome. Fertil Steril. 2009;91:723–6.
28. Smith C, Coyle M, Norman R. Influence of acupuncture stimulation on pregnancy rates for women undergoing embryo transfer. Fertil Steril. 2006;85:1352–8.
29. So E, Ng E, Wong Y, Lau E, Yeung W, Ho P. A randomized double blind comparison of real and placebo acupuncture in IVF treatment. Hum Reprod. 2009; 24:341–8.
30. Andersen D, Lossl K, Andersen A, Fürbringer J, Bach H, Simonsen J, et al. Acupuncture on the day of embryo transfer: a randomized controlled trial of 635 patients. Reprod Biomed Online. 2010;21:366–72.
31. Zhang R, Feng X-J, Guan Q, Cui W, Zheng Y, Sun W, et al. Increase of success rate for women undergoing embryo transfer by transcutaneous electrical acupoint stimulation: a prospective randomized placebo-controlled study. Fertil Steril. 2011;96:912–6.
32. Manheimer E, Zhang G, Udoff L, Haramati A, Langenberg P, Berman B, et al. Effects of acupuncture on rates of pregnancy and live birth among women undergoing in vitro fertilization: a systematic review and meta-analysis. BMJ. 2008;336:545–9.
33. El-Toukhy T, Sunkara S, Khairy M, Dyer R, Khalaf Y, Coomarasamy A. A systematic review and meta-analysis of acupuncture in *in vitro* fertilisation. BJOG. 2008;115:1203–13.
34. Cheong Y, Nardo L, Rutherford T, Ledger W. Acupuncture and herbal medicine in in vitro fertilization: a review of the evidence for clinical practice. Hum Fertil. 2010;13:3–12.

Stress and ART

13

Alice Domar and Jill Gross

Introduction

The vast majority of people who have difficulty conceiving will experience some level of stress. The process of pursuing a diagnosis of any medical condition is inherently stressful and when the source of this condition is related to our innate biological need to procreate, coupled with the cultural expectation to produce children, the resulting level of psychological stress can be overwhelming. The interplay between stress and infertility has led to the current conundrum facing the infertility patient and the medical team. Does infertility cause stress? Does stress cause infertility? What are the implications of patient stress on the success of treatment? These questions have been and continue to be the focus of intense research and debate.

Recent research has specifically focused on this relationship with significant implications for the patient, physician, and treatment team. Stress greatly impacts the likelihood that a patient will enter and continue treatment, the overall disposition of the patient (stress creates a patient population that could be regarded as difficult and miserable to treat) and the outcome of that treatment reflected in pregnancy rates. Therefore, it is of paramount importance that the relationship between stress and the assisted reproductive technologies (ARTs) be fully appreciated in order to successfully treat and support the patient. This chapter covers the prevalence of stress in the infertility population, defines the stressors, and considers the types and impact of psychological interventions on the outcome of infertility treatment. The goal of this chapter is to give the treatment team an overview of the importance of the complex interplay of psychological stress on the physical well-being of the patient and its effect on successful infertility treatment.

A. Domar, Ph.D. (✉)
The Domar Center, Boston IVF, 130 Second Avenue, Waltham, MA 02451, USA
e-mail: domar@domarcenter.com

J. Gross, M.S.
Boston IVF, 130 Second Avenue, Waltham, MA 02451, USA
e-mail: jill.gross@bostonivf.com

Prevalence of Stress in the Infertility Population

Confronting a failure in one's capacity to reproduce can easily overcome typical coping mechanisms in most people. In a study by Freeman et al. approximately half of infertility patients reported infertility as the "most stressful experience of their life," testing even the strongest of coping mechanisms [1]. Another study by Mahlstedt et al. found that infertility itself was described as a stressful or very stressful experience by 80% of infertile couples [2]. It is important to remember that well before the patient's initial consultation the patient typically presents with a history of infertility that

E.S. Ginsburg and C. Racowsky (eds.), *In Vitro Fertilization: A Comprehensive Guide*,
DOI 10.1007/978-1-4419-9848-4_13, © Springer Science+Business Media New York 2012

has been persistent for at least 6 months, and sometimes years, during which time stress levels are increasing. This fact illustrates that patients have a high "baseline" level of stress even before beginning the demanding series of tests and medical procedures typical of infertility diagnosis and treatment. This high level of chronic stress can lead to depression and anxiety. A study by Chen et al. concluded that of 112 infertile women entering an ART clinic who underwent a structured psychiatric interview prior to their first consult with a physician, 40% had a diagnosable psychiatric disorder. Generalized anxiety disorder was the most common (23.3%) followed by major depression (17%) and dysthymic disorder (low-grade chronic depression) (9.8%) [3]. Another study on couples with infertility reported comparable results: 25% of women and 9% of men reported clinically elevated scores on a measure of anxiety [4]. The recurring cycle of hope, elation, and disappointment created by months of infertility treatment can have a substantial negative psychological impact on both the individual and the couple. A similar study by Volgsten et al. found psychiatric disorders present in 30.8% of females and 10.2% of males undergoing IVF treatment. Anxiety disorders were the most common diagnosis: 14.8% of females and 4.9% of males were determined to be suffering from anxiety. Major depression was also common, with 10.9% of females and 5.1% of males presenting with symptoms [5].

Depression and Anxiety

Highly emotional responses are expected when a patient presents with a serious medical condition, but when the patient presents with a condition such as infertility that is not life threatening, it can be difficult to fully appreciate the profound psychological effect it may have on the patient. In fact, psychological factors such as depression and anxiety in women experiencing infertility have been found to be similar to those of women with terminal illnesses such as heart disease, HIV+ status, or metastatic cancer [6]. Despite the inherent physical invasiveness of IVF, most patients report the procedure as more of a psychological stressor than a physical one [7]. Specifically, the most stressful period of IVF is consistently reported as the 2-week interval between embryo transfer and the pregnancy test even though this period has no additional physical intervention—no regular office visits or additional procedures [8].

Even the USA legal system has acknowledged the seriousness of infertility within the context of disabilities. The inability to conceive has been defined as a major condition by the US Supreme court under the Americans with Disabilities Act. Bragdon v. Abbott, 524 U.S. 624 (1998) (majority opinion). The court found that reproduction was a major life activity and conditions that interfere with reproduction can be severely debilitating. This psychological stress is consistent around the globe, as other studies have described significant increases in negative affect and anxiety in samples on infertile persons from other parts of the world. Mahajan et al. compared infertile groups to control groups in India and found as the period of infertility persisted, negative affect and anxiety continued to rise [9].

In addition to anxiety and depression, other psychiatric disorders have been found to be more prevalent in the infertile population, further documenting the psychological disorders that the infertility population experiences. Sbaragli et al. conducted a psychological assessment of 70 fertile and 81 infertile couples and found, in addition to depression and anxiety, a significant occurrence (18%) of binge eating disorder among the infertile group and none among the assessed fertile group [10]. In another study by Freizinger et al. past or present eating disorders were found in 20.7% of the infertile participants, five times higher than would be expected in the general population. It is interesting to note that none of the participants in this study disclosed their eating disorder to their health care provider, indicating that this is a very difficult population to identify and treat [11]. It is hypothesized that the lack of control that the patient experiences in their infertility diagnosis and treatment can manifest itself as an eating disorder characterized by practicing overt control over food intake.

Relationship Issues

In addition to psychiatric symptoms, infertility distress can create discord in a couple's relationship which paradoxically, can be the very relationship identified as a helpful coping mechanism for managing the stress. Infertility is considered a life crisis and has an impact on both the individuals and the partnership. While women tend to have high levels of distress from the beginning of the evaluation through the treatment, men also experience acute stress from the treatment demands [12, 13]. The intense treatment schedules surrounding infertility treatment, and the timed (not spontaneous) nature of intercourse, can lead to a decreased desire for intimacy. Male sexual distress, specifically erectile dysfunction, ejaculatory disorders, loss of libido, and a decrease in the frequency of intercourse, has been associated with lengthy diagnosis and treatment of infertility [14]. In a study by Peterson et al. it was found that couples were more likely to experience marital satisfaction if the partners perceived equal levels of infertility stress in each other. An incongruence of the intense need for parenthood was associated with low marital satisfaction and depression in women [15]. Consequently, communication about specific stressors and the emotional investment in parenthood are very important in maintaining a strong relationship which can help relieve stress. Marital strength is noted as one of the strongest predictors of treatment longevity as relational strain was frequently reported as the reason for premature discontinuation from treatment [16–20]. The prevalence of stress in the infertile population is well documented throughout the diagnosis and treatment cycle. The specific stressors can vary somewhat, but most have a cumulative effect. That is, if a patient or couple experiences many stressors at once without sufficient coping mechanisms, the resulting stress can be severely debilitating. It is therefore important to understand the different types of stressors to accurately assess the present state of your patient.

Stressors: Social, Loss of Control, Biological, and Financial

Social Stressors: Family and Friends

The stressors experienced by the infertility patient can be obvious and well known to both patient and practitioner, or more covert, but all elicit a profound effect on the overall treatment experience, duration, and outcome. One of the most obvious and seemingly innocuous stressors is the verbal pressure to conceive by family and friends. This social pressure can be overwhelming, especially in some religious and tight knit communities, to the point of becoming debilitating to relationships within the community and the couple itself. Some cultures may overtly ostracize those who cannot conceive or may allow a man to divorce his wife based on her infertility [21]. The infertility diagnosis is not only a medical diagnosis, but it also defines a social condition in that childlessness is deemed unacceptable in many societies. A study conducted by Noorbala et al. on Iranian infertile couples states that "as in many oriental countries, the extended family type is dominant in Iran, with relatives providing opinions and comments" [22]. Furthermore, an additional study by Noorbala et al. found a total of 81.3% of surveyed infertile participants reported that the main stressor in their lives was relatives' comments about their infertility [23]. Thus, paradoxically, the very support system, family and friends, that can be beneficial for the couple, can also be the most intense source of stress. Over time, the couple chooses not to participate in the social activities within their community, avoiding the questions but also the support that could be beneficial. Even in western nations such as the USA, parenthood provides access to certain social circles and exclusion from these groups is both painful and isolating. Understandably, women describe the most difficult aspect of infertility as being in the presence of women who are pregnant or have infants; attempting to avoid these stressful triggers leads to the social isolation which can exacerbate the level and severity of stress [24].

Menning describes the infertile couple as being in a state of mourning over the loss of unrealized potential in the unborn child, and the couple or individual passes through all the known stages of grief (state of shock, denial, anger and isolation, and finally acceptance) [25]. Some individuals in the couples' lives may have difficulty acknowledging the grieving process as they may not understand the loss of something that never existed. This leads again to yet greater isolation and deterioration of the psychological state [26].

Loss of Control as a Stressor

The loss of unrealized potential and the loss of control over one's future identity generate an additional stressor. Particularly in the modern world, individuals expect to have some level of control over their future and what roles they will undertake in society. There is an assumption that birth control will control our reproductive future and most assume this control includes an ability to conceive as soon as the birth control is removed. One of the most difficult situations to handle is the loss of control resulting from infertility [24]. Experiencing a lack of control over one's own body and reproductive choice can result in anger and confusion. The unrealized identity as "mother," "dad," or "parent" can raise core identity issues resulting in diminished self-worth and damaged self-esteem [27]. The inherent impact of this perceived loss of control may manifest itself by imbalance, being so focused on becoming a parent that all other goals become superseded by the need to have a baby, further deteriorating social connections even career goals. "For many couples, their infertility becomes the focal point of daily discourse and tasks, often to the exclusion of other important aspects of life" [24].

Biological Stressors

Waiting to conceive creates additional problems because as the biological processes of the body ages, fertility is reduced [28]. The social pressure for a woman to succeed in a career is also strong in some contemporary societies, especially in highly educated groups. This situation may compel women into postponing the attempt to conceive until after a career is established or after schooling is finished. A survey of university students in Sweden revealed that about half of the women reported that they intended to wait to have children until after the age of 35 [29]. In this scenario, the couple is likely to face a "biological clock" stressor in addition to the pressure presented by family and friends.

Financial Stressors

Finances can have a significant impact on the stress a couple experiences during infertility diagnostic testing and treatment. While some insurance providers cover the cost of consultation, diagnosis, and treatment, many do not. Therefore, the choice to pursue a family through the ARTs is not only an emotional one but also can pose financial challenges. The couple that has waited to conceive until they are financially stable may very well find themselves in danger of financial ruin in order to conceive. The typical ART process, including consultation, diagnosis, medications, and treatment can cost many thousands of dollars for one attempt at conception, frequently with less than a 50% chance of being successful. Obviously, cost alone is a very difficult burden to bear but the addition of time taken off work for clinic visits is additionally stressful. Schenker describes the investigation into infertility as highly stressful because of the disturbance in day-to-day functioning from the repeated office visits, blood tests, and frequent ultrasound examinations in addition to several painful procedures such as hysterosalpingography (HSG), laparoscopy, and hysteroscopy. All of which are "time consuming and affect other aspects of life such as work and social activities" [26].

Impact of Psychological Intervention on the Outcome of Infertility Treatment

Sources of stress and the resulting severity will vary somewhat, depending on the coping mechanisms, social support, and the length of time the couple has attempted conception. While some individuals and couples will have strong coping strategies in place prior to treatment, some patients will need additional help securing resources and the skills to cope with the chronic stress which accompanies infertility treatment. Some patients will present as having strong coping mechanisms but as treatment and treatment failure persists, the coping mechanisms begin to weaken. Therefore, it is imperative that the practitioner continually assess the patient's present coping strategies as these can be very fluid with the treatment course.

Psychological stress can have a profound impact on physical and emotional health regardless of fertility, but the impact of stress reduction on infertility patients has, as of yet, been inadequately researched. Reducing the psychological burden on the patient can create a more pleasant infertility experience for both the patient and the staff, resulting in more positive feelings, or at least fewer negative experiences, for both. Theoretically, this creates an environment conducive to continuing treatment until a successful outcome has been attained. As stated before, stress is a common occurrence during the treatment process and a study by Domar et al. states that 39% of patients who prematurely dropout of treatment do so because of reported psychological stress [30]. Boivin et al. state that treatment discontinuation is frequently linked to three factors: fear and negative treatment attitudes, psychological and emotional factors, and relational strain [31]. Similar conclusions were made by Domar et al. and Rajkhowa et al. in two separate studies. Employing self-report questionnaires, these studies found that the most frequent reason for ending treatment was stress, specifically the stress on the couple's relationship followed by being too anxious and depressed to continue treatment [30, 32]. Consequently, psychological and psychosocial treatment has been noted as an essential element in the treatment of infertility, particularly with the most invasive of all treatments, ART. It can be concluded that stress has an effect on fertility if only because patients may discontinue infertility treatment before success, the implications of which are profound on the patient and the infertility treatment team. In "willingness to pay" studies, it has been found that the infertile patient experiences some mental health benefits from undergoing infertility treatment with or without a live birth solely because the treatment reduces feelings of regret as the couple has a sense that they have done everything possible to secure a birth. It can also negatively impact the treatment team when the patient opts to prematurely end treatment, because the team may feel regret that they were not able to provide a successful pregnancy within the context of everything they could do [31]. For these reasons, it is imperative that the patient remain in treatment as long as reasonably necessary to ensure physical and psychological health. In order to create an atmosphere where this is possible, it is necessary to address and reduce stress levels in the patient.

The Effectiveness of Psychological Interventions

The ability to reduce psychological stress in infertility patients will yield benefit on multiple fronts. Several studies have examined the effectiveness of various approaches to reduce stress. In a meta-analysis of the literature on psychosocial interventions Boivin et al. state that about half of the studies employing interventions to reduce stress were successful, of particular note, these interventions uniformly reduced infertility-specific distress. It is hypothesized that when stress is reduced among patients undergoing infertility treatment, the tendency to end treatment prematurely will likewise be reduced, thereby increasing the chances that a patient will successfully end treatment with a baby. Additionally, Boivin found that psychosocial interventions were successful in reducing stress and had a positive impact on pregnancy rates not just treatment longevity [33]. Another study by Ramezanzadeh et al. found a combination of psychotherapy and antidepressant medication on depressed infertile patients yielded a significantly higher pregnancy rate in the intervention group (47.1%) when compared to the control group (7.1%) [34]. This underscores the importance of including psychosocial resources in order to produce the best and most successful care for the patient.

Types of Effective Psychosocial Therapy

Several studies have found specific types of psychosocial interventions to be effective in reducing the stress of patients participating in infertility treatment [35–37]. Some of the most common highly researched therapies for infertility distress include cognitive behavioral therapy (CBT), relaxation training, behavioral modification, and group education/support.

Cognitive behavioral therapy (CBT) was designed by Aaron Beck and has been widely used to treat many different psychological issues. CBT is based upon the premise that maladaptive thought patterns are the cause of psychological pain and by restructuring the negative thoughts, the patient can change the resulting negative feelings. The negative thoughts shape the patient's reality, creating a self-fulfilling prophecy in which the patient can only focus on the events that confirm the negative thoughts (i.e., a failed IVF attempt) as opposed to the other very real facts that can give hope (a normal FSH level, several frozen good quality embryos). Sole attention to the negative aspects allows the mind to spiral into hopelessness and loss of control leading to depression and anxiety. Through several sessions, CBT critically examines defective thought patterns that create the psychological pain and teaches the patient techniques to restructure the thoughts to allow for a paradigm shift into hopefulness. The effectiveness of this technique has been well researched. A study by Faramarzi et al. randomly assigned 89 depressed infertile women in Iran to three groups: receiving CBT, antidepressant drug therapy, or no intervention. The CBT group participated in ten sessions of therapy providing relaxation training and cognitive restructuring typical of CBT. 79.3% of the women in the CBT group were free of depression, while drug therapy provided relief for 50% of women and only 10% of the control group experienced relief [37].

Research has uncovered additional effective means for treating distress symptoms in patients undergoing infertility treatment, including a cognitive behavioral approach specifically designed for those participating in infertility treatment. The first mind/body program for infertility was developed in 1987 using a combination of approaches including cognitive strategies, group support, relaxation techniques, and stress management with the goal of teaching basic skills for reducing distress. Participation in the mind/body program resulted in significant decreases in psychological symptoms such as depression, anxiety, and hostility in addition to decreases in physical symptoms such as fatigue, headaches, insomnia, and abdominal pain [38]. Of particular note, an additional study published in 2011 found a positive effect on pregnancy rates in IVF patients randomized to participate in a mind/body program. Domar et al. found that significantly higher pregnancy rates occurred in patients randomly assigned to attend a 10 week mind/body program as compared with those assigned to the control group. Fifty-two percent of the women who attended more than half of the mind/body program were pregnant in their second IVF cycle, compared to a pregnancy rate of 20% in the control group [39]. Additional research further illustrates that effective interventions consisting of at least five sessions of counseling, education, and group support results in less depression and anxiety and an increase in life satisfaction. In the control group undergoing infertility treatment with no psychosocial treatment, no such improvements were seen [40, 41]. The aforementioned meta-analysis by Boivin found that interventions including a cognitive and educational component, focusing on teaching coping skills and providing information were more effective than traditional counseling or supportive interventions, the latter emphasizing emotional expression [33]. It has been acknowledged that traditional counseling may be more effective in a population with chronic mental health issues. The infertile population experiences depression and anxiety acutely in correspondence with their infertility diagnosis and otherwise experiences strong mental health which may account for the lack of effectiveness of traditional psychotherapy [35]. Importantly, an additional randomized controlled study by Domar et al. found that patients participating in counseling interventions emphasizing emotional expression experienced significantly higher pregnancy rates and lower levels of psychological symptoms than the control subjects [36]. Psychosocial interventions have been found to have a significant effect on reducing distress in the infertility population through mind/body programs emphasizing cognitive behavioral techniques, relaxation training, group support, and education. It is through these resources that the treatment staff can support the patient participating in infertility treatment, and ensure the most positive outcome of treatment.

Does Stress Cause Infertility?

The effect stress has on fertility itself is an intensely debated topic. A recent study concluded that the likelihood of conception in women that have just started attempting pregnancy was negatively affected by distress [42]. Another study revealed strong evidence supporting the notion that stress affects pregnancy outcome. Klonoff-Cohen found that subjects who expressed the lowest baseline level of distress were 93% more likely to have a live birth when compared to subjects who reported the highest baseline level of distress [43]. However, some studies ended with the opposite conclusion. A recent meta-analysis of 14 studies indicated that there is no relationship between distress and pregnancy [44]. It is notable that the 14 studies reviewed represented roughly half of the studies available at the time, and in these studies, distress was only ascertained at one point in time and this point varied from 3 months prior to cycle start to early in the cycle. In addition, another study found that stress may have a positive effect on pregnancy. Domar et al. concluded that a moderate level of stress prior to IVF treatment resulted in higher pregnancy rates, as long as the stress was reduced during the course of treatment [45]. This conclusion follows the Yerkes-Dodson Law in psychology stating that there exists an optimum level of stress—not too much and not too little. Consequently, these studies illustrate the need for further research to determine the effect that psychological stress has on fertility.

Summary

It is widely accepted that patients who go through infertility treatment experience high levels of depression and anxiety as well as stress. The types and severity of emotional distress will vary with the individual patient and couple. It is important to recognize the relationship that exists between infertility and stress, and the different stressors, in order to fully and successfully treat the patient. This chapter has reviewed some of the most widely researched psychosocial interventions that have been found to be effective in reducing stress, and encourages use of these interventions. No matter how stress is reduced, reduction will help create a positive experience for both the patients and the treatment team involved in infertility diagnosis and treatment.

Acknowledgment The authors would like to thank Kristin Rooney for her assistance with this chapter.

References

1. Freeman EW, Boxer AS, Rickels K, Tureck R, Mastoinni L. Psychological evaluation and support in a program of in vitro fertilization and embryo transfer. Fertil Steril. 1985;43:48–53.
2. Mahlstedt PP, Macduff S, Bemstein J. Emotional factors and the in vitro fertilization and embryo transfer process. J In Vitro Fert Embryo Transf. 1987;4(4): 232–6.
3. Chen TH, Chang SP, Tsai CF, et al. Prevalence of depressive and anxiety disorders in an assisted reproductive technique clinic. Hum Reprod. 2004; 19(10):2313–8.

4. Anderson KM, Sharpe M, Rattray A, Irvine DS. Distress and concerns in couples referred to an infertility specialist. J Psychosom Res. 2003;54(4):353–5.
5. Volgsten H, Skoog Svanberg A, Ekselius L, Lundkvist O, Sundstrom Poromaa I. Prevalence of psychiatric disorders in infertile women and men undergoing in vitro fertilization treatment. Hum Reprod. 2008; 23(9):2056–63.
6. Domar AD, Zuttermeisiter PC, Friedman R. The psychological impact of infertility: a comparison to women with other medical conditions. J Psychosom Obstet Gynaecol. 1993;14:45–52.
7. Eugster A, Vingerhoets AJ. Psychological aspects of in vitro fertilization: a review. Soc Sci Med. 1999; 48:575–89.
8. Benyamini Y, Gozlan M, Kokia E. Variability in the difficulties experienced by women undergoing infertility treatments. Fertil Steril. 2005;83(2):275–83.
9. Mahajan NN, Turnbull DA, Davies MJ, Jundal UN, Briggs NE, Taplin JE. Adjustment to infertility: the role of intrapersonal and interpersonal resources/vulnerabilities. Hum Reprod. 2009;24(4):906–12.
10. Sbaragli C, Morgante G, Goracci A, Hofkens T, DeLeo V, Castrogiovanni P. Infertility and psychiatric morbidity. Fertil Steril. 2008;90(6):2107–11.
11. Freizinger M, Franko DL, Dacey M, Okun B, Domar AD. The prevalence of eating disorders in infertile women. Fertil Steril. 2010;93(1):72–8.
12. Edelmann RJ, Humphrey M, Owens DJ. The meaning of parenthood and couple's reactions to male infertility. Br J Med Psychol. 1994;67(Pt 3):291–9.
13. Daniluk JC. Gender and infertility. In: Leiblum SR, editor. Infertility, psychological issues and counseling strategies. New York: Wiley; 1997. p. 103–35.
14. Lenzi A, Lonbardo F, Salacone P, Gandini L, Jannini EA. Stress, sexual dysfunctions, and male infertility. J Endocrinol Invest. 2003;26(3 Suppl):72–6.
15. Peterson BD, Newton CR, Rosen KH. Examining congruence between partners' perceived infertility-related stress and its relationship to marital adjustment and depression in infertile couples. Fam Process. 2003;42(1):59–70.
16. Brandes M, van der Steen JO, Bokdam SB, Hamilton CJ, de Bruin JP, Nelen WL, Kremer JA. When and why do subfertile couples discontinue their fertility care? A longitudinal cohort study in a secondary care subfertility population. Hum Reprod. 2009;24: 3127–35.
17. Van den Broeck U, Holvoet L, Enzlin P, Bakelants E, Demyttenaere K, D'Hooghe T. Reasons for dropout in infertility treatment. Gynecol Obstet Invest. 2009;68: 58–64.
18. Strauss B, Hepp U, Staeding G, Mettler L. Psychological characteristics of infertile couples: can they predict pregnancy and treatment persistence? J Comm Appl Soc Psychol. 1998;8:289–301.
19. Verhagen TE, Dumoulin JC, Evers JL, Land JA. What is the most accurate estimate of pregnancy rates in IVF dropouts? Hum Reprod. 2008;23:1793–9.
20. Daniluk JC. Reconstructing their lives: a longitudinal, qualitative analysis of the transition to biological childlessness for infertile couples. J Couns Devel. 2001;79:439–49.
21. World Health Organization. Current practices and controversies in assisted reproduction. Report of a meeting on Medical, ethical and social aspects of assisted reproduction, Geneva, Switzerland, 64; 2001
22. Noorbala AA, Ramazanzadeh F, Malekafzali H, Abedinia N, Forooshani AR, Shariat M, Jafarabadi M. Effects of a psychological intervention on depression in infertile couples. Int J Gynaecol Obstet. 2008; 101(3):251.
23. Noorbala AA, Ramazanzadeh F, Abedinia N, Bagheri SA, Jafarabadi M. Study of psychiatric disorders among fertile and infertile women and some predisposing factors. J Fam Reprod Health. 2007;1(1): 6–11.
24. Domar AD, Seibel MM. Emotional aspects of infertility. In: Seibel MM, editor. Infertility: a comprehensive text. Stamford, CT: Appleton & Lange; 1997. p. 29–44.
25. Menning ECK. Effect of infertility on psychosexual function. Br Med J. 1975;5:295.
26. Schenker JG, Meirow D, Schenker E. Stress and human reproduction. European Journal of Obstetics &Gynecology and Reproductive Biology. 1992; 45(1):1–8.
27. Greil A. Not yet pregnant: infertile couples in contemporary America. London: Rutgers University Press; 1991.
28. Gordon JD, Dimattina M. 100 Questions and answers about infertility. Jones and Bartlett Publishers Inc: Sudbury, MA; 2008. p. 114.
29. Lampic C, Svanberg AS, Karlström P, Tydén T. Fertility awareness, intentions concerning childbearing, and attitudes towards parenthood among female and male academics. Hum Reprod. 2006;21(2):558–64.
30. Domar AD, Smith K, Conboy L, Iannone M, Alper M. A prospective investigation into the reasons why insured United States patients drop out of in vitro fertilization treatment. Fertil Steril. 2010;94(4): 1457–9.
31. Boivin J, Domar AD, Shapiro D, Fauser B, Verhaak CM. Tackling burden in ART: an integrated approach for fertility clinic staff. Hum Reprod. 2012;27(4): 941–50.
32. Rajkhowa M, McConnell A, Thomas GE. Reasons for discontinuation of IVF treatment: a questionnaire study. Hum Reprod. 2006;21:358.
33. Boivin J. A review of psychosocial interventions in infertility. Soc Sci Med. 2003;57(12):2325–41.
34. Ramezanzadeh F, Noorbala AA, Abedinia N, Rahimi Forooshani A, Naghizadeh MM. Psychiatric intervention improved pregnancy rates in infertile couples. Malays J Med Sci. 2011;18(1):16–24.
35. Hammerli K, Znoj H, Barth J. The efficacy of psychological interventions for infertile patients: a meta-analysis examining mental health and pregnancy rate. Hum Repro. 2009;15(3):279–95.
36. Domar AD, Clapp D, Slawsby E, Kessel B, Orav J, Freizinger M. The impact of group psychological interventions on distress in infertile women. Health Psychol. 2000;19(6):568–75.
37. Faramarzi M, Alipor A, Esmaelzadeh S, Kheirkhah F, Poladi K, Pash H. Treatment of depression and

anxiety in infertile women: cognitive behavioral therapy versus fluoxetine. J Affect Disord. 2007;108(1): 159–64.
38. Domar AD, Siebel MM, Benson H. The mind/body program for infertility: a new behavioral treatment approach for women with infertility. Fertil Steril. 1990;53(2):246–9.
39. Domar AD, Rooney KL, Wiegand B, Orav EJ, Alper MM, Berger BM, Nikolovski J. Impact of a group mind/body intervention on pregnancy rates in IVF patients. Fertil Steril. 2011;95(7):2269–73.
40. Hosaka T, Matsubayashi H, Sugiyama Y, et al. Effect of psychiatric group intervention on natural-killer cell activity and pregnancy rate. Gen Hosp Psychiatry. 2002;24(5):353–6.
41. Terzioglu F. Investigation into effectiveness of counseling on assisted reproductive techniques in Turkey. J Psychosom Obstet Gynaecol. 2001; 22(3):133–41.
42. Louis GMB, et al. Stress reduces conception probabilities across the fertile window: evidence in support of relaxation. Fertil Steril. 2011;95(7):2184–9.
43. Klonoff-Cohen H, Chu E, Natarajan L, Sieber W. A prospective study of stress among women undergoing in vitro fertilization or gamete intrafallopian transfer. Fertil Steril. 2001;71:675–87.
44. Boivin J, Griffiths E, Venetis CA. Emotional distress in infertile women and failure of assisted reproductive technologies: meta-analysis of prospective psychosocial studies. BMJ. 2011;342:223.
45. Domar AD, Backman K, Wiegand B, Friscia D, Orav EJ, Nikolovski J. The relationship between stress and IVF outcome. Paper presented at the annual meeting of ASRM. Denver, CO; 2010

Fertility Preservation

14

Pascale Jadoul, Marie-Madeleine Dolmans,
and Jacques Donnez

Introduction

With the development of combination chemotherapy and radiotherapy for the treatment of malignancies, prognoses have dramatically improved, shifting the area of focus towards preventing posttreatment complications, such as infertility. At the same time, the last decade has seen significant progress in the field of fertility preservation. Several methods are now available to safeguard fertility, and it is the oncologist's and the reproductive endocrinologist's ethical and moral responsibility to discuss these issues with all girls and women with reproductive potential, who are subjected to potentially gonadotoxic therapy.

Indications for Fertility Preservation

Fertility preservation may be required for both oncological and non-oncological indications.

P. Jadoul, M.D. • M.-M. Dolmans, M.D., Ph.D.(✉)
• J. Donnez, M.D., Ph.D.
Department of Gynecology, Cliniques Universitaires Saint-Luc and pôle de Recherche en Cognicologié Institut de recherche Experimentale at clinique, Université Catholique de Louvain, Brussels 1200, Belgium
e-mail: pascale.jadoul@uclouvain.be; marie-madeleine.dolmans@uclouvain.be; jacques.donnez@gmail.com

Oncological Indications

Cancer treatment is the most frequent cause of ovarian damage in women. Both chemo- and radiotherapy may result in ovarian damage.

Chemotherapy

Ovaries are very sensitive to cytotoxic treatment, especially to alkylating agents (e.g., cyclophosphamide, busulfan, melphalan, chlorambucil, dacarbazine, procarbazine, ifosfamide, thiotepa, and nitrogen mustard), which are classified as high risk for gonadal dysfunction (for review, see [1]) (Table 14.1). Cyclophosphamide is the agent most commonly implicated in causing damage to oocytes and granulosa cells in a dose-dependent manner [2].

Follicular destruction induced by alkylating agents generally results in loss of both endocrine and reproductive function, depending on the dose and age of the patient. For example, Larsen et al. [3] reported a fourfold increased risk of POF in teenagers treated for cancer, and the risk increased by a factor of 27 in women between 21 and 25 years of age. Complete amenorrhea was reported after a dose of 5 g of cyclophosphamide in women over 40 years of age, and after doses of 9 and 20 g in women of 30–40 and 20–30 years of age, respectively [4]. A combination of various chemotherapeutic agents further increases gonadal toxicity. After MOPP/ABV [Mustargen (mechlorethamine—nitrogen mustard), Oncovin (vincristine—plant alkaloid), Procarbazine (alkylating agent), Prednisone/

E.S. Ginsburg and C. Racowsky (eds.), *In Vitro Fertilization: A Comprehensive Guide*,
DOI 10.1007/978-1-4419-9848-4_14, © Springer Science+Business Media New York 2012

Table 14.1 Gonadotoxicity of cytotoxic agents

High risk	Intermediate risk	Low/no risk
Cyclophosphamide	Adriamycin (doxorubicin)	Methotrexate
Busulfan	Cisplatin	Bleomycin
Melphalan	Carboplatin	5-Fluorouracil
Cholarambucil		Actinomycin D
Dacarbazine		Mercaptopurine
Procarbazine		Vincristine
Ifosfamide		
Thiotepa		
Nitrogen mustard		

Adriamycin (doxorubicin), Bleomycin (antibiotic), Vinblastine (plant alkaloid)] hybrid chemotherapy, Schilsky et al. [5] found that amenorrhea developed in 89 and 20% of patients over and under 25 years of age at the time of treatment, respectively. The median age of patients who became amenorrheic after therapy was significantly higher than that of patients who maintained normal menses (26 years vs. 20 years; $p=0.008$).

The mechanisms by which chemotherapy impairs ovarian function have not yet been completely elucidated. Besides direct destruction of primordial oocytes [6, 7], vascular damage and fibrosis may contribute to follicular loss [7]. Another potential mechanism of primordial oocyte loss is explained by the burnout theory. When exposed to chemotherapy, growing follicles are destroyed and, as a consequence, inhibitory paracrine factors like anti-Müllerian hormone are decreased. These changes induce continuous recruitment of primordial follicles "burning out" the ovarian reserve.

Radiotherapy

Gonadal damage by radiotherapy mainly depends on total irradiation dose and age at irradiation, with very little hope of persistent ovarian function after 10 Gy of radiotherapy. A model has been developed to predict the age of menopause onset according to radiation dose and age at irradiation [8]. This model has the great virtue of showing that even if ovarian function is maintained after irradiation, the risk of POF is nevertheless high. On the other hand, when chemotherapy is associated with radiotherapy, as is usually the case, this model often overestimates the age of menopause onset and omits the additional deleterious effects of combined chemotherapy.

In addition to ovarian injury, total body irradiation (TBI) may cause damage to uterine vascular and muscular structures, resulting in diminished uterine blood flow, reduced uterine volume, decreased endometrial thickness, and loss of distensibility. When analyzing reports on pregnancy after bone marrow transplantation (BMT) [9–12], it appears that for women who conceive, there is an increased risk of preterm delivery (PTD) and low birth weight in women who have previously undergone BMT, and that the increased risk of PTD is more pronounced after TBI [12, 13]. Irradiation affecting the uterus in childhood and adolescence is associated with a higher incidence of spontaneous miscarriage and intrauterine growth retardation [13, 14]. The extent of the impact of radiation on the uterus may be less pronounced if administered after puberty. Women exposed to pelvic radiation after puberty have a larger uterus and a greater likelihood of live birth than those exposed prior to puberty [15].

Non-oncological Indications (Table 14.2)

Certain benign conditions, such as myelodysplasia, aplastic anemia, thalassemia, drepanocytosis, and multiple sclerosis, as well as severe rheumatic diseases, like Wegener's syndrome, polyarthritis, and systemic lupus erythematosus, may also necessitate administration of high doses

Table 14.2 Nonmalignant pathologies with risk of premature ovarian failure

Bone marrow transplantation
Sickle cell anemia
Thalassemia major
Aplastic anemia
Autoimmune diseases unresponsive to immunosuppressive therapy
Autoimmune diseases requiring chemotherapy
Systemic lupus erythematosus
Rheumatoid arthritis
Behçet's disease
Wegener's disease
Multiple sclerosis
Ovarian pathologies
Recurrent ovarian cysts
Ovarian torsion
Endocrine or genetic diseases
Turner syndrome
Galactosemia
Family history of premature ovarian failure

of chemotherapy with or without BMT. In these patients too, fertility preservation options should be contemplated.

Repeat ovarian surgery, especially for endometriomas, may be associated with POF.

POF may also be related to endocrine or genetic diseases, such as galactosemia and Turner syndrome. Although 30% of girls with Turner syndrome undergo spontaneous pubertal development, only 2–5% experience spontaneous menses with the potential to achieve pregnancy without medical intervention [16]. Ovarian function appears to be preserved for longer in patients with mosaic Turner syndrome [16, 17]. Cryopreservation of ovarian tissue has therefore been proposed to girls with Turner syndrome, especially those with the mosaic type [1, 16, 18, 19].

Options for Fertility Preservation

Several options have been proposed for the preservation of fertility in cancer patients. The choice of the most suitable strategy depends on different parameters, such as age, type of gonadotoxic treatment, timing of chemotherapy, partner status, and risks related to the technique. Fertility counseling should be adapted to individual patients and based on a thorough knowledge of the efficacy, risks, and technical aspects associated with the different fertility preservation methods. The most important issue to consider is ensuring that the intervention does not harm the patient or alter her prognosis by significantly delaying cancer treatment.

Medical Therapy

On the basis of observations that premenarchal girls are less affected by gonadotoxic treatments, oral contraceptives and gonadotropin-releasing hormone agonists (GnRHa) have been used to create a hypogonadotropic state, with low follicle-stimulating hormone (FSH) and luteinizing hormone (LH) concentrations causing decreased follicular recruitment. However, no protective effect of oral contraceptives has been identified [20–22], and serious doubts remain about the efficacy of GnRHa. Initial studies showing a protective effect were nonrandomized, with small patient numbers and historical controls, and used menstruation, not fertility, as an endpoint measure. Although meta-analyses [23–26] and three randomized controlled trials (RCTs) showed a protective effect of GnRH agonists [27–29], a third RCT in women with Hodgkin's lymphoma treated with highly gonadotoxic regimens was recently prematurely halted due to lack of protection [30]. The recent ZORO study reported no significant difference in the restoration of spontaneous cycles and hormone profiles after GnRHa cotreatment compared with controls in patients up to 45 years of age treated for breast cancer [31].

At present, the only clear advantage of hormone treatment is prevention of uterine bleeding, which is especially important in women with hematological malignancies or those undergoing myelosuppressive therapy who may experience severe menorrhagia requiring transfusion due to low platelet counts. The findings of ongoing RCTs in the UK and the US need to be taken into account before any definitive conclusions can be reached. In the meantime, this approach is not recommended.

Other molecules are under investigation for fertility preservation. These molecules could directly prevent DNA damage caused by chemotherapeutic agents on gonads without interfering with their efficiency. In mice, oocytes lacking the gene for acid sphingomyelinase or wildtype oocytes treated with sphingosine-1 phosphate resisted apoptosis induced through anti-cancer therapy [32]. Sphingosine 1-phosphate also preserved fertility in irradiated female mice without propagating genomic damage to offspring [33]. Other experiments in mice show that AS101, a nontoxic immunomodulator, can specifically protect against cyclophosphamide-induced damage in the testes [34].

In Vitro Fertilization and Embryo Cryopreservation

In vitro fertilization (IVF) followed by cryopreservation of embryos is a well established procedure for fertility preservation. Several issues should nevertheless be discussed when considering this technique for fertility preservation purposes.

Fertility Preservation Outcomes

The latest findings from the Society for Assisted Reproductive Technology and the European IVF Monitoring Program report a pregnancy rate of 34% following frozen-thawed embryo transfer in women under 35 years of age and an overall pregnancy rate of 19% [35, 36]. However, there are few published studies on pregnancy rates after IVF carried out as an emergency procedure in cancer patients. In most studies, the mean number of oocytes retrieved and embryos obtained in women undergoing IVF before chemotherapy is not different from women undergoing routine IVF [37–39], although the duration of stimulation and gonadotropin doses may be increased [40]. A recent meta-analysis on ovarian response to stimulation for fertility preservation in women with cancer [41] found that slightly fewer mature oocytes were obtained from women with cancer, but stimulation durations and fertilization rates did not differ between women with or without cancer. An average of 9–10 oocytes [42] and 6 embryos [39] (60% fertilization rate) [43, 44] may be expected, but this is variable and dependent on a woman's ovarian reserve and age, and ovulation-induction protocol chosen.

IVF Protocols

A classic IVF cycle starts during the early follicular phase and takes approximately 2–5 weeks. This delay before cancer treatment could potentially alter the prognosis, so it is essential to have the oncologist's approval before discussing this option with the patient. However, luteal phase IVF is now feasible, reducing the delay before chemotherapy. Follicular recruitment occurs in waves, so it is possible to stimulate recruitment of a new wave of oocytes even after ovulation. Preliminary results suggest that this timing may yield similar results to follicular phase IVF [45].

Emergency IVF should not be proposed after a first course of chemotherapy. Indeed, the number of embryos obtained is very low [46] and concerns have been raised about the quality of embryos derived from oocytes harvested after recent exposure to chemotherapy and the risks of increased congenital malformations [47].

Protocols using GnRH antagonists should be favored, as they are associated with a lower risk of ovarian hyperstimulation syndrome (OHSS) [44], and there is no wait to ensure downregulation has occurred prior to the start of ovulation induction.

In some hormone-dependent cancers (e.g., breast cancer, endometriod ovarian cancer, endometrial cancer), elevated estrogen levels associated with ovarian stimulation and IVF might have a deleterious effect on the disease or on treatment efficacy [42]. Stimulation protocols using tamoxifen and aromatase inhibitors alone or in combination with exogenous FSH have thus been proposed to women suffering from breast cancer [48]. Stimulation protocols using letrozole alongside gonadotropins are currently preferred over tamoxifen protocols, as treatment with letrozole has been shown to be associated with a higher number of retrieved and fertilized oocytes, and lower circulating estradiol levels, compared to tamoxifen protocols [49]. Moreover, short-term (2 year) follow-up of breast cancer patients undergoing ovarian stimulation with letrozole for fertility preservation has not shown any detrimental effects on survival [50]. However, as breast cancers may recur 20 years later, long-term follow-up data are needed.

Further improvements in letrozole stimulation protocols have been reported. Triggering oocyte maturation with GnRHa instead of human chorionic gonadotropin (hCG) decreases estradiol exposure after trigger more rapidly, further reducing the risk of OHSS, a known complication of controlled ovarian stimulation [51]. Although aromatase inhibitors are contraindicated during pregnancy, data indicate that fertility treatments with letrozole are safe and that letrozole use before conception is not associated with increased risks for the fetus [52].

As far as the actual cryopreservation technique is concerned, there is no statistical difference between pregnancy rates after slow freezing or vitrification of embryos [53], although vitrification might prove to be more effective in the future, particularly when blastocysts are frozen. At present, the method of choice should be determined by the assisted reproductive technology (ART) center itself based on its own experience and statistics.

Limitations of IVF and Embryo Cryopreservation

Besides the previously mentioned risks of delay in cancer treatment and potential stimulation of estrogen-dependent tumors, embryo cryopreservation is mostly reserved for adult women with a partner. However, living with cancer, enduring oncological treatment, and being a cancer survivor are all psychologically very demanding. Even when a relationship appears secure, it is impossible to guarantee that this will remain the case. Other techniques that preserve the patient's own fertility should therefore be proposed in addition to embryo cryopreservation.

IVF and Cryopreservation of Mature Oocytes

Cryopreservation of oocytes obtained by ovulation induction and oocyte retrieval for future use in IVF represents an alternative method for fertility preservation, especially in women without a partner.

The first birth after human oocyte cryopreservation was reported back in 1986 [54]. However, low oocyte survival rates and low fertility potential due to problematic freezing processes (slow freezing) were impediments to successful reproduction, with live birth rates of just 2% per oocyte [55]. Vitrification protocols have since greatly improved upon these results. In a meta-analysis conducted by Cobo and Diaz in 2011, vitrification methods were shown to yield higher fertilization, cleavage, and embryo quality rates than slow freezing in egg donors [56].

In experienced hands, vitrified oocytes obtained after IVF in a non-oncological population yield 80–95% survival rates after thawing, 75% fertilization rates, clinical pregnancy rates per cycle of 45–65% and live birth rates of 40% [35, 57]. Pregnancy rates in centers specialized in egg donation are similar with fresh and vitrified oocytes [58]. Despite concerns being raised about the toxicity of high doses of cryoprotectants needed for vitrification of oocytes, no increase in congenital anomalies was observed in a series of more than 1,000 infants born following oocyte vitrification [59, 60].

The first live birth achieved after vitrification of mature oocytes before cancer treatment was reported in 2007 [61]. However, success rates of vitrification of mature oocytes in the context of cancer are much less well documented. Very little has been published on pregnancy rates, making it difficult to give any clear idea of likely success rates when discussing this alternative with women prior to cancer treatment.

In Vitro Maturation for Oocyte or Embryo Cryopreservation

Immature oocytes can be collected during unstimulated cycles for fertility preservation. The speed of the technique, absence of elevated estrogen levels and OHSS risks, and possibility of application to oocytes obtained during ovarian tissue sampling for cryopreservation [62–64] make this technique very attractive for women suffering from cancer. In vitro maturation (IVM) has become an effective treatment option for many infertile women, especially with polycystic ovaries, resulting in the birth of over 2,000 healthy infants without any increase in fetal abnormalities or miscarriage rates in comparable subjects [35]. However, despite satisfactory pregnancy rates, overall pregnancy rates remain lower than those achieved in IVF cycles using in vivo matured oocytes [65].

In experienced centers, women undergoing IVM before cancer treatment can expect retrieval of 8–17 immature oocytes, maturation rates of 50–60% and fertilization rates of 60–70% [66, 67]. HCG is administered when the largest follicle seen on ultrasound measures 12 mm, and oocytes are collected approximately 36 h after HCG injection [67]. Compared to the 2–5 weeks required for a stimulated IVF cycle, immature oocyte retrieval can be done within 2–10 days. Immature oocytes can even be collected during the luteal phase, with similar results to follicular phase retrieval [35, 66]. The process of luteal phase retrieval is performed either 36 h after hCG administration, or after a few days of gonadotropin administration followed by hCG administration. However, to our knowledge, no pregnancies have been reported after fertilization of in vitro-matured oocytes harvested and vitrified before cancer therapy.

Ovarian Cortex Cryopreservation

Harvesting and cryopreservation of ovarian tissue before sterilizing chemo- and/or radiotherapy have been increasingly implemented and documented during the past decade. The main aim of this strategy is to reimplant ovarian tissue in case of POF, and its major advantage is that it is applicable in prepubertal girls [68] and women who cannot delay the start of chemotherapy. The first live birth obtained using this technique was published in 2004 [69]. At least 18 pregnancies have since been described after reimplantation of frozen-thawed ovarian tissue [70–72], with estimated pregnancy rates of 30%. Analysis of the literature yields a wealth of information that can be used when counseling such patients.

Ovarian Tissue Cryopreservation

Important Points That Should Be Included in the Research Protocol

- Ovarian tissue harvesting can be performed by laparoscopy at any age, without postponing chemotherapy. A maximum age limit of 35–37 years is recommended. All pregnancies but one achieved by this technique were in women who had had their ovarian tissue cryopreserved before the age of 30.
- The risks of general anesthesia must be assessed, particularly in patients with mediastinal masses.
- The quantity of ovarian tissue removed should be influenced by the expected probability of POF (i.e., biopsy of a portion of the ovarian cortex of one ovary vs. oophorectomy). At the time of ovarian sampling, once the tissue is in the laboratory, visible follicles can be aspirated and IVM performed [62–64].
- Biopsies should be histologically evaluated to exclude tumor cells and confirm the presence of follicles.
- Removed ovarian tissue should be transported on ice. If necessary, transport is feasible over an extended period of time (up to 24 h) [70, 73].
- The most efficient method of cryopreservation at present appears to be slow freezing.

Ovarian Tissue Reimplantation

- The oncologist's approval should be obtained before proceeding with ovarian tissue reimplantation. All pregnancies achieved after reimplantation of frozen–thawed ovarian tissue occurred after orthotopic reimplantation (i.e., reimplantation into the original site where the ovary was located). Orthotopic ovarian tissue reimplantation can be performed by laparoscopy or laparotomy, and the choice of technique depends on the individual surgeon's skill and experience. In the largest reported series [71], a peritoneal window

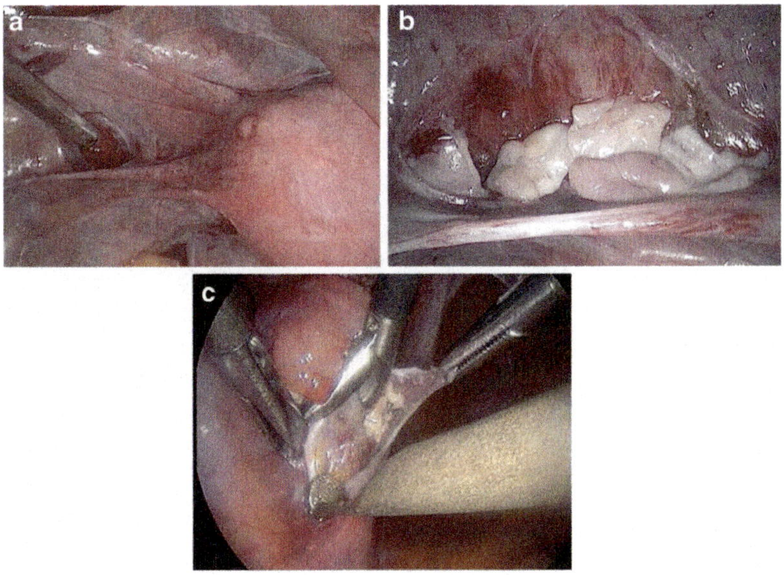

Fig. 14.1 Ovarian cortex reimplantation in a peritoneal pocket. (**a**) Peritoneal pocket in the broad ligament. (**b**) Large pieces of ovarian cortex placed in the peritoneal pocket. (**c**) Small cubes of ovarian cortex placed in a peritoneal pocket under the fallopian tube

(Fig. 14.1) created close to the ovarian hilus and the ovarian medulla (Fig. 14.2) both appear to be equally efficient sites of reimplantation. Large strips (8–10 mm×5 mm) and small cubes (2×2 mm) of tissue both restore ovarian function. Restoration of ovarian function occurs 3½–6½ months after reimplantation, and takes longer in patients who underwent chemotherapy before cryopreservation than in those who did not. Persistence of restored ovarian function has been described for up to 5 years. This duration is shorter in women who received chemotherapy before cryopreservation, and longer in patients younger at the time of cryopreservation. Several women have obtained more than one pregnancy after ovarian tissue reimplantation. More than 50% of women who achieved pregnancy were able to conceive naturally.

- In women undergoing IVF, an increased rate of empty follicle syndrome (as high as 29–35%) was observed [73–75]. No congenital anomalies have so far been encountered in children born using this technique. A significant concern is the possibility of ovarian tissue contamination by malignant cells. In case of Hodgkin's and non-Hodgkin's lymphoma, the risk is minimal, if not nonexistent. In case of leukemia, malignant cells may be present in the bloodstream, running the risk of being transferred [76–78]. Whenever there is a theoretical risk that the frozen tissue may contain malignant cells, all available tests to exclude minimal residual disease should be performed. Besides histological evaluation, analyses by PCR and xenografting to nude mice are available options. Meirow et al. [77] recently identified chronic myeloid leukemia (CML) cells in frozen-thawed ovarian tissue from a patient with the disease using reverse transcription quantitative real-time polymerase chain reaction (RT-qPCR), which proved positive for BCR-ABL1 transcripts. This avoided transplantation of the stored tissue.

In a recent study by our team [76], histology failed to detect malignant cells in fresh and frozen ovarian tissue from CML and acute lymphoblastic leukemia (ALL) patients. However, using disease-specific PCR techniques, we found

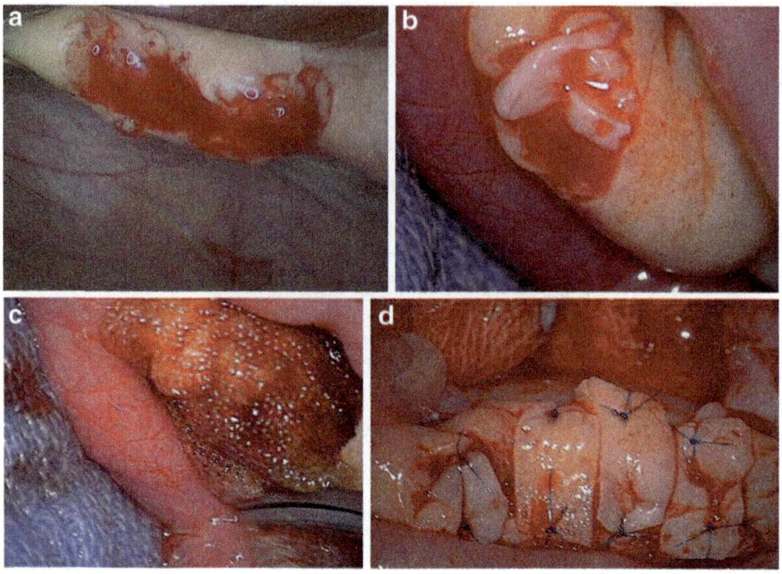

Fig. 14.2 Ovarian cortex reimplantation on the ovarian medulla. (**a**) The cortex of the native atrophic ovary is removed. (**b**) Small strips of thawed ovarian cortex are placed on the medulla. (**c**) The ovary is covered with Interceed (Johnson and Johnson, New Brunswick, USA) to prevent the strips from sliding. (**d**) Larger pieces of thawed ovarian cortex can be sutured to the medulla

contamination of ovarian tissue by leukemic cells in respectively 33 and 70% of CML and ALL patients. Indeed, tissue from two out of six CML patients proved positive for BCR-ABL1 by RT-qPCR. Among the 12 ALL patients, 10 had available molecular markers and seven of them showed positive leukemic markers in their ovarian tissue (translocations or rearrangement genes). This study demonstrated that RT-qPCR was able to detect ovarian contamination by malignant cells in acute as well as chronic leukemia, while histology failed to do so.

What to Do if Cancer Cells Are or May Well Be Present in Ovarian Tissue

In case of risk of contamination, ovarian reimplantation should be avoided. To avoid possible reimplantation of malignant cells (in case of leukemia, for example), two approaches are possible:

1. Reimplantation of isolated follicles in an artificial ovary or scaffold [71, 76, 79].
2. IVM of primordial follicles [80–82].

The first approach involves grafting isolated follicles enzymatically purified from frozen-thawed ovarian tissue [83, 84]. Research is currently under way to design a scaffold to act as an effective support for these follicles. Creation of an artificial ovary [71, 76, 79] is a further avenue warranting ongoing investigation, with the potential to solve all these issues in the future.

IVM of follicles within pieces of cryopreserved ovarian tissue is another way of circumventing this problem, but has not yet yielded pregnancies. Protocols for long-term in vitro culture of human ovarian cortical tissue are nevertheless being developed [80, 82, 85]. It was recently demonstrated that it is possible to achieve accelerated maturation and development of primordial and primary follicles using a two-step culture system [82]. Follicles were shown to maintain bidirectional communication between somatic cells and germ cells, creating an environment conducive to oocyte growth and normal steroid production [86]. Our preliminary results indicate that alginate hydrogels may be a suitable system for in vitro culture of isolated human preantral follicles. A total of 159 small preantral follicles from frozen-thawed tissue were incubated in a 3D system (alginate hydrogel). After 7 days, all of them showed an increase in size, with a survival rate of 90% (oocyte and all granulosa cells viable) [79].

The next frontier will be maturation of oocytes grown in vitro up to metaphase II, fertilization and embryo development, and adaptation of these techniques to primordial follicles and cryopreserved tissues. Significantly accelerated growth of in vitro-cultured oocytes and follicles from primordial to antral stages has been extensively studied [87]. Preantral follicles were obtained on day 6 and then cultured after nonenzymatic isolation for a further 4 days in individual culture medium. Early follicular recruitment was achieved following activin A supplementation in two-step serum- and stroma-free culture [82]. A dose-dependent activin A effect, combined or not with FSH, was shown to inhibit or promote follicle activation and to preserve morphology in both human [82, 88] and bovine [89] experiments.

Ovariopexy and Ovarian Transposition

When radiotherapy is indicated, ovariopexy or ovarian transposition can be proposed in order to displace the ovaries away from the radiation field. In case of craniospinal irradiation, the ovary can be fixed laterally as far as possible from the spine. In case of pelvic irradiation, the ovary can be moved outside the pelvis, which may require section of the utero-ovarian ligament and fallopian tube. The ovary is then anchored, as high as possible, to the anterior abdominal wall, laterally in the paracolic gutter. Titanium clips are placed on the two opposite borders of the ovary to allow radiological identification prior to radiotherapy. The success of preservation of ovarian function by means of ovarian transposition prior to radiotherapy ranges from 16 to 90% [90–93].

Success rates are affected by the degree of scatter radiation, vascular compromise, patient age, radiation dose, and use (or not) of concomitant chemotherapy [94]. When the ovaries are transposed to an abdominal position, spontaneous pregnancy may not be possible unless a second procedure is performed to relocate the ovaries back to the pelvis. Furthermore, should these patients require IVF in the future, oocyte retrieval may be technically more challenging (see Chap. 4 on Oocyte Retrieval for procedure for transabdominal oocyte retrieval). Candidates for ovarian transposition should therefore be selected carefully, taking into account all variables that may affect its success rate. Ovarian cryopreservation should be performed at the same time as transposition, even in the absence of highly gonadotoxic chemotherapy.

Ethical Issues

The two most important ethical issues to consider are to ensure that the intervention does not harm the patient by dangerously delaying cancer treatment and that no remnant cells are reintroduced by subsequent transplantation. Taking these points into account, we agree with Dudzinski [95] that policies to protect the patient's future rights to her gametes should be developed, as well as policies addressing the disposition of the gametes if the patient dies.

Although an adolescent is more vulnerable when consent is sought in the rush to begin chemotherapy, she must be mature enough to understand the risks and benefits of the procedure. Consent must then be discussed extensively, the discussion including both the adolescent patient and her parents, to minimize the risk of conflict of interest or inadvertent caution [96]. Respecting the code of good practice, all patients who may become infertile have the right to receive proper consideration of their interests for future possibilities in the field of ovarian function preservation. Case selection should be carried out on the basis of a multidisciplinary staff discussion including oncologists, gynecologists, biologists, psychologists and pediatricians. Counseling should be given and informed consent obtained from the patient. Cancer treatment takes priority over potential restoration of fertility, but offering the chance to preserve fertility may greatly enhance quality of life for cancer survivors.

In 2012, we believe it is our ethical responsibility to propose cryopreservation of ovarian tissue to all adolescents and young women under IRB protocols, who have to undergo chemotherapy with alkylating agents. If a program does not provide the option of ovarian tissue cryopreservation, practitioners who treat women with cancer should be familiar with programs that do, so that referral may be suggested. Indeed, is it ethical to simply accept the existing discrepancy between males and females with regard to their chances of preserving their fertility following cancer treatment?

Conclusions

Fertility counseling should be given to all women with reproductive potential and parents of all girls subjected to potentially gonadotoxic treatment. The counseling should be adapted to individual patient needs and based on thorough knowledge of the efficacy, risks and technical aspects of the different fertility preservation options. All applicable methods should be discussed in the counseling sessions and, whenever possible, different techniques should be combined to increase the chances of future pregnancy. Primary care physicians and oncologists need to be made aware of the available fertility preservation options in order to prevent loss of valuable time and allow referral to ART centers that offer fertility preservation alternatives.

In addition, social, legal and ethical issues should be taken into account, though these may vary from country to country. The two most important ethical issues to consider are ensuring that the intervention does not harm the patient by dangerously postponing cancer treatment and that no remnant cells are reintroduced by subsequent transplantation. Finally, it is mandatory to give the patient clear information on the expected results and possible risks of the procedures.

References

1. Donnez J, Martinez-Madrid B, Jadoul P, Van Langendonckt A, Demylle D, Dolmans MM. Ovarian tissue cryopreservation and transplantation: a review. Hum Reprod Update. 2006;12:519–35.
2. Meirow D, Lewis H, Nugent D, Epstein M. Subclinical depletion of primordial follicular reserve in mice treated with cyclophosphamide: clinical importance and proposed accurate investigative tool. Hum Reprod. 1999;14:1903–7.
3. Larsen EC, Muller J, Schmiegelow K, Rechnitzer C, Andersen AN. Reduced ovarian function in long-term survivors of radiation- and chemotherapy treated childhood cancer. J Clin Endocrinol Metab. 2003;88: 5307–14.
4. Shalet SM. Effects of cancer chemotherapy on gonadal function of patients. Cancer Treat Rev. 1980;7: 141–52.
5. Schilsky RL, Sherins RJ, Hubbard SM, Wesley MN, Young RC, DeVita VT. Long-term follow up of ovarian function in women treated with MOPP chemotherapy for Hodgkin's disease. Am J Med. 1981;71:552–6.
6. Familiari G, Caggiati A, Nottola SA, Ermimi M, di Benedetto MR, Motta PM. Ultrastructure of human ovarian primordial follicles after combination chemotherapy for Hodgkin's disease. Hum Reprod. 1993;8(12):2080–7.
7. Meirow D, Dor J, Kaufman B, Shrim A, Rabinovici J, Schiff E, Raanani H, Levron J, Fridman E. Cortical fibrosis and blood-vessels damage in human ovaries exposed to chemotherapy. Potential mechanisms of ovarian injury. Hum Reprod. 2007;22(6):1626–33.
8. Wallace WH, Thomson AB, Saran F, Kelsey TW. Predicting age of ovarian failure after radiation to a field that includes the ovaries. Int J Radiat Oncol Biol Phys. 2005;62:738–44.
9. Carter A, Robison LL, Francisco L, Smith D, Grant M, Baker KS, Gurney JG, McGlave PB, Weisdorf DJ, Forman SJ, Bhatia S. Prevalence of conception and pregnancy outcomes after hematopoietic cell transplantation: report from the Bone Marrow Transplant Survivor Study. Bone Marrow Transplant. 2006; 37:1023–9.
10. Loren AW, Chow E, Jacobsohn DA, Gilleece M, Halter J, Joshi S, Wang Z, Sobocinski KA, Gupta V, Hale GA, Marks DI, Stadtmauer EA, Apperley J, Cahn JY, Schouten HC, Lazarus HM, Savani BN, McCarthy PL, Jakubowski AA, Kamani NR, Hayes-Lattin B, Maziarz RT, Warwick AB, Sorror ML, Bolwell BJ, Socié G, Wingard JR, Rizzo JD, Majhail NS. Pregnancy after hematopoietic cell transplantation: a report from the late effects working committee of the Center for International Blood and Marrow Transplant Research (CIBMTR). Biol Blood Marrow Transplant. 2011;17:157–66.
11. Salooja N, Szydlo RM, Socie G, Rio B, Chatterjee R, Ljungman P, Van Lint MT, Powles R, Jackson G, Hinterberger-Fischer M, Kolb HJ, Apperley JF, Late Effects Working Party of the European Group for Blood and Marrow Transplantation. Pregnancy outcomes after peripheral blood or bone marrow transplantation: a retrospective survey. Lancet. 2001; 358:271–6.
12. Sanders JE, Hawley J, Levy W, Gooley T, Buckner CD, Deeg HJ, Doney K, Storb R, Sullivan K, Witherspoon R, Appelbaum FR. Pregnancies following high-dose cyclophosphamide with or without high-dose busulfan or total-body irradiation and bone marrow transplantation. Blood. 1996;87:3045–52.
13. Wallace WHB, Thomson AB, Kelsey TW. The radiosensitivity of the human oocyte. Hum Reprod. 2003;18:117–21.
14. Critchley HO, Wallace WHB, Shalet SM, Mamtora H, Higginson J, Anderson DC. Abdominal irradiation in childhood; the potential for pregnancy. Br J Obstet Gynaecol. 1992;99:392–4.

15. Bath LE, Wallace WH, Critchley HO. Late effects of the treatment of childhood cancer on the female reproductive system and the potential for fertility preservation. Br J Obstet Gynaecol. 2002;109:107–14.
16. Saenger P, Wikland KA, Conway GS, Davenport M, Gravholt CH, Hintz R, Hovatta O, Hultcrantz M, Landin-Wilhelmsen K, Lin A, et al. Fifth International Symposium on Turner Syndrome. Recommendations for the diagnosis and management of Turner syndrome. J Clin Endocrinol Metab. 2001;86:3061–9.
17. Pasquino AM, Passeri F, Pucarelli I, Segni M, Municchi G. Spontaneous pubertal development in Turner's syndrome. Italian Study Group for Turner's Syndrome. J Clin Endocrinol Metab. 1997;82: 1810–3.
18. Borgström B, Hreinsson J, Rasmussen C, Sheikhi M, Fried G, Keros V, Fridström M, Hovatta O. Fertility preservation in girls with turner syndrome: prognostic signs of the presence of ovarian follicles. J Clin Endocrinol Metab. 2009;94:74–80.
19. Oktay K, Oktem O. Fertility preservation medicine: A new field in the care of young cancer survivors. Pediatr Blood Cancer. 2009;53(2):267–73.
20. Longhi A, Pignotti E, Versari M, Asta S, Bacci G. Effect of oral contraceptive on ovarian function in young females undergoing neoadjuvant chemotherapy treatment for osteosarcoma. Oncol Rep. 2003;10(1):151–5.
21. van der Kaaij MA, van Echten-Arends J, Simons AH, Kluin-Nelemans HC. Fertility preservation after chemotherapy for Hodgkin lymphoma. Hematol Oncol. 2010;28(4):168–79.
22. Whitehead E, Shalet SM, Blackledge G, Todd I, Crowther D, Beardwell CG. The effect of combination chemotherapy on ovarian function in women treated for Hodgkin's disease. Cancer. 1983;52(6):988–93.
23. Bedaiwy MA, Abou-Setta AM, Desai N, Hurd W, Starks D, El-Nashar SA, Al-Inany HG, Falcone T. Gonadotropin-releasing hormone analog cotreatment for preservation of ovarian function during gonadotoxic chemotherapy: a systematic review and meta-analysis. Fertil Steril. 2011;95(3):906–14.
24. Ben-Aharon I, Gafter-Gvili A, Leibovici L, Stemmer SM. Pharmacological interventions for fertility preservation during chemotherapy: a systematic review and meta-analysis. Breast Cancer Res Treat. 2010;122(3):803–11.
25. Clowse ME, Behera MA, Anders CK, Copland S, Coffman CJ, Leppert PC, Bastian LA. Ovarian preservation by GnRH agonists during chemotherapy: a meta-analysis. J Womens Health (Larchmt). 2009;18(3):311–9.
26. Kim SS, Lee JR, Jee BC, Suh CS, Kim SH, Ting A, Petroff B. Use of hormonal protection for chemotherapy-induced gonadotoxicity. Clin Obstet Gynecol. 2010;53(4):740–52.
27. Badawy A, Elnashar A, El-Ashry M, Shahat M. Gonadotropin-releasing hormone agonists for prevention of chemotherapy-induced ovarian damage: prospective randomized study. Fertil Steril. 2009;91(3):694–7.
28. del Mastro L, Boni L, Michelotti A, Gamucci T, Olmeo N, Gori S, Giordano M, Garrone O, Pronzato P, Bighin C, Levaggi A, Giraudi S, Cresti N, Magnolfi E, Scotto T, Vecchio C, Venturini M. Effect of the gonadotropin-releasing hormone analogue triptorelin on the occurrence of chemotherapy-induced early menopause in premenopausal women with breast cancer: a randomised trial. J Am Med Assoc. 2011;30(3):269–76.
29. Sverrisdottir A, Nystedt M, Johansson H, Fornander T. Adjuvant goserelin and ovarian preservation in chemotherapy treated patients with early breast cancer: results from a randomized trial. Breast Cancer Res Treat. 2009;117(3):561–7.
30. Behringer K, Wildt L, Mueller H, Mattle V, Ganitis P, van den Hoonaard B, Ott HW, Hofer S, Pluetschow A, Diehl V, Engert A, Borchmann P, German Hodgkin Study Group. No protection of the ovarian follicle pool with the use of GnRH-analogues or oral contraceptives in young women treated with escalated BEACOPP for advanced-stage Hodgkin lymphoma. Final results of a phase II trial from the German Hodgkin Study Group. Ann Oncol. 2010;21(10): 2052–60.
31. Gerber B, von Minckwitz C, Stehle H, Reimer T, Felberbaum R, Maass N, Fischer D, Sommer HL, Conrad B, Ortmann O, Fehm T, Rezai M, Mehta K, Loibl S, German Breast Group Investigators. Effect of luteinizing hormone-releasing hormone agonist on ovarian function after modern adjuvant breast cancer chemotherapy: the GBG 37 ZORO study. J Clin Oncol. 2011;29(17):2334–41.
32. Morita Y, Perez I, Perez F, Miranda S, Ehleiter D, Haimovitz-Friedman A, Fuks Z, Xie Z, Reed JC, Schuchman EH, Kolesnick RN, Tilly JL. Oocyte apoptosis is suppressed by disruption of the acid sphingomyelinase gene or by sphingosine 1-phosphate therapy. Nat Med. 2000;6(10):1109–14.
33. Paris F, Perez GI, Fuks Z, Haimovitz-Friedman A, Nguyen H, Bose M, Ilagan A, Hunt PA, Morgan WF, Tilly JL, Kolesnick R. Sphingosine 1-phosphate preserves fertility in irradiated female mice without propagating genomic damage in offspring. Nat Med. 2002;8(9):901–2.
34. Carmely A, Meirow D, Perets A, Albeck M, Bartoov B, Sredni B. Protective effect of the immunomodulator AS101 against cyclophosphamide-induced testicular damage in mice. Hum Reprod. 2009;24(6):1322–9. Epub 2009 Feb 24.
35. Ata B, Chian RC, Tan SL. Cryopreservation of oocytes and embryos for fertility preservation for female cancer patients. Best Pract Res Clin Obstet Gynaecol. 2010;24(1):101–12.
36. Nyboe Andersen A, Goossens V, Bhattacharya S, Ferraretti AP, Kupka MS, de Mouzon J, Nygren KG, European IVF-monitoring (EIM) Consortium, for the

European Society of Human Reproduction and Embryology (ESHRE). Assisted reproductive technology and intrauterine inseminations in Europe, 2005: results generated from European registers by ESHRE: ESHRE. The European IVF Monitoring Programme (EIM), for the European Society of Human Reproduction and Embryology (ESHRE). Hum Reprod. 2009;24(6):1267–87.

37. Das M, Shehata F, Moria A, Holzer H, Son WY, Tulandi T. Ovarian reserve, response to gonadotropins, and oocyte maturity in women with malignancy. Fertil Steril. 2011;96(1):122–5.
38. Knopman JM, Noyes N, Talebian S, Krey LC, Grifo JA, Licciardi F. Women with cancer undergoing ART for fertility preservation: a cohort study of their response to exogenous gonadotropins. Fertil Steril. 2009;91(4 Suppl):1476–8.
39. Robertson AD, Missmer SA, Ginsburg ES. Embryo yield after in vitro fertilization in women undergoing embryo banking for fertility preservation before chemotherapy. Fertil Steril. 2011;95(2):588–91.
40. Quintero RB, Helmer A, Huang JQ, Westphal LM. Ovarian stimulation for fertility preservation in patients with cancer. Fertil Steril. 2010;93(3):865–8.
41. Friedler S, Koc O, Gidoni Y, Raziel A, Ron-El R. Ovarian response to stimulation for fertility preservation in women with malignant disease: a systematic review and meta-analysis. Fertil Steril. 2012;97(1):125–33.
42. Anderson RA, Wallace WH. Fertility preservation in girls and young women. Clin Endocrinol (Oxf). 2011;75(4):409–19.
43. Leader A, Lishner M, Michaeli J, Revel A. Fertility considerations and preservation in haemato-oncology patients undergoing treatment. Br J Haematol. 2011;153(3):291–308.
44. von Wolff M, Montag M, Dittrich R, Denschlag D, Nawroth F, Lawrenz B. Fertility preservation in women-a practical guide to preservation techniques and therapeutic strategies in breast cancer, Hodgkin's lymphoma and borderline ovarian tumours by the fertility preservation network FertiPROTEKT. Arch Gynecol Obstet. 2011;284(2):427–35.
45. von Wolff M, Thaler CJ, Frambach T, Zeeb C, Lawrenz B, Popovici RM, Strowitzki T. Ovarian stimulation to cryopreserve fertilized oocytes in cancer patients can be started in the luteal phase. Fertil Steril. 2009;92(4):1360–5.
46. Dolmans MM, Demylle D, Martinez-Madrid B, Donnez J. Efficacy of in vitro fertilization after chemotherapy. Fertil Steril. 2005;83(4):897–901.
47. Meirow D, Schiff E. Appraisal of chemotherapy effects on reproductive outcome according to animal studies and clinical data. J Natl Cancer Inst Monogr. 2005;34:21–5.
48. Oktay K, Hourvitz A, Sahin G, Oktem O, Safro B, Cil A, Bang H. Letrozole reduces estrogen and gonadotropin exposure in women with breast cancer undergoing ovarian stimulation before chemotherapy. J Clin Endocrinol Metab. 2006;91(10):3885–90.
49. Oktay K, Buyuk E, Libertella N, Akar M, Rosenwaks Z. Fertility preservation in breast cancer patients: a prospective controlled comparison of ovarian stimulation with tamoxifen and letrozole for embryo cryopreservation. J Clin Oncol. 2005;23(19):4347–53.
50. Azim AA, Costantini-Ferrando M, Oktay K. Safety of fertility preservation by ovarian stimulation with letrozole and gonadotropins in patients with breast cancer: a prospective controlled study. J Clin Oncol. 2008;26(16):2630–5.
51. Oktay K, Turkcuoglu I, Rodriguez-Wallberg KA. GnRH agonist trigger for women with breast cancer undergoing fertility preservation by aromatase inhibitor/FSH stimulation. Reprod Biomed Online. 2010;20(6):783–8.
52. Tulandi T, et al. Congenital malformations among 911 newborns conceived after infertility treatment with letrozole or clomiphene citrate. Fertil Steril. 2006;85(6):1761–5.
53. Kolibianakis EM, Venetis CA, Tarlatzis BC. Cryopreservation of human embryos by vitrification or slow freezing: which one is better? Curr Opin Obstet Gynecol. 2009;21(3):270–4.
54. Chen C. Pregnancy after human oocyte cryopreservation. Lancet. 1986;1:884–6.
55. Oktay K, Cil AP, Bang H. Efficiency of oocyte cryopreservation: a meta-analysis. Fertil Steril. 2006;86(1):70–80.
56. Cobo A, Diaz C. Clinical application of oocyte vitrification: a systematic review and meta-analysis of randomized controlled trials. Fertil Steril. 2011;96(2):277–85.
57. Cobo A, Domingo J, Pérez S, Crespo J, Remohí J, Pellicer A. Vitrification: an effective new approach to oocyte banking and preserving fertility in cancer patients. Clin Transl Oncol. 2008;10(5):268–73.
58. Cobo A, Meseguer M, Remohí J, Pellicer A. Use of cryo-banked oocytes in an ovum donation programme: a prospective, randomized, controlled, clinical trial. Hum Reprod. 2010;25(9):2239–46.
59. Chian RC, Huang JY, Tan SL, Lucena E, Saa A, Rojas A, Ruvalcaba Castellón LA, García Amador MI, Montoya Sarmiento JE. Obstetric and perinatal outcome in 200 infants conceived from vitrified oocytes. Reprod Biomed Online. 2008;16(5):608–10.
60. Noyes N, Porcu E, Borini A. Over 900 oocyte cryopreservation babies born with no apparent increase in congenital anomalies. Reprod Biomed Online. 2009;18(6):769–76.
61. Yang D, Brown SE, Nguyen K, Reddy V, Brubaker C, Winslow KL. Live birth after the transfer of human embryos developed from cryopreserved oocytes harvested before cancer treatment. Fertil Steril. 2007;87(6):1469e1–4.
62. Fasano G, Moffa F, Dechène J, Englert Y, Demeestere I. Vitrification of in vitro matured oocytes collected from antral follicles at the time of ovarian tissue

cryopreservation. Reprod Biol Endocrinol. 2011;23:9–15.
63. Huang JY, Tulandi T, Holzer H, Tan SL, Chian RC. Combining ovarian tissue cryobanking with retrieval of immature oocytes followed by in vitro maturation and vitrification: an additional strategy of fertility preservation. Fertil Steril. 2008;89(3):567–72.
64. Revel A, Revel-Vilk S, Aizenman E, Porat-Katz A, Safran A, Ben-Meir A, Weintraub M, Shapira M, Achache H, Laufer N. At what age can human oocytes be obtained? Fertil Steril. 2009;92(2):458–63.
65. Chian RC, Buckett WM, Tan SL. In-vitro maturation of human oocytes. Reprod Biomed Online. 2004;8(2):148–66.
66. Maman E, Meirow D, Brengauz M, Raanani H, Dor J, Hourvitz A. Luteal phase oocyte retrieval and in vitro maturation is an optional procedure for urgent fertility preservation. Fertil Steril. 2011;95(1):64–7.
67. Moria A, Das M, Shehata F, Holzer H, Son WY, Tulandi T. Ovarian reserve and oocyte maturity in women with malignancy undergoing in vitro maturation treatment. Fertil Steril. 2011;95(5):1621–3.
68. Jadoul P, Dolmans MM, Donnez J. Fertility preservation in girls during childhood: is it feasible, efficient and safe and to whom should it be proposed? Hum Reprod Update. 2010;16(6):617–30.
69. Donnez J, Dolmans MM, Demylle D, Jadoul P, Pirard C, Squifflet J, Martinez-Madrid B, van Langendonckt A. Livebirth after orthotopic transplantation of cryopreserved ovarian tissue. Lancet. 2004;364(9443):1405–10.
70. Dittrich R, Lotz L, Keck G, Hoffmann I, Mueller A, Beckmann MW, van der Ven H, Montag M. Live birth after ovarian tissue autotransplantation following overnight transportation before cryopreservation. Fertil Steril. 2011;97(2):387–90.
71. Donnez J, Silber S, Andersen CY, Demeestere I, Piver P, Meirow D, Pellicer A, Dolmans MM. Children born after autotransplantation of cryopreserved ovarian tissue. A review of 13 live births. Ann Med. 2011;43(6):437–50.
72. Revel A, Laufer N, Ben Meir A, Lebovich M, Mitrani E. Micro-organ ovarian transplantation enables pregnancy: a case report. Hum Reprod. 2011;26:1097–103.
73. Andersen CY, Rosendahl M, Byskov AG, Loft A, Ottosen C, Dueholm M, Schmidt KL, Andersen AN, Ernst E. Two successful pregnancies following autotransplantation of frozen/thawed ovarian tissue. Hum Reprod. 2008;23(10):2266–72.
74. Dolmans MM, Donnez J, Camboni A, Demylle D, Amorim C, Van Langendonckt A, Pirard C. IVF outcome in patients with orthotopically transplanted ovarian tissue. Hum Reprod. 2009;24(11):2778–87.
75. Meirow D, Levron J, Eldar-Geva T, Hardan I, Fridman E, Zalel Y, Schiff E, Dor J. Pregnancy after transplantation of cryopreserved ovarian tissue in a patient with ovarian failure after chemotherapy. N Engl J Med. 2005;353(3):318–21.
76. Dolmans MM, Marinescu C, Saussoy P, Van Langendonckt A, Amorim C, Donnez J. Reimplantation of cryopreserved ovarian tissue from patients with acute lymphoblastic leukemia is not safe. Blood. 2010;116:2908–14.
77. Meirow D, Hardan I, Dor J, Fridman E, Elizur S, Ra'anani H, Sluyusarevsky E, Amariglio N, Schiff E, Rechavi G, Nagler A, Ben Yehuda D. Searching for evidence of disease and malignant cell contamination in ovarian tissue stored from hematologic cancer patients. Hum Reprod. 2008;23:1007–13.
78. Rosendahl M, Andersen MK, Ralfkiaer E, Kjeldsen L, Andersen MK, Andersen CY. Evidence of residual disease in cryopreserved ovarian cortex from female patients with leukemia. Fertil Steril. 2010;94:2186–90.
79. Amorim CA, Van Langendonckt A, David A, Dolmans MM, Donnez J. Survival of human pre-antral follicles after cryopreservation of ovarian tissue, follicular isolation and in vitro culture in a calcium alginate matrix. Hum Reprod. 2009;24:92–9.
80. Hovatta O, Wright C, Krausz T, Hardy K, Winston RML. Human primordial, primary and secondary ovarian follicles in long-term culture: effect of partial isolation. Hum Reprod. 1999;14:2519–24.
81. Hovatta O. Cryopreservation and culture of human ovarian cortical tissue containing early follicles. Review. Eur J Obstet Gynecol Reprod Biol. 2004;113:S50–4.
82. Telfer EE, McLaughlin M, Ding C, Thong KJ. A two-step serum-free culture system supports development of human oocytes from primordial follicles in the presence of activin. Hum Reprod. 2008;23:1151–8.
83. Dolmans MM, Martinez-Madrid B, Gadisseux E, Guiot Y, Yuan WY, Torre A, Camboni A, Van Langendonckt A, Donnez J. Short-term transplantation of isolated human ovarian follicles and cortical tissue into nude mice. Reproduction. 2007;134:253–62.
84. Dolmans MM, Yuan WY, Camboni A, Torre A, Van Langendonckt A, Martinez-Madrid B, Donnez J. Development of antral follicles after xenografting of isolated small human preantral follicles. Reprod Biomed Online. 2008;16:705–11.
85. Abir R, Franks S, Mobberley MA, Moore PA, Margara RA, Winston RM. Mechanical isolation and in vitro growth of preawntral and small antral human follicles. Fertil Steril. 1997;68:682–8.
86. Jeruss JS, Woodruff TK. Preservation of fertility in patients with cancer. N Engl J Med. 2009;360:902–11.
87. Telfer EE, McLaughlin M. In vitro development of ovarian follicles. Semin Reprod Med. 2011;29:15–23.
88. Ding CC, Thong KJ, Krishna A, Telfer EE. Activin A inhibits activation of human primordial follicles in vitro. J Assist Reprod Genet. 2010;27:141–7.
89. McLaughlin M, Telfer EE. Oocyte development in bovine primordial follicles is promoted by activin and

FSV within a two-step serum-free culture. Reproduction. 2010;139(6):971–8. Epub 2010 mar 5.
90. Aubard Y, Piver P, Pech JC, Galinat S, Teissier MP. Ovarian tissue cryopreservation and gynecologic oncology: a review. Eur J Obstet Gynecol Reprod Biol. 2001;97:5–14.
91. Morice P, Juncker L, Rey A, El-Hassan J, Haie-Meder C, Castaigne D. Ovarian transposition for patients with cervical carcinoma treated by radiosurgical combination. Fertil Steril. 2000;74:743–8.
92. Scott SM, Schlaff W. Laparoscopic medial oophoropexy prior to radiation therapy in an adolescent with Hodgkin's disease. J Pediatr Adolesc Gynecol. 2005;18:355–7.
93. Thibaud E, Ramirez M, Brauner R, Flamant F, Zucker JM, Fekete C, Rappaport R. Preservation of ovarian function by ovarian transposition performed before pelvic irradiation during childhood. J Pediatr. 1992;121:880–4.
94. Sonmezer M, Oktay K. Fertility preservation in female patients. Hum Reprod Update. 2004;10:251–66.
95. Dudzinski DM. Ethical issues in fertility preservation for adolescent cancer survivors: oocyte and ovarian tissue cryopreservation. J Pediatr Adolesc Gynecol. 2004;17:97–102.
96. Bukovsky A. Can ovarian infertility be treated with bone marrow- or ovary-derived germ cells? Reprod Biol Endocrinol. 2005;3:36.
97. Carely A, Meirow D, Peretz A, Albeck m, Bartoov B, Sredni (2009). Protective effect of the immunomodulator AS101 against cyclophosphmide-induced testicular damage in mice. Jun;24(6):1322–9.

Ongoing Quality Assessment/ Improvement in Clinical IVF

15

Charles L. Bormann and Catherine Racowsky

Introduction

The overriding goal in all medical fields is to provide the highest level of care to each patient. In an infertility clinic, this is largely measured by the program's success rate, particularly by the delivery rate. Thus, the overall goal is to maximize the possibility of every couple conceiving a healthy singleton pregnancy. Until that goal is achieved, there will always be room for improvement, and even if that point is reached, a strong total quality management (QM) system must be in place in order to maintain that success. Towards that end, there are numerous variables that go into each in vitro fertilization (IVF) cycle that must be monitored and maintained.

When a clinic experiences any decrease in success it is common for both the clinical team (physicians and nurses) to question the laboratory for these declines and, likewise, for the laboratory staff to question performance in the clinic. In an ideal infertility practice, both the clinical staff and laboratory staff will have strong quality management systems in place which, when combined with collegial and open communication, will help identify the root cause of a decline in success rates.

It would be bold to suggest that the laboratory is exclusively responsible for any changes in success rates of a clinic. There are clearly many clinical variables that impact success, such as patient stimulations, egg retrieval efficiency, and embryo transfer expertise. However, performance of the laboratory is a critical component of an infertility program. As such, each IVF laboratory is obligated to maintain consistency in performance and to strive for continuous improvement through an effective quality management program. In the USA, the Clinical Laboratory Improvement Amendments of 1988 (CLIA 88) mandates that all laboratories implement a quality management program that monitors and evaluates the overall quality of laboratory services [1].

In this chapter, we first define quality control, quality assurance, and quality improvement, and then describe four major areas of quality management that must be adhered to in order to ensure performance standards are maintained, patient safety is ensured, and overall care to patients is of the highest quality. Finally, we consider the design of trials focused on quality improvement.

C.L. Bormann, Ph.D. (✉)
Department of Obstetrics, Gynecology, and Reproductive Biology, Brigham and Women's Hospital, Harvard Medical School, 75 Francis Street, ASB 1+3, Room 082, Boston, MA 02115, USA
e-mail: cbormann@partners.org

C. Racowsky, Ph.D.
Division of Reproductive Endocrinology and Infertility, Department of Obstetrics and Gynecology, Brigham and Women's Hospital, Boston, MA 02115, USA
e-mail: cracowsky@partners.org

E.S. Ginsburg and C. Racowsky (eds.), *In Vitro Fertilization: A Comprehensive Guide*, DOI 10.1007/978-1-4419-9848-4_15,

General Principles of Quality Management

Definitions

Quality control (*QC*): Quality control is focused on collection of data, and therefore involves measures and activities undertaken to control the quality of products, methods, equipment, and the environment to ensure that the laboratory is functioning correctly. These activities should be undertaken at regular and defined intervals to prevent ongoing undetected problems that lead to a compromise in patient care [2]. Accordingly, QC activities should run concurrently with laboratory activities to ensure that the laboratory produces the same results every time [3].

Quality assurance (*QA*): In general terms, QA is defined as the entirety of systematic activities implemented within a quality management system that are necessary to provide adequate confidence that a product or service will satisfy its required quality characteristics [4]. In a laboratory, QA is the comprehensive program to monitor and to evaluate the entire process that goes on within the laboratory. This includes all activities and programs intended to ensure or improve the performance of the laboratory and therefore the quality of care to patients. Quality assurance includes both analyses of the QC data that are collected, as well as measures such as record keeping, maintaining up-to-date comprehensive laboratory manuals, routine evaluation and education of laboratory staff, results reporting, treatment auditing, incident reporting, proficiency testing, as well establishing the protocols for QC methodology [2, 3]. Most QA activities run concurrently with laboratory procedures as an integral part of daily work, although those involving QC data review and analyses are typically performed retrospectively [3].

Quality improvement (*QI*): QI is the process used to enhance all phases of the laboratory performance and so differs from QA because QA is designed to find problems/errors and correct them. QI includes those procedures that are incorporated into the lab in an effort to improve a specific aspect of the lab [3].

Total quality management (*TQM*): Total Quality Management is an all-encompassing concept that integrates quality control, quality assurance, and quality improvement. It is more of a philosophy than a model. The objective of TQM is to strive continuously to improve every aspect of a service and to provide an optimal product as efficiently as possible. This requires continuous scrutiny of all components of the QC, QA, and QI programs. Keck and colleagues [2] identified 14 important elements that make up a TQM program (Table 15.1).

The Plan-Do-Check-Act Cycle

Continuous measurement and feedback are crucial elements in a TQM Program [2]. One of the most simplified and most recognizable models utilized to identify and test process changes is the "Plan-Do-Check-Act" or PDCA Cycle (Fig. 15.1), sometimes referred to as the Shewhart or Deming Cycle [4, 5]. This model is recognizable to most scientists, as it follows the same principles as the scientific method. The model can be applied to all aspects of QC/QA/QI and can serve as a guide for monitoring a laboratory's performance and for making quality improvements. Once the area for monitoring or improvement has been identified, these four basic steps (plan, do, check, and act) can be followed to test process changes.

1. *Plan*: This is the step where objectives are established, whether it be to identify a problem or implement an improvement. Expected outcomes should be established and appropriate indicators for measurement are identified. When possible, it is best for the focus to be narrowed, with effects tested on a small scale. This approach will help eliminate compounding variables [6, 7].
2. *Do*: At this step, the action is taken to implement the plan or execute a new process. This step involves preparation of criteria, data col-

Table 15.1 The elements comprising a total quality improvement program

1	Appropriately educated and trained personnel with training records
2	Complete listing of all technical procedures formed
3	Housekeeping procedures: cleaning and decontamination procedures
4	Correct operation, calibration, and maintenance of all instruments with manuals and logbook records
5	Adequate and current procedure policy and safety manuals
6	Consistent and proper execution of appropriate techniques and methods
7	Proper documentation, record keeping, and reporting of results
8	Thorough description of specimen collection and handling, including verification procedures for patient identification and chain of custody
9	Safety procedures, including appropriate storage of materials
10	Infection control measures
11	Documentation of suppliers and sources of chemicals and supplies, with dates of receipt/expiry
12	System for appraisal of test performance correction of deficiencies and implementation of advances and improvements
13	Quality materials, tested with bioassays when appropriate
14	Quality assurance programs

From Keck et al. [2]

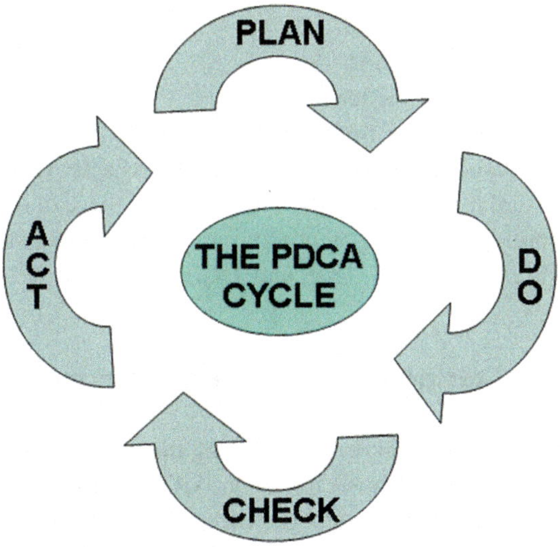

Fig 15.1 The Plan-Do-Check-Act or "PDCA" cycle. This cycle illustrates the process for continuous measurement, monitoring, and feedback in a Total Quality Management Program

lection, measurements, charting, and analysis, i.e., QC activities [6, 7].

3. *Check*: During this step, the results collected in the "Do" step are analyzed and compared against expected outcomes previously established in the "Plan" phase of the cycle. This step is used to detect any differences or deviations in the implementation of the plan and also to look at the appropriateness and completeness of the plan. Results from these analyses may also influence the way in which the "Do" step is executed for future measurements [6, 7].
4. *Act*: During this final step, all significant differences between the actual and planned results are closely scrutinized. Each of these differences is analyzed for their root causes and corrective actions are put into place to improve the process.

When progression through the above four steps does not result in the need to improve, the objective of the previously implemented PDCA should be refined for use in the next iteration of the cycle. Alternatively, the plan can shift to a new focus at a different stage of the process [6, 7].

Patient and Tissue Identification

The importance of patient and tissue identification in the IVF laboratory cannot be overstated. In the field of assisted reproduction, there is no room for mistakes. From a patient's perspective, going through IVF can be a very vulnerable experience. These patients entrust the laboratory with the care of their gametes and embryos. While this responsibility may be routine for laboratory staff, the idea of relinquishing this care and control may feel very unnatural and stressful for couples. These fears can be overwhelming when the possibility of any type of identification error within a clinic or laboratory is considered. Unfortunately, errors such as using the wrong sperm for insemination [8] or transfer of the wrong embryos [9, 10] have been reported in our field. In such dire incidents, there was a clear breakdown in verification of patient identification. The possibility of misidentifying or mixing up a sample is probably the single greatest concern for any IVF laboratory.

Regulatory Requirements for Patient and Tissue Identification

The College of American Pathologists (CAP) has developed detailed regulations for patient identification during specimen collection and handling in the IVF laboratory. These regulations are incorporated into the General Laboratory Checklist [11] and the Reproductive Laboratory Checklist [12]. The most salient of these regulations include the requirements for two patient identifiers (e.g., patient name, date of birth, hospital number, social security number, requisition number, accession number), a written policy regarding correction of information on specimen labels, a chain-of-custody protocol for all reproductive gametes or embryos, and a "time-out" prior to an egg retrieval and embryo transfer procedure.

Identification Checkpoints: Protocol Development

Each laboratory must identify all points along the way in which patient identification is required and by whom. One very effective way of identifying such checkpoints is to create a process map or flowchart for all steps of IVF. Several excellent examples and illustrations of such process mapping can be found in David Mortimer's textbook, "Quality and Risk Management in the IVF Laboratory" [4]. This textbook describes how to build both simple and complex process maps, and how to develop flowcharts, top-down and swim-lane process maps and textual top-down process maps for the IVF laboratory. With such process maps, one can pinpoint exact points in the IVF process that patient identification needs to be verified (Table 15.2).

Once the points of patient identification have been ascertained, the laboratory can establish checklists to monitor the chain of custody of each sample and to ensure that misidentification does not occur. Use of checklists in extremely complex processes, such as those performed in the IVF laboratory, help reduce or greatly eliminate procedural drift and the possibility of errors [13]. Therefore, it is strongly recommended that checklists are developed for the following procedures:

- Sperm receiving/processing
- Oocyte retrieval
- Insemination/ICSI
- Embryo transfer

The authors find that such checklists in their own laboratory are extremely useful as active and visual reminders for the completion of these daily routines, which potentially carry very high risk (Figs. 15.2, 15.3, 15.4, and 15.5) [7].

Monitoring the Identification Process

There is natural drift in the way most operations are performed however, in an ART laboratory, it is critical that protocol or procedural drift is readily identified and corrected. This is particularly true for patient and tissue identification where there is absolutely no room for error; the processes must be watertight and stable at all times. Therefore, ongoing monitoring of the utilization and effectiveness of the patient identification process is essential. Without such a monitoring system in place, a failure in the process may occur that could be disastrous.

Depending upon the goal of the monitoring, an entire checklist can be analyzed or just a specified section. For example, one way to monitor the success of the insemination checklist is to

Table 15.2 Steps in the IVF laboratory requiring patient and tissue identification.

Procedural step	Suggested identification steps				
Sperm collection	Cup label	Patient ID at drop off	Chain of custody	Lab receiving	
Sperm prep	Cup ID	Gradient tube ID	Wash tube ID	Final prep ID	
Oocyte collection	Time out patient ID	Retrieval tubes ID	Retrieval dishes ID	IM dish ID	Incubator ID
IVF	Incubator ID	Sperm ID	Oocyte ID	Incubator ID	
ICSI	Incubator ID	Egg cleaning ID	ICSI dish ID	Sperm ID	Incubator ID
IVF fertilization check	Incubator ID	Fert dish ID	Wash dish ID	Culture dish ID	Incubator ID
ICSI fertilization check	Incubator ID	Culture dish ID	Incubator ID		
Embryo grading	Incubator ID	Culture dish ID	Incubator ID		
Assisted hatching/biopsy	Incubator ID	Culture dish/embryo ID	Incubator ID		
Embryo transfer	Patient ID	Incubator ID	Culture dish ID	Transfer dish ID	Incubator ID
Cryopreservation	Straw ID	Cane ID	Freeze dish ID	Incubator ID	Culture dish ID

TEMPLATE FOR SEMEN VERIFICATION/REQUISITION

Female Label	Partner Label

PHYSICIAN REQUESTING THE TEST: ______________________________

Directions for collecting a semen specimen are posted on the wall of the lounge. Please read them and carefully follow all directions. After collecting your specimen, please give your specimen to the unit receptionist.

WRITE YOUR NAME ON THE LABEL PROVIDED AND PLACE THIS ON THE SPECIMEN CUP
UNLABELLED CONTAINERS WILL NOT BE PROCESSED

PATIENT TO COMPLETE THE FOLLOWING

DATE/TIME COLLECTED: ______________ DAYS SINCE LAST EJACULATION: ________

This sample has been collected as follows (please explain any changes on the comments line)

SPECIMEN COLLECTED FOR: Fresh ART cycle Comments:______________

METHOD OF COLLECTION: Ejaculation Comments:______________

COLLECTION VESSEL: Sterile Specimen Cup (provided) Comments:______________

ENTIRE SAMPLE COLLECTED? Yes If no, 1st or 2nd portion lost (circle) Comments:______________

SAMPLE STORED AT ROOMP TEMP AFTER COLLECTION? Yes Comments:______________

PLEASE LIST ANY MEDICATIONS YOU ARE ON: ______________

IF YOU HAVE HAD MEDICAL CONDITION CHANGES IN PAST 60 DAYS, PLEASE EXPLAIN:

____

Do you or your partner currently smoke cigarettes? I do ________ My partner does________

If so, how many packs per day? I smoke ________packs My partner smokes ______packs

OTHER COMMENTS: ______________________________

I certify that this is my sample to be used for inseminating the eggs of my partner as indicated above:

Signature: ______________________ Date: ______________

STAFF TO COMPLETE: Do not accept the sample if: mislabeled, illegible, or the patient has not completed this form

Picture ID'd		(y/n)	Comments:
Sample Labeled Correctly:		(y/n)	Comments:
Received Intact?		(y/n)	Vessel appears sterile and tightly capped)

Date/Time Received: Received by:

______________________________ Chain of custody #1

______________________________ Chain of custody #2

______________________________ Chain of custody #3

Case Identifier (ER Date-Case#) ______________

Comments

Fig. 15.2 An example of a Semen Verification/Requisition form. This form is used in the IVF laboratory at Brigham and Women's Hospital, Boston, MA

perform regular audits on the relevant documented steps and sign-offs for a specified series of patient charts. Any identified deviation from protocol must be immediately addressed with a written Incident Report, root cause analysis, and corrective action to prevent repeat of such an incident.

Another beneficial way to measure and confirm effectiveness of patient and sample identification protocols is to perform mock cases. These dem-

TEMPLATE FOR CHECKLIST FOR OOCYTE RETRIEVAL

(Retrieval embryologist must check all boxes, initial patient chart after each confirmation performed, and also initial below to confirm check completion)

Patient ID Sticker	Partner ID Sticker

HOOD SETUP

- [ ] Hood surface and microscope stage area clean
- [ ] Dissecting microscope turned on with oculars and focus adjusted ready for use
- [ ] Numbered Petri dishes present and pre-warmed in hood
- [ ] At least 2 fire-polished, smooth tipped Pasteur pipettes available with pipettor or pipette bulb at hand
- [ ] 1ml syringes with needles, and Ultra Fine Sharpie by microscope

RETRIEVAL INCUBATOR

- [ ] Only contains unlabeled dishes (on top shelf) and dishes labeled with ID's of the patient being retrieved
- [ ] Patient last name and Case ID confirmed on dishes to be used for the retrieval
- [ ] Dish ID confirmed, and confirmation documented by embryologist doing the retrieval, by initialing on Egg Retrieval Sheet
- [ ] ID of dishes confirmed by second embryologist and confirmation documented by initialing on Egg Retrieval Sheet

SURGICAL PAUSE

- [ ] Retrieval embryologist present at surgical pause which includes 2 identifiers, the planned procedure stated and confirmation of written physician orders in chart
- [ ] Visual confirmation of patient ID from her hospital bracelet
- [ ] Documented confirmation of patient ID by initialing on the Egg Retrieval Sheet

PROCEDURE

- [ ] All oocyte-cumulus complexes (OCCs) collected and set-up in labeled dishes per protocol

  Any unlabelled ("spare") dishes used?
  - [ ] No
  - [ ] Yes, then:
    - [ ] Dishes checked for absence of any OCCs before use
    - [ ] Dishes labeled with patient last name and Case # immediately after placement of OCCs
- [ ] OCC tallies confirmed, number of OCCs in each dish recorded on the lids
- [ ] Final egg tally recorded on Oocyte/Embryo Sheet
- [ ] Dishes with OCCs set up in a culture incubator with the Incubator and Shelf Number recorded on the Oocyte/Embryo Sheet (e.g. 17-3 for Incubator #17, Shelf #3).
- [ ] No OCCs in any remaining dishes in Retrieval Incubator
- [ ] Lids of any remaining dishes labeled with pt IDs replaced with new, clean lids; dishes placed on top shelf
- [ ] Chart updated
- [ ] Hood wiped down with Multiclean and UV light turned on for at least 10 minutes

Initials: ______________________

Fig. 15.3 A template for the Checklist for Oocyte Retrievals. This form is used in the IVF laboratory at Brigham and Women's Hospital, Boston, MA

TEMPLATE FOR CHECKLIST FOR INSEMINATION/ICSI *(circle as appropriate)*

(Insemination/ICSI embryologist must checkall boxes, initial patient chart after each confirmation performed, and then initial below to confirm check completion)

Patient ID Sticker	Partner ID Sticker

HOOD SETUP

- ☐ Hood surface and microscope stage area clean of any 1ml pipettes or used pipette tips
- ☐ Dissecting microscope turned on with oculars and focus adjusted ready for use
- ☐ Hood clear of any dishes containing OCCs
- ☐ Hood clear of any micro-vials containing sperm
- ☐ Hood clear of any used pipette tips
- ☐ Pipettor WITHOUTpipette tip attached, rack, and 1ml unused sterile pipette at hand

CHART AND INCUBATOR CHECK

Immediately before removing sperm from incubator:

- ☐ Double sign-off by two staff on Oocyte/Embryo Sheet that no tip on pipette
- ☐ Link between Incubator/Shelf #'s (e.g. 17-3 for Incubator #17, Shelf #3) to Name and Case# on Oocyte/Embryo Sheet, cross-checked and matched against incubator board.

IVF INSEMINATION

- ☐ Confirmed double sign-off on Oocyte/Embryo Sheet of inseminate volume indicated on Sperm Prep Sheet and pipettor adjusted to that volume
- ☐ Patient name and Case# re-confirmed against Incubator/Shelf location
- ☐ Confirmation by two staff of sperm micro-vial ID linkage with name and Case# on patient chart whose OCCs are to be inseminated
- ☐ Patient name and Case# confirmed on all dishes
- ☐ Inseminate mixed with 1 ml pipette attached to blue pipettor and pipette discarded
- ☐ 1st dish inseminated and checked for sperm concentration under inverted scope, any adjustments made if necessary and remaining OCCs inseminated per protocol
- ☐ Dishes containing inseminated OCCs returned to their home Incubator/Shelf #
- ☐ Sperm micro-vial discarded
- ☐ Insemination volume, and date/time insemination done documented and initialed on Oocyte/Embryo Sheet
- ☐ Chart placed in dedicated station for fertilization check

ICSI

- ☐ Patient name and Case# re-confirmed against Incubator/Shelf location
- ☐ Confirmation by two staff of sperm micro-vial ID linkage with name and Case# on patient chart whose OCCs are to be injected
- ☐ Sperm drop in ICSI dish loaded with patient sperm
- ☐ Oocytes injected per protocol and then oocytes returned to their home Incubator/Shelf #
- ☐ Date/time ICSI recorded and Oocyte/Embryo Sheet initialed
- ☐ Any sperm needed for day 1 injections?
  - ☐ No: Sperm discarded ☐ Yes: Sperm micro-vial in incubator
- ☐ Chart placed in dedicated station for fertilization check

Initials: ____________________

Fig. 15.4 A template for the Checklist for Insemination or Intracytoplasmic Sperm Injection (ICSI). This form is used in the IVF laboratory at Brigham and Women's Hospital, Boston, MA

TEMPLATE FOR CHECKLIST FOR EMBRYO TRANSFER

(Embryologist assisting with the transfer must checkall boxes, initial patient chart after each confirmation performed, and then initial below to confirm check completion)

Patient ID Sticker	Partner ID Sticker

HOOD SETUP

- ☐ Hood surface and microscope stage area clean
- ☐ Dissecting microscope turned on with oculars and focus adjusted ready for use
- ☐ HEPES dishes prepared and pre-warmed in hood per protocol
- ☐ Stripper with new tip attached

PAPERWORK AND INCUBATOR CHECK

- ☐ Information relating to number of embryos to transfer recorded on Oocyte/Embryo Sheet
- ☐ No dishes in the Transfer Incubator

PREPARATION OF EMBRYOS FOR TRANSFER

- ☐ Link between Incubator/Shelf #'s (e.g. 17-3 for Incubator #17, Shelf #3) to Name and Case# on Oocyte/Embryo Sheet, cross-checked and matched against incubator board
- ☐ Patient name and Case# re-confirmed against Incubator/Shelf location
- ☐ Dishes relocated to Transfer Incubator
- ☐ Patient name and Case# re-confirmed by physician performing the transfer
- ☐ Documented confirmation of embryo ID by inserting initials in "Emb's ID" box on the Oocyte/Embryo Sheet

SURGICAL PAUSE

- ☐ Present at surgical pause, which includes pt 2 identifiers, the planned procedure stated and as written in physician orders and confirmation of number of embryos to be transferred
- ☐ Documented confirmation of patient ID from hospital bracelet and with verbal patient confirmation by inserting initials in"Pt ID" box on the Oocyte/Embryo Sheet
- ☐ Verbal confirmation with patient regarding number of embryos to transfer

PROCEDURE

- ☐ Transfer catheter loaded with embryos and passed off to physician per protocol
- ☐ If difficulty with transfer, embryos returned to original culture dish
- ☐ After transfer, catheter immediately rinsed to confirm absence of embryos
- ☐ Any remaining selected embryos re-loaded and passed off to physician
- ☐ Embryos destined for freezing?
  - ☐ No: All dishes checked and then discarded
  - ☐ Yes, then:
    - ☐ Dishes returned to "home" Incubator and Shelf; Cryo person notified
- ☐ Chart updated and placed at appropriate station per protocol

Initials: ______________________

Fig. 15.5 A template for the Checklist for Embryo Transfers. This form is used in the IVF laboratory at Brigham and Women's Hospital, Boston, MA

onstrations should mimic the laboratory's process of receiving sperm samples, frozen tissues, egg retrievals, and should be performed for all steps involved with each of the protocols including routine insemination, ICSI, PGD, embryo transfer, embryo cryopreservation and embryo disposition. The laboratory should label all paperwork, collection containers, incubators, dishes, etc., as if they were handling a real case. These demonstrations should include all embryology team members so that each member can participate during each step of the identification process.

It is during these mock cases that problems and areas of confusion can be most readily identified, discussed, and corrected. Such mocks also provide an opportunity to reinforce the importance of all the patient identification checkpoints; a designated person should take notes as these will be used as the measurement for monitoring the identification process.

During mock cases, one may learn that some embryologists label dishes differently from others or that some have a more difficult time reading different color markers or names written with a diamond cutter. During these trials, one may also learn that some team members only read names from the dish lids and not the bottom of the dish or that they are verifying a patient's name from laboratory notes (eraser board) instead of directly from their medical record.

Supply Management

Human embryos exhibit plasticity, which allows them to develop in a variety of culture environments. However, they are exquisitely sensitive to suboptimal or compromised conditions which, in turn, may result in impaired development and potentially compromised pregnancy outcomes [14, 15]. The toxicity of supplies used for human embryo culture has been well-documented [3, 16, 17] and recent reports provide evidence that quality of supplies remains variable [18–23]. Therefore, it is critical that all materials and reagents used for handling gametes or culturing embryos in a clinical IVF laboratory are tested for toxicity.

Standards for Supply Management

The International Organization for Standardization, (ISO), and the Fertility Clinic Success Rate and Certification Act (FCSRCA) model program in the USA, each spell out standards for a comprehensive quality management program, including those relevant to supply management. CAP follows the principles and standards of these organizations and serves as a model for Good Laboratory Practices for IVF laboratories. Commercial suppliers provide Certificates of Analyses for all IVF-specific products. Nevertheless, to meet the requirements of the above organizations, the IVF laboratory must have required standards for supply management (Appendix 1).

Bioassays for Supply QC

The two assays most utilized for assessing toxicity in contact materials are the human sperm survival assay, and the mouse embryo assay (Table 15.3) [3, 26]. In this context, "contact materials" are, quite literally, any materials with which gametes or embryos come into contact and include culture media, supplies and equipment.

The strength of a bioassay is dependent on the sensitivity of the assay and the standards set for determining "pass" for a test material. If the bioassay is too robust with, for example, all embryos in the mouse assay routinely reaching the blastocyst stage, it may make it very difficult to detect subtle changes or toxicity in the culture environment. Conversely, if the assay is too sensitive such that the control conditions intermittently and unpredictably do not pass the test, then one loses the ability to assess acceptability of the so-called "contact" material in the assay.

The manner in which contact materials are tested is critically important. Ideally, each material should be evaluated in the same manner that it is used clinically, but this is frequently not possible. Moreover, evaluation of several samples from each lot might increase the likelihood of identifying toxicity within the lot. For example, in 2010, we identified toxicity in a lot of oil that

Table 15.3 The distribution of IVF laboratories according to the bioassay used

Testing year	Shipment number/year	One-cell mouse bioassay	Two-cell mouse bioassay	Human sperm bioassay	Hamster sperm bioassay
2008	1	62	142	142	2
	2	65	134	138	0
2009	1	67	140	140	0
	2	57	125	143	0
2010	1	56	114	135	3
	2	51	120	145	1
2011	1	53	118	146	2
	2	58	119	134	2
2012	1	48	108	128	2
Mean	–	57	124	139	1
% of Total	–	18% (517/2,900)	39% (1,120/2,900)	43% (1,251/2,900)	<1% (12/2,900)

The data show the number of laboratories reporting results for each bioassay to the American Association of Bioanalysts Proficiency Testing Service, Brownsville, TX, 2008–2012 (http://www.aab-pts.org/statistical-summaries/2012-statistical-summaries)
Adapted from Boone et al. [3]

was only identifiable in some bottles within the lot. Based on this result, we now test oil using a sample from pooled aliquots taken from all bottles in a lot. Regardless of the manner in which contact materials are tested, protocols for each material should be established and adhered to consistently from one bioassay to another.

The Sperm Motility Bioassay

In this assay, the motility of sperm after exposure to a test condition followed by culture (typically 24 or 48 h) is compared with that of sperm cultured in control conditions [26, 27, 28]. Any test condition associated with a percentage motility below a preset minimum threshold for acceptable performance is re-tested. Contact materials that fail to pass the second test are not used in the laboratory.

The Mouse Embryo Bioassay

The mouse embryo assay (MEA) is the most widely used bioassay for QC of clinical IVF supplies [3, 29–31]. In the 1980s, the MEA was considered to be performing acceptably providing the control embryos progressed through two cell divisions to reach the 4-cell stage. Thus, if embryos cultured in a test "contact" condition reached the 4-cell stage, it was assumed that that contact material did not contain a high concentration of toxins [32]. However, with improvements in culture systems, the assay endpoints have been expanded, and bioassays are now considerably more sensitive. Some very sensitive mouse bioassays only utilize mouse embryos derived from IVF [33–35] while others measure the number of live pups born to assess the strength of their bioassay [36, 37].

The sensitivity of the MEA is inversely proportional to the age of the embryos at recovery, i.e., 1-cell embryos are more susceptible to their environment than embryos collected at the 2-cell stage [29]. A major criticism of the 2-cell MEA is that it lacks sensitivity [8, 29, 38, 40]. The sensitivity can, however, be improved if in vivo-derived zygotes are collected from a uterine flush, and only those that have reached the 2-cell stage are used in the bioassay [30]. Furthermore, removal of the zona pellucida further increases the sensitivity of the embryo to toxins in the culture environment [41].

The strain of mouse also affects the sensitivity of the MEA. Several commercial suppliers perform additional testing beyond the scope of their Certificate of Analysis using an outbred or inbred strain of mouse. This is in part because of the general consensus that embryos from these strains are more sensitive to adverse conditions than those from F1 hybrid mice, and thus may be a more appropriate model for human embryos [16, 42]. Moreover, Byers and colleagues compared ten different strains of mice and found significant differences regarding the response of mice to superovulation, with different strains producing different numbers of oocytes, varying rates of fertilization, and variances in the ability of embryos to be cryopreserved and even to produce pups [43]. Given the great variability among strains, it is important that each lab carefully selects a strain that will allow them to detect toxicity in their QC assay, and that the same strain is consistently used to allow for meaningful inter-assay comparisons [3].

One other major consideration in establishing a sensitive mouse bioassay is the selection of the media and conditions used for the assay. To strengthen the sensitivity of the MEA, the assay should be performed in simplified media, as those more complex (e.g., Ham's F-10) contain amino acids which may chelate potential embryotoxins and mask possible toxins [44–46]. Additionally, MEA assays should be performed in protein-free media as serum or serum albumin can chelate toxins such as heavy metal ions, and mask potential negative effects from the media [46].

An example of a well established and sensitive MEA for testing embryo toxicity is shown in Appendix 2 [46]. A minimum number of embryos should be cultured in each treatment group to enable reliable conclusions to be drawn. Moreover, attention must be paid to the timing of embryo grading, the final stage of development to be used for analysis and the denominator/percentage of development deemed acceptable. As a rule, if test products routinely pass the MEA or the percent development far exceeds the minimum acceptable rate, the sensitivity of the assay should be adjusted by, for example, tightening the acceptable range.

Sperm or Mouse Bioassay?

There is no consensus regarding which of these bioassays is superior for detecting toxicity of IVF contact materials [21]. While the sperm assay is much cheaper and easier to run, some argue that it is less suitable than the MEA which at least uses embryos from a mammalian species. However, mouse embryos are much less sensitive to toxicity than human embryos. In our own lab, we use the MEA as our first-line QC bioassay, but will occasionally use the sperm assay.

Equipment

A critical aspect of setting up an ART laboratory is the selection of appropriate equipment. Laboratory personnel are frequently contacted by sales representatives who promote each product as being "state of the art" with additional promises of customer and patient satisfaction. It is the responsibility of the Laboratory Director to determine which products best meet the needs of the program. Each equipment purchase must be scrutinized for cost, usability, biological relevance, and its ability to be properly controlled and maintained. All equipment from pipettors, embryo work station hoods to laboratory HVAC systems fall under these standards.

Selecting the Right Culture Incubator

The embryo culture incubator is arguably the most important piece of equipment in an ART laboratory as deviations from acceptable performance will affect implantation rates. For this reason, selection of the right incubator is of paramount importance. A multitude of questions need to be considered when selecting the most suitable incubator to meet the needs of a practice (see Appendix 3 for a detailed list). Similar lists and thought processes should be considered when making any significant equipment purchase in an ART laboratory.

The laboratory director must consider both the size of the IVF practice and the laboratory space when selecting incubators. If incubators need to accommodate more than one patient at a given time, there must be considerations for the number of shelves in an incubator as well as the incubator's rate of gas and temperature recovery between door openings. For instance, if incubators are going to be accessed frequently, it may be more beneficial to select water-jacketed incubators with infrared CO_2 sensors, as these incubators will maintain their temperatures better and will quickly adjust to the appropriate CO_2 environment during active use. The downside of these incubators is that they are more expensive and can require more maintenance than those that are not water-jacketed or that utilize a thermal conductivity (TC) sensor for monitoring CO_2. The conditions in which the embryos are cultured also play a big role in incubator selection. Programs that wish to culture embryos under low oxygen tension need to select incubators that are compatible with nitrogen sources or mixed gas tanks or have adequate space if they decide to culture in low oxygen chambers. Other considerations include: the ability to integrate into the clinic's alarm system, the ability to calibrate and adjust incubator parameters, the ease of collecting daily QC measurements, the required maintenance for the incubator and, finally, the cost of the incubator and its and annual maintenance charges.

Table 15.4 Preventative maintenance schedule for incubators

Incubator activity	Frequency performed
Water pans sterilized and replaced	Biweekly
Fan doors to prevent styrene buildup	Biweekly
Wipe down incubator shelves	Monthly
Oil sink for VOCs exchanged	Monthly
Full cleaning and sterilization of incubator	Semi-annually
Change incubator filters and tubing	Annually
Preventative maintenance and service	Annually or as needed

Equipment Selection and Maintenance

All equipment must be validated for acceptable performance before being implemented for clinical use. In addition, a separate QC protocol must be established for each item and ongoing QC and routine maintenance is mandatory. Protocols should not only follow the manufacturer's guidelines for operation and maintenance, but also include the frequency of QC assessment, (e.g., daily, weekly, monthly, or annually), the thresholds and tolerance limits, the corrective measures, and all records of QC analyses (see Appendix 4).

The laboratory should always maintain copies of equipment manuals and make them readily available to all laboratory staff. It is the responsibility of the staff to identify and document any unusual trends observed during routine QC monitoring and notify the supervisor and/or the laboratory director. Likewise, actions should include requests for technical assistance from the manufacture to ensure appropriate repair; any malfunctioning equipment should be removed from lab operations. Equipment maintenance must be performed by qualified individuals or companies that are able to repair and certify equipment to the specifications established by the unit's manufacturer.

Each piece of laboratory equipment must be fully serviced and cleaned on an established routine basis. The frequency of this preventative maintenance should be based on the volume and usage in the laboratory. For example, a laboratory using a micromanipulator ten times a day needs more frequent maintenance than a clinic utilizing a micromanipulator once a week. This preventive maintenance is designed to prevent breakdowns, reduce or eliminate operational drift and extend the life of equipment.

It is critical that each laboratory establish a schedule for maintaining and cleaning equipment (see Table 15.4). The simplest way to monitor completion of these activities is to include them on a laboratory calendar or on a permanent QC log with each activity recorded with a date and a laboratory staff member's initials once completed. This record can serve as a visual reminder that the activity was completed and can also be used to monitor that the assigned maintenance activity is being properly completed within the defined timeframe. A routine audit of the maintenance and cleaning activities should be performed to ensure strict adherence to laboratory procedures.

Table 15.5 Incubator QC activity log

Parameter	Frequency	Target	Acceptable range	Corrective action
CO_2	Daily while in use	Based on pH of culture media	Adjusted by pH ± 1%	Adjust when out of range for 2 consecutive days
O_2	Weekly	5%	±1%	Adjust when out of range for 2 consecutive days
Humidity	Daily while in use	95%	≥70%	Add sterile water
Temperature	Daily while in use	37°C	36.7–37.0°C	Adjust when out of range for 2 consecutive days
pH	Weekly	Based on media specifications	Based on media specifications	Adjust CO_2 when out of range 2 consecutive days
Alarm check	Monthly	Email and phone notification	100%	Contact IT support
CO_2 tanks	Daily	Full back-up supply	≥1,500 psi in primary tank	Order new tanks
Liquid N_2	Daily	Full back-up supply	≥1 Available for use	Order new tanks
N_2 tanks	Daily	Full back-up supply	≥1,500 psi	Order new tanks
1-Cell MEA	Semi-annual	≥70% Blastocyst development	≥70% Blastocyst development	Clean and sterilize incubator, repeat MEA

The incubator is the most vigilantly monitored piece of equipment in the ART laboratory. Each incubator must be monitored on a daily basis using an independent measuring device. In addition, successful operation is dependent on many outside pieces of equipment such as N_2 and CO_2 gas tanks and manifolds, alarm systems, back-up power generators as well as all devices used to calibrate and measure the incubator's settings. For this reason, it is important to establish a routine for monitoring incubator QC activities using an activity log that stipulates acceptable ranges for each parameter being measured (Table 15.5). Clear instructions must be available for making corrective actions when measurements fall outside an acceptable range.

Data Analysis and Quality Improvement

Data analysis is a crucial part of an effective IVF laboratory QM program. Routine review of identified key indicators are important to ensure proper laboratory functioning and, perhaps more importantly, to identify potential problems to permit timely correction. In fact, this is the primary reason for data analysis: to achieve early identification of factors that could negatively impact laboratory function which, in turn, allows timely insight into targets for corrective action.

Frequency of Data Analysis

The frequency of data analysis will depend on a number of factors including program volume and the QA indicator being monitored. In programs with low cycle numbers, it is tricky to draw meaningful conclusions while attempting to troubleshoot. However, at least monthly review is recommended. In larger programs biweekly or even weekly assessment of a subset of indicators should be performed. For laboratories that batch cycles, assessment of QC data points should be performed shortly after completion of each cycle batch to enable timely detection of possible adverse trends and to permit corrective actions prior to the next patient series.

Key Laboratory Indicators

The most important aspect of QA data analysis is identification of key indicators or endpoint variables that will provide meaningful insight

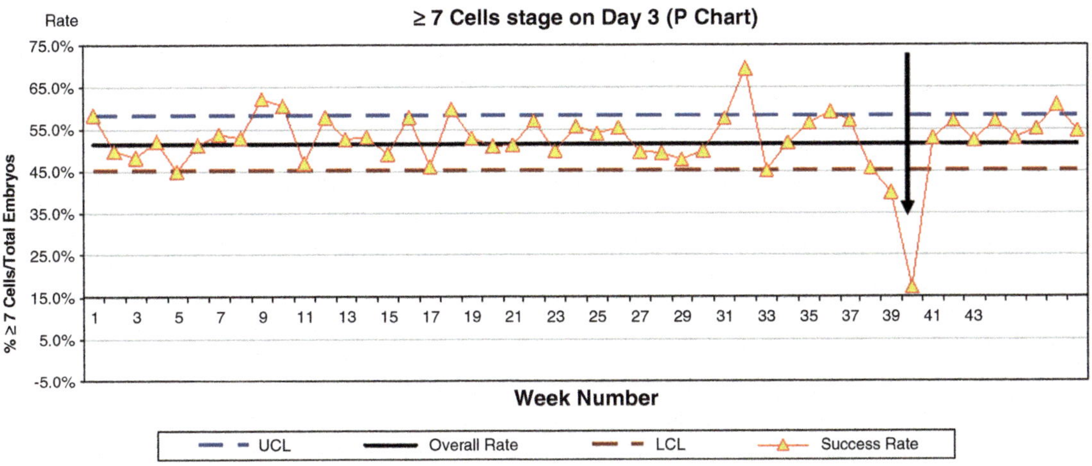

Fig. 15.6 A P-chart for tracking embryo quality. In this example, the percentage of embryos with ≥7-cells is plotted weekly and assessed to identify outliers that fall below the lower 95% confidence limit. The % of ≥7-cell embryos is shown as fluctuating within the upper confidence limit (UCL) and lower confidence limit (LCL) through Week #38, but as falling below the LCL in Week #39, followed by a substantial decrease in Week #40 (indicated by *arrow*). If intervention was effective, recovery in performance would occur, as shown in this theoretical example for Week #41

into laboratory functioning. While the key indicators may vary among laboratories, some are routinely assessed and considered standard. These include the following:

Oocytes retrieved: Tracking the number of oocytes retrieved, and, more importantly, the number of mature oocytes retrieved, gives some insight into, respectively, efficiency of embryologists finding oocytes and the effectiveness of the stimulation protocols used.

Fertilization rates: This is a particularly useful indicator that provides real-time insight into variance in laboratory performance in addition, possibly, to changes in stimulation protocols. Fertilization rates from both standard IVF and ICSI should be evaluated with data stratified by the andrologists preparing the sperm, and the embryologists inseminating or injecting the oocytes. Assessment of 2PN, 3PN, 1PN, and 0PN rate/mature oocyte should be determined, as well as the degeneration rate from ICSI.

Day 2 cleavage: The rate of embryo development is a predictive indicator of embryo quality. The number of 4-cell embryos on day 2 is a common indicator of quality of the culture system. Additionally, assessment of multinucleation in day 2 cleavage embryos may provide insight into nuances of culture system efficacy. High rates of multinucleation could indicate problems with the culture system [47].

Day 3 embryo development: The number of cells on day 3 gives considerable insight into performance of the culture system as failure to undergo embryonic genome activation will be reflected in arrest at around the 4- to 6-cell stage. Human embryos developing along the normal timeline should have progressed to the 7- to 8-cell stage [48]. Therefore, the percentage of 2PN zygotes with ≥7-cell embryos provides a useful marker of overall embryo quality. In our program, we use a performance chart (P-chart) to monitor this variable on a weekly basis with deviations below the 95% confidence interval being a trigger for a QA investigation (Fig. 15.6). In addition to cleavage rate, subjective grading scales assessing fragmentation and cell symmetry are also employed [49, 50]. The incidence of high-quality 8-cell embryos exhibiting early compaction may also be a sign of a high-performing culturing system [51].

Day 5 blastocyst formation: Early blastocyst formation on day 5 is an excellent marker of culture system efficiency; transfer of blastocysts formed on day 5 results in higher implantation rates compared with those from blastocysts formed on day 6 [52, 53].

Day 5/6 blastocyst formation and embryo freezing: Tracking total blastocyst formation, as well as quality of blastocysts as evidenced by those that meet a minimal freeze criteria helps give insight into quality of the culture system. Low rates of blastocyst formation or high rates of degeneration after 6 days of culture indicate sub-optimal conditions may exist [53–55].

Cryo-survival: Tracking cell survival following cryopreservation/thawing of cleavage stage embryos is an important marker of technical efficiency of a cryopreservation program. Though success rates may vary based on stage of embryo frozen [53–55] as well as method of cryopreservation (slow-rate vs. vitrification) [53], a specified minimum survival rate should be established for each laboratory.

Pregnancy, implantation and live birth outcomes: The clinical outcome of an IVF cycle is perhaps the best indicator of system efficiency with implantation rates providing the most robust and timely marker of embryo quality. Assessment of pregnancy rates per physician performing the transfer is critical. If decreases in pregnancy rate per transfer for a particular clinician are identified, and ensuring that embryo quality and patient characteristics were equivalent to those of other clinicians, it is our policy to alert the Medical Director for investigation and potential corrective action.

Thresholds

Quality assurance data review and examination of key indicators is a useless exercise unless meaningful threshold values are identified. These thresholds can initially be set based on national or peer/published data. However, individualized thresholds should eventually be set based on the performance of each laboratory. Thresholds should not be set too low, as the goal is constantly to improve outcomes. A useful approach when starting a QA program is to compare current means and standard deviations of selected performance indicators with those from an optimized program or published data. Threshold values can then be adjusted over time as the program is fine-tuned.

Methodology

Paramount to a comprehensive QA program is establishment and upkeep of a thorough database. While a simple spreadsheet may suffice for smaller programs, specialized software, such as that which is commercially available, may be more appropriate for larger programs. Ideally, data entry should be a shared responsibility among the team so as to encourage all members of the laboratory to take an interest in the QM program. This, in turn, helps reinforce the importance of the exercise. Importantly, just as too little data can render analysis a pointless exercise, large amounts of data must be analyzed appropriately (e.g., with multiple logistic regression analyses to control for potential confounders). Over-analysis of small numbers of cycles can monopolize time, offer very little additional insight and should be avoided. As illustrated by the P-chart discussed above (Fig. 15.6), one useful method of tracking trends is to graph outcomes at regulator intervals, rather than simply summarizing data in tabular form. Data can then be easily presented to the group for review and discussion of corrective actions as necessary.

Regulation in the IVF Laboratory

The 2010 Reproductive Laboratory CAP Checklist [12] lists the following requirements for recording IVF laboratory outcome data:

1. Laboratory records are generated for each individual patient's treatment cycle and a copy is retained in the laboratory to include the following as applicable.

   (a) Results of oocyte retrieval procedure
   (b) Semen analysis before and after processing
   (c) Outcome of insemination (e.g., fertilization)
   (d) Outcome of any culture (e.g., cleavage)
   (e) Relative timing of protocol events (incubation hours, etc.)
2. The laboratory at least annually reviews clinical outcome in relation to all data collected.
   (a) The laboratory must keep statistical records and review the clinical outcome in relation to this data. The frequency of these reviews should be appropriate to the size of the laboratory and the number of patient cycles, but must be documented at least annually.

Routine data analysis should be considered a critical component of a comprehensive QM program. Currently, reporting in the US of assisted reproductive technology outcomes is mandated by the 1992 Fertility Clinic Success Rate and Certification Act. The Society for Assisted Reproductive Technology (SART) monitors its member clinics annually. Recently, SART has proactively taken steps to ensure compliance with its requirements and has included quality of outcome parameters to the oversight process. These guidelines were established to assist clinics in identifying where quality can be improved. Governing bodies, such as SART and the CDC, are passing stricter regulations and imposing sanctions on laboratories that do not meet or exceed key threshold outcome indicators. Below is a list of the categories evaluated by SART:

1. Outcomes of two standard deviations (SD) below SART mean for Live Births per cycle (LB/cycle) in fresh, nondonor cycles for women under age 38 (combined two lower age categories).
2. Triplet (or greater number) rate of 2SD above the SART mean for women under age 38 (combined two lower age categories) in fresh, nondonor cycles or in recipients of donated eggs of any age.
3. Transfer of >3 embryos on average in women under age 35.
4. Any transfer of five or more embryos in women under age 35 without adequate clinical justification.

Programs found deficient in any of these areas are subject to disciplinary actions ranging from a warning to losing their SART membership status [56].

Quality Improvement Trials

The introduction of any new product or protocol into the clinical IVF laboratory should be undertaken with great care, recognizing that compromise to patient care should be kept to an absolute minimum. There are two main designs for QI trials:

Randomization of Patients

In this design, the patients themselves are randomized to the two conditions: either the standard, currently used protocol in the lab or the intervention arm. The advantage of this approach is that one can track the developmental fate of the embryos transferred and therefore obtain comparative implantation rates for the two treatment groups. The disadvantages of this design are: (1) the possible compromise to patient care if any risks to the intervention treatment are unknown; and (2) the time required to recruit sufficient numbers of patients to demonstrate any significance.

Randomization Within Patients

In this design, the gametes or embryos for each patient are randomized between the two treatment groups. If, for example, a new type of fertilization medium is being evaluated, the oocytes are randomized at retrieval using a coin toss to determine which ovary will provide the oocytes for each treatment arm. Conversely, if a new culture medium is being evaluated, zygotes are randomized at the fertilization check, again using a coin toss. To reduce the likelihood of any compromise to patient care, the typical inclusion criteria for such trials in our laboratory are patients <37 years with a minimum of ten follicles on the day of hCG trigger.

The advantage of this type of design is that one is not putting "all the eggs in one basket."

Moreover, as the patient is serving as her own control, a matched pair analysis can be performed allowing effective comparisons of embryo quality between the two treatment groups. The main disadvantage of this approach is that embryo implantation potential can only be tracked in cases of no implantation or when either a singleton is conceived with transfer of a single embryo, or dizygotic twins occur after transfer of two embryos.

Summary

A comprehensive and effective QM program must be in place in the IVF laboratory in order to maximize the possibility that every couple conceives with a healthy pregnancy. With this goal in mind, each program must not only strictly adhere to its defined protocols for QC and QA, but must also strive for constant improvement through QI activities. By using the basic steps of the PDCA cycle, each area defined in a QM program can be effectively managed to help provide consistent, optimal conditions for gametes and embryo culture and ultimately to ensure the best care for patients. An operational environment in the IVF laboratory must exist so that all team members realize that constant surveillance through QC and QA programs is not a process of finger pointing but, rather, is a proactive process that identifies problems and defines the necessary corrective actions needed to resolve them.

Appendix 1: Requirements for Supply Management in the IVF Laboratory

1. Maintenance of records of the batch or lot number, date of receipt and date placed in use of all reagents and media.
2. Reagents and solutions are properly labeled, as applicable and appropriate, with the following elements [12].
   (a) Content and quantity, concentration of titer
   (b) Storage requirements
   (c) Date of prepared or reconstituted by laboratory
   (d) Expiration date
3. All reagents are used within their indicated expiration date [12].
4. Explicit procedures for media preparation and modification are documented [12].
5. For each batch of culture media prepared in-house, the quality of the media, including pH, osmolarity and culture suitability using an appropriate bioassay system should be confirmed [24].
6. Media storage and expiration requirements are documented [12].
7. The laboratory has a documented method for quality control of media [12].
   (a) Culture media must be able to support the viability of gametes and/or the growth of embryos. Media must be evaluated using a bioassay system such as the one or two cell mouse embryo culture assay or a sperm motility assay. If culture media or protein supplement is modified or prepared in-house, there must be documentation that it has been tested on site. Commercial media must be used within the labeled expiration period. Documentation of quality control testing using an appropriate bioassay system must always be supplied by the manufacturer and retained for quality control records. The media quality control process must include steps to document the acceptability of the receiving conditions for transported commercial media [12, 25].
8. The laboratory tests and documents the quality of the contact material using a bioassay [12]. Materials pretested by the manufacturer with an appropriate bioassay system do not require further in-house testing. Documentation of testing performed by the manufacturer must be retained as part of the quality control records [12].

Appendix 2: One-Cell Mouse Bioassay Protocol

Super ovulation: Inject 4 to 6-week-old virgin females with 5–10 i.u. pregnant mare serum (PMS), followed 48 h later with 5–10 i.u. human chorionic gonadotropin (hCG). Place females with males immediately following the hCG injection; mating is assessed the following morning by the presence of a vaginal plug.

Embryo collection: Sacrifice females around 10 AM on the day of plug, excise the oviducts and place in warm collecting medium in a Petri dish. After tearing open the ampullary region of the oviduct close to the cumulus mass cluster, the cluster is expelled under positive pressure into the medium containing hyaluronidase (1 mg/ml). The cumulus masses are disaggregated after about 1 min, leaving denuded zygotes. Wash the embryos in collecting medium then and then once in the culture medium before placing them into culture. Embryos from each female should be allocated equally to each treatment group in order to overcome any donor variation.

Embryo culture: Place embryos into protein-free culture media that was pre-equilibrated overnight in a 6% CO_2 atmosphere. Culture embryos in groups of 10 in 20 μl drops of medium under an oil overlay at 37°C for 96 h.

MEA assessment: Assess embryo development in the afternoon of Day 4 and record the stage of development to determine the % of embryos that formed blastocysts. Ideally, culture the embryos for an additional 24 h to obtain the number of hatched blastocysts; in addition, obtain the total blastocyst cell count for each blastocyst using an inverted microscope.

Below is an example of acceptable criteria for using a 1-cell assay:

1. There must be 20 1-cell embryos in each treatment.
2. When evaluated at 96 h, the controls must yield ≥70% expanded blastocysts to pass:
   (a) Expanded blastocysts ÷ 1 − cell embryos = % expanded blastocysts
3. The average total expanded blastocyst cell count must be ≥80 cells.
4. Items whose treatments pass the mouse assay are suitable for use in human embryo culture.
5. Those treatments that fail are tested again; if a treatment fails the assay twice, it is not considered further for use in the IVF laboratory.

Adapted from [46]

Appendix 3: Questions to Ask When Selecting an Incubator for Your Laboratory

(a) What size incubator do you need?
  - How large is your lab space?
    - Do you have room for stackable incubators?
    - Do you have room for benchtop incubators?

(b) What is the patient volume for your lab?
  - How many patients will you place in one incubator at a time?
    - How many patients will you place on a shelf?
  - What about any program growth?

(c) Do you need additional space for more advanced technologies?
  - Time lapse video recording?
  - Microfluidic embryo culture?
  - Real-time bioanalyses of embryos?

What Is the Set Up and Flow for Your Culture System?

- What size are your dishes?
  - Do you place them within a larger dish or on a platform during culture?
- Do you perform all steps of IVF in one incubator?
- Do you euse the same incubator for both dish equilibration and culture?
- How many oocytes/embryos do you place in a dish?
  - For IVM?
  - For IVF/ICSI?
  - For Embryo Culture?
- How often do you change dishes for embryo culture?
  - No media changes?
  - Daily?
  - Every 2 days?
  - After 3 days?

What Kind of Atmosphere Do You Plan to Use for Your Culture System?

- What will be the O_2 Tension (atmospheric or low O_2)?
- What will be the N_2 source?
  - N_2 Generator?
  - N_2 Cylinders?
  - Liquid N_2 Vapor?
  - Mixed gas tanks?

How Do You Plan to Regulate the Incubator Atmosphere?

- What is your preference for measuring CO_2?
  - Infrared (IR) sensor?
  - Thermal Conductivity (TC) sensor?
- How do you want your incubator insulated?
  - Air jacketed?
  - Water jacketed?
- Do you want internal doors for your incubator?
  - How many?
- How is the access to the water pan?

What Level of External Monitoring Do You Require?

(a) What readings are on the digital display?
  - CO_2?
  - O_2?
  - Temperature?
  - Humidity?

(b) Can each of these parameters be adjusted?

(c) Can you set your own critical limits for each parameter being measured?
  - How sensitive can you establish these limits?
    - ±1.0° or 0.1°?
    - ±1.0% or 0.1%?

(d) How is the access to sampling ports?

(e) Can this incubator be integrated with your external alarm system?

(f) Can this incubator be placed on a back-up generator?
  - What happens to the internal atmosphere when the incubator switches to a generator?
    - Does the incubator also need to be placed on a UPS machine?

What Is Required for the Maintenance of the Incubator?

- How often do you need to clean the incubator?
  - Can the incubator easily be taken apart and cleaned?
- How often do probes need to be replaced?
- How often do filters need to be replaced?

How Much Does the Incubator Cost?

- How much does it cost for preventative maintenance?
- What type of warranty does the incubator come with?
- What's the proximity of the distributer?
  - How fast can I have a problem addressed by a technician?
  - How much are technical fees?

What Are Other Considerations for Purchasing an Incubator?

- Have other successful IVF programs used this incubator for embryo culture?
  - Have you contacted these programs for references?
  - How are their statistics?
- How user-friendly is the incubator?

Appendix 4: College of American Pathologist Guidelines for the Maintenance and Quality Control of Equipment

Following installation and validation of your equipment, it is imperative that there is continuous monitoring while in clinical use. Close monitoring of equipment helps to ensure its performance is maintained and that problems are detected as they occur. The 2010 Reproductive

Laboratory CAP Checklist [12] lists the following requirements for maintaining general lab equipment and incubators:

1. There is documentation of monthly evaluation of instrument maintenance and function, including temperatures of refrigerators/freezers in which reagents or patient specimens are kept.
2. There is a schedule or system available at the instrument for the regular checking of the critical operating characteristics for all instruments in use.
   (a) This must include, but is not limited to electronic, mechanical, and operational checks. The procedure and schedule must be as thorough and as frequent as specified by the manufacturer. There must be a routine plan or schedule available at the instrument for the regular checking of the critical operating characteristics of all the instruments in use. The laboratory should have an organized system for monitoring and maintaining all instruments. Function checks should be designed to check the critical operating characteristics to detect drift, instability, or malfunction, before the problem is allowed to affect test results. All servicing and repairs should be documented.
3. There is documentation of checks of incubator function each day of use using an independent measuring device for the following.
   (a) Temperature of incubators
   (b) Gas concentrations in incubators
   - In lieu of measuring daily gas concentrations, the laboratory may verify acceptable incubator culture conditions by monitoring and documenting daily checks for pH. Alternatively, laboratories using premixed gas may retain the manufacturer's certificate of analysis as documentation of acceptable QC records instead of performing independent measurements
4. Acceptable limits of temperature, humidity, gas content, and/or pH are defined.
5. The laboratory has a method to detect and prevent incubator gas failure.
6. The laboratory's incubator for embryos and gametes has emergency backup power, and it is tested at least quarterly.
7. All critical incubator, storage, refrigeration, and freezing units are monitored and checked each day of use.
8. The laboratory's incubator for embryos and gametes has emergency backup power, and it is tested at least quarterly.
9. Incubator alarms are monitored 24 h/day (either remote or in the laboratory).
   (a) Alarm systems, if used, must be checked at least annually. Audible alarms are only effective if someone is able to respond to the difficulty and is trained to follow the appropriate methodology to correct the problem or take alternative measures.

References

1. Boone DJ. Literature review of research related to the clinical laboratory improvement amendments of 1988. *Arch Pathol Lab Med.* 1992;116:681–693.
2. Keck CS, Sjöblom C, Fischer R, Baukloh V, Alper M. David K. Gardner, Ariel Weissman, Colin M. Howles and Zeev Shoham, Quality management in reproductive medicine. In: David K. Gardner, Ariel Weissman, Colin M. Howles and Zeev Shoham, editors. Textbook of assisted reproductive technologies. 3rd ed. United Kingdom: Informa Healthcare; 2009. p. 435–45.
3. Boone WR, Higdon HL, Johnson JE. Quality management issues in the assisted reproduction laboratory. J Reprod Stem Cell Biotechnol. 2010; 1(1):30–107.
4. Mortimer D, Mortimer S. Quality and risk management in the IVF Laboratory. British Columbia: Cambridge University Press; 2005.
5. Hutchison D. Total quality management in the clinical laboratory. Milwaukee, WI: ASQC Quality Press; 1994.
6. ISO 9001. Quality management systems—requirements. Geneva: International Standardization Organization; 2008.
7. Moen R, Norman C. Evolution of the PDCA cycle. Associates in process improvement; 2011. p. 1–11. http://pkpinc.com/files/NA01MoenNormanFullpaper.pdf. Accessed 12 June 2012.
8. Pomeroy KO, Racowsky C. Patient and tissue identification in the assisted reproductive technology laboratory. Semin Reprod Med. 2012;30(3):173–81.
9. Bender S, Geirsson RT, Kosunen E. Trends in teenage fertility, abortion, and pregnancy rates in Iceland compared with other Nordic countries, 1976–1999. Acta Obstet Gynecol Scand. 2003; 82(1):38–47.

10. Newman A. Visiting rights denied in embryo mix-up case. New York Times; 2000. http://www.nytimes.com/2000/10/27/myregion/visiting-rights-denied-in-embryo-mix-up-case.html. Accessed 14 June 2012.
11. College of American Pathologists. Laboratory general checklist. Northfield, IL: College of American Pathologists; 2010.
12. College of American Pathologists. Reproductive laboratory checklist. Northfield, IL: College of American Pathologists; 2010.
13. Gwande A. The checklist manifesto: how to get things right. New York, NY: Metropolitan Books, a division of Henry Holt and Company, LLC; 2009.
14. Gardner DK. Changes in requirements and utilization of nutrients during mammalian preimplantation embryo development and their significance in embryo culture. Theriogenology. 1998;49(1):83–102.
15. Lane M, Gardner DK. Understanding cellular disruptions during early embryo development that perturb viability and fetal development. Reprod Fertil Dev. 2005;17(3):371–8.
16. Gardner DK, Reed L, Linck D, Sheehan C, Lane M. Quality control in human in vitro fertilization. Semin Reprod Med. 2005;23(4):319–24.
17. van den Bergh M, Baszo I, Biramane J, Bertrand E, Devreker F, Englert Y. Quality control in IVF with mouse bioassays: a four years' experience. J Assist Reprod Genet. 1996;13(9):733–8.
18. Otsuki J, Nagai Y, Chiba K. Peroxidation of mineral oil used in droplet culture is detrimental to fertilization and embryo development. Fertil Steril. 2007; 88(3):741–3.
19. Otsuki J, Nagai Y, Chiba K. Damage of embryo development caused by peroxidized mineral oil and its association with albumin in culture. Fertil Steril. 2009;91(5):1745–9.
20. Sifer C, Pont JC, Porcher R, Martin-Pont B, Benzacken B, Wolf JP. A prospective randomized study to compare four different mineral oils used to culture human embryos in IVF/ICSI treatments. Eur J Obstet Gynecol Reprod Biol. 2009;147:52–6.
21. Lierman S, De Sutter P, Dhont M, Van der Elst J. Double-quality control reveals high-level toxicity in gloves used for operator protection in assisted reproductive technology. Fertil Steril. 2007;88(4 Suppl): 1266–72.
22. Punt-van der Zalm JP, Hendriks JC, Westphal JR, Kremer JA, Teerenstra S, Wetzels AM. Toxicity testing of human assisted reproduction devices using the mouse embryo assay. Reprod Biomed Online. 2009;18(4):529–35.
23. Morbeck DE. Importance of supply integrity for in vitro fertilization and embryo culture. Semin Reprod Med. 2012;30(3):182–90.
24. Schalue TK, Keel BA. Embryology laboratory management. H.C.L.D. General Knowledge Examination Study Guide, vol. 21. Saint Louis, MO: American Board of Bioanalysts; 2006. p. 1–49.
25. Revised guidelines for human embryology and andrology laboratories. Fertil Steril. 2008:S45–59.
26. American Association of Bioanalysts: proficiency testing service. Brownsville, TX; 2012. http://www.aab-pts.org/statistical-summaries/2012-statistical-summaries. Accessed 16 June 2012.
27. Claassens OE, Wehr JB, Harrison KL. Optimizing sensitivity of the human sperm motility assay for embryo toxicity testing. Hum Reprod. 2000;15(7): 1586–91.
28. De Jonge CJ, Centola GM, Reed ML, Shabanowitz RB, Simon SD, Quinn P. Human sperm survival assay as a bioassay for the assisted reproductive technologies laboratory. J Androl. 2003;24(1):16–8.
29. Davidson A, Vermesh M, Lobo RA, Paulson RJ. Mouse embryo culture as quality control for human in vitro fertilization: the one-cell versus the two-cell model. Fertil Steril. 1988;49(3):516–21.
30. Hershlag A, Feng HL, Scholl GS. Betadine (povidone-iodine) is toxic to murine embryogenesis. Fertil Steril. 2003;79(5):1249–50.
31. Fleetham JA, Pattinson HA, Mortimer D. The mouse embryo culture system: improving the sensitivity for use as a quality control assay for human in vitro fertilization. Fertil Steril. 1993;59(1):192–6.
32. Lee BE, Boone WR, Brackelsberg PO, Carmichael RA. Development of screening systems for evaluation of materials used in mammalian embryo transfer. Theriogenology. 1988;30(3):605–12.
33. Gianfortoni JG, Andresen PJ, Cieslak JM. In vitro and in vivo fertilization and embryo development in the murine model: comparison of sensitivity and outcome. Fertil Steril. 1987;48:106.
34. Han HD, Kiessling AA. In vivo development of transferred mouse embryos conceived in vitro in simple and complex media. Fertil Steril. 1988;50(1):159–63.
35. Jackson KV, Kiessling AA. Fertilization and cleavage of mouse oocytes exposed to the conditions of human oocyte retrieval for in vitro fertilization. Fertil Steril. 1989;51(4):675–81.
36. Mahadevan MM, Fleetham J, Church RB, Taylor PJ. Growth of mouse embryos in bicarbonate media buffered by carbon dioxide, hepes, or phosphate. J In Vitro Fert Embryo Transf. 1986;3(5):304–8.
37. Whitten WK, Biggers JD. Complete development in vitro of the pre-implantation stages of the mouse in a simple chemically defined medium. J Reprod Fertil. 1968;17(2):399–401.
38. Davidson A, Vermesh M, Lobo RA, Paulson RJ. The temporal effects of changes in in vitro fertilization culture media on the one-cell mouse embryo system. J In Vitro Fert Embryo Transf. 1988;5(3):149–52.
39. Quinn P, Warnes GM, Kerin JF, Kirby C. Culture factors in relation to the success of human in vitro fertilization and embryo transfer. Fertil Steril. 1984; 41(2):202–9.
40. John DP, Kiessling AA. Improved pronuclear mouse embryo development over an extended pH range in Ham's F-10 medium without protein. Fertil Steril. 1988;49(1):150–5.
41. Fleming TP, Pratt HPM, Braude PR. The use of mouse preimplantation embryos for quality control of culture

reagents in human in vitro fertilization programs: a cautionary note. Fertil Steril. 1987;47:858–60.

42. Bavister BD. Culture of preimplantation embryos: facts and artifacts. Hum Reprod Update. 1995;1(2): 91–148.
43. Byers SL, Payson SJ, Taft RA. Performance of ten inbred mouse strains following assisted reproductive technologies (ARTs). Theriogenology. 2006;65(9): 1716–26.
44. Fissore RA, Jackson KV, Kiessling AA. Mouse zygote development in culture medium without protein in the presence of ethylenediaminetetraacetic acid. Biol Reprod. 1989;41:835–41.
45. Flood LP, Shirley B. Reduction of embryotoxicity by protein in embryo culture media. Mol Reprod Dev. 1991;30(3):226–31.
46. Gardner DK, Lane M. Embryo culture systems. In: Gardner DK, editor. In vitro fertilization: a practical approach. Informa Healthcare: New York; 2007. p. 221–82.
47. Van Royen E, Mangelschots K, Vercruyssen M, De Neubourg D, Valkenburg M, Ryckaert G, et al. Multinucleation in cleavage stage embryos. Hum Reprod. 2003;18(5):1062–9.
48. Edwards RG, Purdy JM, Steptoe PC, Walters DE. The growth of human preimplantation embryos in vitro. Am J Obstet Gynecol. 1981;141(4):408–16.
49. Racowsky C, Vernon M, Mayer J, Ball GD, Behr B, Pomeroy KO, et al. Standardization of grading embryo morphology. Fertil Steril. 2010;94(3):1152–3.
50. Alpha Scientists in Reproductive Medicine and ESHRE Special Interest Group of Embryology, 2011. Istanbul consensus workshop on embryo assessment: proceedings of an expert meeting. Reprod Biomed Online. 2011;22(6):632–46.
51. Skiadas CC, Jackson KV, Racowsky C. Early compaction on day 3 may be associated with increased implantation potential. Fertil Steril. 2006;86(5): 1386–91.
52. Shapiro BS, Daneshmand ST, Garner FC, Aguirre M, Ross R. Contrasting patterns in in vitro fertilization pregnancy rates among fresh autologous, fresh oocyte donor, and cryopreserved cycles with the use of day 5 or day 6 blastocysts may reflect differences in embryo-endometrium synchrony. Fertil Steril. 2008;89(1):20–6.
53. Liebermann J, Tucker MJ. Comparison of vitrification and conventional cryopreservation of day 5 and day 6 blastocysts during clinical application. Fertil Steril. 2006;86(1):20–6.
54. Levens ED, Whitcomb BW, Hennessy S, James AN, Yauger BJ, Larsen FW. Blastocyst development rate impacts outcome in cryopreserved blastocyst transfer cycles. Fertil Steril. 2008;90(6):2138–43.
55. Noyes N, Reh A, McCaffrey C, Tan O, Krey L. Impact of developmental stage at cryopreservation and transfer on clinical outcome of frozen embryo cycles. Reprod Biomed Online. 2009;19 Suppl 3:9–15.
56. Practice Committee of the American Society fro Reproductive Medicine; Practice Committee of the Society for Assisted Reproductive Technology. Guidelines on the number of embryos transferred. Fertil Steril. 2009; 92(5):1518–9.

Regulation and Legal Concerns in IVF

16

G. David Adamson

Introduction

The regulation of any social activity is exceedingly complex because of the numerous stakeholders involved. Furthermore, regulations mandate legal requirements with societal sanctions if stakeholders do not meet those requirements. This necessarily creates concerns regarding potential sanctions because they can have financial and other serious consequences for the individuals affected.

Since Louise Brown was born in 1978, in vitro fertilization (IVF) has evolved extensively. IVF is defined as an ART procedure that involves extracorporeal fertilization [1]. Assisted reproductive technologies (ART) is defined as all treatments or procedures that include the in vitro handling of both human oocytes and sperm or of embryos for the purpose of establishing a pregnancy. This includes, but is not limited to, IVF, gamete intrafallopian transfer, zygote intrafallopian transfer, tubal embryo transfer, gamete and embryo cryopreservation, oocyte and embryo donation, and gestational surrogacy. It also includes intracytoplasmic sperm injection (ICSI), preimplantation genetic diagnosis/screening (PGD/S) and assisted hatching (AH). ART does not include assisted insemination ("artificial insemination") using sperm from either a woman's partner or a sperm donor [1]. For the purposes of this chapter IVF and ART terms will be used synonymously.

G.D. Adamson, M.D. (✉)
Fertility Physicians of Northern California,
2581 Samaritan Drive, Suite 301, San Jose,
CA 95124, USA
e-mail: gdadamson@arcfertility.com

The regulation of IVF began early after its inception. The UK and Australia both had early interventions in ART with government-appointed panels, reports with recommendations, and subsequent regulations. These regulations and laws both limited and enabled different aspects of the development of IVF. Other countries soon followed with a variety of laws but the development of professional guidelines also began. The USA has been a leader in this regard but many other countries have also developed guidelines [2, 3].

It is important to differentiate between regulations and guidelines [4]. Regulations are created by federal or state authorities and are associated with formal state sanctions, such as loss of medical license, fines, or prison sentences. Guidelines are developed by professional organizations and are usually only associated with professional sanctions, such as requirement for participation in a quality assurance program or loss of membership in the professional organization. Such sanctions do not carry the weight of the state. Blended models with regulations based on professionally developed guidelines are also present in some federal, state, and provincial jurisdictions. Furthermore, some countries have federally developed guidelines without legislation, but these guidelines are universally adopted. The different models seem to have the potential for both success and failure; success being defined as a model that enjoys generally wide support of patients, professionals, and the public. Some

E.S. Ginsburg and C. Racowsky (eds.), *In Vitro Fertilization: A Comprehensive Guide*,
DOI 10.1007/978-1-4419-9848-4_16, © Springer Science+Business Media New York 2012

regulatory models appear to be generally successful and some do not, and some guideline models have been generally successful while others have not.

Many countries have neither regulations nor guidelines. This appears to be the least successful model, particularly because very little is known regarding ART activity in such jurisdictions. If it is not possible to measure healthcare activity it is not possible to improve it. This chapter will address some of the contemporary issues surrounding regulations, guidelines, and legal concerns with respect to IVF.

Factors Affecting Regulation of IVF

Approximately five million babies have been born worldwide as a result of ART procedures. In many developed countries between 1 and 5% of babies are born as a result of IVF [5].

The significant role of IVF in reproduction places it in the mainstream of medicine. Recognition of this important role has been confirmed by the awarding of the Nobel Prize to Robert Edwards, whose pioneering work led to the birth of Louise Brown. Furthermore, many of the recent technological developments in ART are at the forefront of science, including somatic cell nuclear transfer ("cloning"), PGD/S, oocyte cryopreservation for cancer management and reproductive "insurance," as well as the use of donor sperm, oocytes, and embryos (third party reproduction).

Medicine generally is a social activity that affects individuals in personal ways and, therefore, is highly regulated. Nevertheless, because it is so personal, there is the potential for conflict among society, patients, health care professionals, other involved entities, regulatory organizations, and even government. This is especially true in reproductive medicine and IVF because it involves reproduction, sexuality, technology, and multiple parties—factors evoking complex responses [4].

Religion

There are, of course, major religious differences among and within countries. The primary reason these religious differences affect regulation is that they create a divergence of opinion on the moral status of the embryo [6]. The moral and legal status of the embryo are interlinked and are often the key to the acceptability of many ART procedures. There can be great legal difficulty in dealing with an entity that is neither a thing nor a person, and on this issue there is great diversity of opinion. Countries with a very strict view of the embryo as a person commonly limit ART technologies either through religious edict, social discouragement, or legislation. For example, Costa Rica is a strictly religious Roman Catholic country and has banned IVF. Some religions have a more permissive view of the moral status of the embryo, while others have a very restrictive and definitive view, e.g., Roman Catholicism. There is much variation within some religions, e.g., different types of Protestantism. For example, some Episcopalians tend to be very liberal with regard to the embryo and others are very conservative, considering it to have the moral status of a person, similar to some southern US Baptists who can be extremely conservative. Some religions tend to be pragmatic, but with specific limitations, e.g., Islam. Among different countries of the same religion, there can be different interpretations of what is morally correct, possible or desirable. Individuals of the same socioeconomic level living in the same country, and having the same religion, can have dramatically different perspectives on the moral status of the embryo and therefore how they feel about IVF and how it should be regulated. Overall, however, religion plays a central role in determining regulation of IVF because it affects individual perspectives, social norms, and availability of IVF services.

Other cultural forces can either reinforce or counterbalance the effect of religions on the availability of ART. Saudi Arabia and Turkey are both Muslim countries, but Saudi Arabia is very conservative and performs a small number of cycles annually compared with Turkey, a far more liberal Muslim country, that performs tens of thousands [5]. Therefore, cultural factors can reinforce or mitigate the religious perspective on the moral status of the embryo and regulation.

Politics

Political factors can also affect policy. For example, Turkey's desire to join the European Union has led to closer communication between Turkey and European countries on the provision of ART services in a manner that is harmonious with that of Europe. A symposium was organized by government and professional representatives in 2009 to develop improvements that could be implemented in documenting IVF services through a Turkish registry. However, as political commitment towards the European Union has waned in the last few years, Turkey has implemented strict regulations forbidding their citizens from traveling abroad for third party reproduction and threatening criminal prosecution of both physicians and patients.

Economics

Economics can affect the regulation of IVF simply because the lack of resources in many developing countries means that other healthcare priorities take precedence. It is in these situations that the risk of abusive practices by financially motivated providers can cause the most harm. Mitigating these problems is a long and difficult process that can be initiated by requirements for reporting the existence of IVF clinics and reporting results to registries. In many countries, the burden of the cost of regulation is passed on to the providers of the service, and then often to the patient. In countries that are sufficiently wealthy, this allows the government to establish quite significant regulation with expenditure of minimal resources. One aspect of this problem, however, is that even well-intentioned and appropriate regulation in principle can become overly expensive and not cost-effective [7]. An additional role of economics is the driving of provider behavior towards desired regulatory outcomes. For example, some countries, e.g., Belgium, link reimbursement to providers and/or patients to adherence to regulations regarding the number of embryos to transfer.

Regulation of IVF can be affected by the health care system. Publicly funded systems generally can find it easier to regulate than mostly private ones. In some countries health care is the responsibility of a province or state and not the federal government. In such countries regulations can vary from jurisdiction to jurisdiction.

Technology

Technology affects regulation. The birth of Dolly, the world's first somatic cell nuclear transfer or cloned animal, had a profound impact on the global view of reproduction and raised many challenging questions with many conflicting perspectives. Somatic cell nuclear transfer (SCNT) or "cloning" has been classified into therapeutic cloning (i.e., the use of SCNT to produce cells and tissues for use to treat disease), which is considered appropriate by many people, and reproductive cloning (i.e., the use of SCNT to create a genetically "identical" individual), which is considered inappropriate use of the technology by almost everyone. ART technologies are also used to create stem cells for both research and potential therapeutic purposes. A resolution was passed by the United Nations prohibiting scientific or other activities to enable reproductive cloning. Some countries, e.g. Singapore, passed regulations promoting the development of such technologies, while others, e.g. the USA, passed regulations generally preventing federal funding of such research.

Societal Changes

Societal changes also affect regulation. Current controversial topics include assisting single adults with IVF and the rights of those with non-heterosexual orientation to become married and have children. Perspectives on issues such as these vary widely among and even within countries and drive much legislation directed at regulating IVF. It is important for IVF practitioners to remain abreast of such social trends and issues so that they can participate in the resolution of these issues in the best interests of their patients.

What is notable is that regulations are dynamic in many countries. The IFFS has published three surveillance documents in the last 12 years, and there are many changes reflected globally in the documents [3]. These changes can be expected in the future as new technology and social trends occur, as genetics plays an even larger role in IVF, and as globalization "flattens" the world.

Regulatory Environment in the USA

There is a widely held but inaccurate perception that ART is unregulated in the USA. In fact, the USA has more regulation than most countries. There are a number of possibilities why this perception has developed: absence of a socialized healthcare system with its attendant controls; absence of a single national regulatory body; limited insurance coverage for infertility services; illegal, immoral, irresponsible, and unethical behavior by a few practitioners; minimal federal involvement in reproductive research; rapid scientific advances; different values and ethical perspectives on reproductive medicine; and a media presentation of reproductive issues that focuses on sensationalism. Regulation of ART in the USA was initially, and remains, fragmented, although efforts at coordination among the different stakeholders have had some success. While the overall process of IVF is highly regulated, reproductive choice for individual women and men remains unregulated. This has become an area of significant social disagreement, however, as stakeholders and society debate, often in the government and media, how best to protect and promote the rights of the individual while at the same time respecting the divergent values of a very heterogeneous society. The issue of reproductive rights vs. responsibility looms large when discussing multiple births, third party reproduction, single parenting, family balancing and genetic diagnosis and screening.

Mandatory Regulations Affecting ART

Numerous general mandatory regulations affect ART either directly and/or indirectly [8]. The Centers for Medicare and Medicaid Services (CMS) are responsible for implementation of the Federal Clinical Laboratory Improvement Act of 1988 (CLIA 88) that governs endocrinology and andrology laboratories performing, respectively, hormonal assays and semen analysis tests for IVF. CMS CLIA 88 inspections can be performed with "deemed status" by individual states. Furthermore, CMS oversees the accreditation of ambulatory surgery centers and provides certification, sometimes through the Accreditation Association for Ambulatory Health Care (AAAHC) which has "deemed status" for such accreditation. The National Institutes of Health (NIH) and federal research regulations cover all human research, including that performed in IVF laboratories. The Food and Drug Administration (FDA) has regulations that govern SCNT, and other federal government laws restrict research on embryos, SCNT and stem cell research. The Federal Trade Commission (FTC) has intervened to sanction ART clinics that marketed or advertised their results in a manner that the FTC considered inappropriate. CMS sets payment levels for all medical services, including those provided by ART centers. Even though Medicare and Medicaid do not pay for IVF, the setting of reimbursement levels in general has a direct effect on payment by insurance companies and others to ART centers. The Department of Health and Human Services (DHHS) has multiple policies that affect ART genetic testing and genetic policy. The Public Health Service Act prohibits human embryo research; the embryo was classified as a "human subject" in 2002. These federal policies have had the primary impact of limiting human embryo research and support for reproductive research, including stem cell research. Importantly, all stakeholders in healthcare must follow the Health Insurance Portability and Accountability Act of 1996 which protects confidential patient information [9]. Practitioners must take remedial actions when patient confidentiality is compromised and can be sanctioned for not following this law. Additionally, all data submitted to the Society for Assisted Reproductive Technology (SART) and the Centers for Disease Control must be protected according to the requirements of Section 308(d) of the PHS Act (42 USC 242m(d)) [10].

There are also many levels of state and institutional regulation that affect ART. For example, states regulate licenses to practice medicine and have removed licenses from ART practitioners for transgressions unique to ART (e.g., not informing a patient that she had a different woman's embryos implanted into her uterus, or transferring too many embryos to a patient). They require licenses for hospitals, operating and procedure rooms in which egg retrievals for IVF are performed. In some states (e.g., New York and California) the state requires an embryology laboratory license. Some states have laws that regulate ART technologies regarding embryo use and research (e.g., Louisiana), surrogacy (e.g., Michigan), sexually transmitted infection screening (e.g., California), informed consent regarding disposition of gametes (e.g., California), or the use of gametes posthumously (e.g., California). Additionally, institutions in which ART is practiced, such as universities, have regulations affecting clinical care, research, ethics, and funding. The requirement for Institutional Review Board (IRB) approval for all research treating human subjects is universal. This includes the universal need for informed consent by patients. So ART clinics in the USA must, in fact, abide by many general regulations in order to provide their services.

Research and ART

Regulation of research in ART has a long and tortuous history in the USA. Since 1975, federal regulations required review and approval of research involving IVF by an Ethical Advisory Board (EAB). In 1979 this body released a report supporting IVF research, but in 1980 the Board was disbanded because political differences over the abortion issue prevented the selection of a chairman. In 1993 the Human Embryo Research Panel recommended that some embryo research (up to 14 days) be acceptable and that other research (e.g., "cloning") not be. In 1994 President Clinton limited the Panel's recommendations and he would not support the "creation of human embryos for research purposes." In 1996 President Clinton signed a "Continuing Resolution" that banned funding for human embryo research. In 2000 the NIH expressed an interest in funding some ART, but only non-embryo, research which has been extremely limited because of the lack of federal funding.

The USA also has mandatory specific regulation of stem cell research, including guidelines established by the NIH in 2000. On August 9, 2001, President George W. Bush announced criteria for federal funding of stem cell research, limiting it to 64 stem cell lines in existence at that time. Subsequently it has been determined that fewer than a dozen of these lines are functional for research, and many scientists and others are critical of this limitation. However, the regulations do not preclude private funding of stem cell research and federal law does not prevent private funding of production of embryos for research purposes. California passed an initiative in 2004 to provide $3 billion over 10 years for stem cell research. One of the requirements is that there is no payment to women for donating their eggs for stem cell research. Efforts to revoke this aspect of the law have been initiated by the California Medical Association. In 2005 the state of Massachusetts passed Senate Bill No. 2039, an Act Relative to Enhancing Regenerative Medicine in the Commonwealth, to encourage stem cell research in their state. Other states have also passed legislation regarding stem cell research.

Somatic cell nuclear transfer (SCNT), commonly referred to as cloning, has been very controversial. After the cloned sheep, Dolly, was born in 1996, the political consequences were such that oversight of SCNT was given to the FDA by Congress. The FDA instructed all ART laboratories that FDA permission by way of a New Drug Application (NDA) is required in order to perform SCNT of any type in humans. To date, several controversial bills have been introduced to Congress, but none have passed both the House of Representatives and the Senate and been signed into law. California passed a pro-therapeutic SCNT bill, SB253, in 2002, as have several other states.

Regulations affecting genetics also impact ART, in an increasing manner, because of the application of PGD/S which is performed by testing cells biopsied from embryos that have been created by IVF. The Department of Health and Human Services (DHHS) oversees genetic tests through the CDC, FDA, CMS, and Office for Human Research Protection (OHRP). CLIA has laboratory oversight and the NIH oversees genetics research activities. The Secretary's Advisory Committee on Genetic Testing (SAGCT) made comprehensive recommendations in 2000 regarding genetics testing. The Health Care Portability and Accountability Act of 1996 restricts use of genetic test data and the Equal Opportunity Commission prohibits discrimination based on genetic tests. State health agencies have additional oversight roles.

The Fertility Clinic Success Rate and Certification Act of 1992 ("Wyden Law")

In the late 1980s it became clear that a mechanism to report results of ART procedures would be useful for both physicians and patients for clinical care and research. Congressman Ron Wyden from Oregon also felt that a reporting system would be important so that consumers (i.e., patients) could make more informed choices about different ART programs. With the support and active participation of the American Society for Reproductive Medicine (ASRM) and its affiliated society, SART, he developed and passed the Fertility Clinic Success Rate and Certification Act of 1992 (FCSRCA), commonly referred to as "the Wyden Law" [11]. This law required annual reporting of clinic-specific success rates; listing of clinics that do not report; development of a model program for certification of embryo laboratories; and promulgation of criteria and procedures for approval of accreditation programs to inspect and certify embryology laboratories.

The FCSRCA has been implemented by the CDC, and currently over 97% of ART programs report their results to them annually, most reporting through SART. The few programs that do not report are listed as "non-reporters." This has not been considered a sufficient penalty to cause them to report. A major criticism of the FCSRCA is that it does not contain serious financial or other sanctions for those who do not report their results. However, the CDC is not a regulatory body and does not have the authority to sanction nonresponders other than to report them as such. The results that are reported are validated annually by randomly selecting approximately 10% of the reporting clinics for on-site visits and chart review with the possibility of contacting patients to confirm the birth outcomes of ART treatment.

The results that are reported by ART clinics are analyzed by the CDC and a sophisticated report is presented on the web [12]. Another significant criticism of the FCSRCA is that the complexity of the data results in patient misinterpretation and inappropriate comparison of one clinic to another. There are many who feel this has resulted in ART clinics competing with each other on the basis of pregnancy rates which, in turn, has contributed to the dramatic increase in multiple births resulting from ART during the 1990s and an inability to reduce the twin pregnancy rate. Much discussion and debate has taken place regarding the balance between information that assists patients as opposed to that which confuses, especially when many confounding variables affect the data.

The CDC did develop a model program for certification of IVF laboratories, but since responsibility for implementing such programs is a state function, no national certification program was actually implemented. However, professional societies and organizations do have standardized embryo laboratory certification programs, and with recent FDA regulatory involvement this is not considered an area of significant deficiency. Since model programs for certification of embryo laboratories were not developed in the states based on the CDC's recommendations, there has also been no promulgation of criteria and procedures for approval of accreditation programs to inspect and certify laboratories as called for in the FCSRCA.

Overall, despite many difficulties in being the first "regulation" directly addressing ART in the USA, the FCSRCA has generally been considered a success by physicians, patients, and the government. Implementation, which has improved over time, has provided useful information to patients, and has been used by SART, the CDC and others for publication of papers regarding ART. The SART/CDC report has provided some of the most detailed and specific data regarding IVF available in the world because it records individual cycles and reports these with identification of the individual ART clinics.

Food and Drug Administration Regulation

The FDA first became involved in ART when Congress gave them the authority to oversee "cloning" in 1996. The FDA first exercised this authority in an obvious way in 2002 when, in response to professional and others' concerns, they sent letters to ART clinics informing them of the need for a New Drug Application (NDA) for cytoplasmic transfer (a technique involving transfer of cytoplasm from the cell of one person to that of another, with the transfer also of some mitochondrial genes) and use of coculture (which involved the use of some animal-sourced products that came into contact with human cells). Subsequently, the FDA began developing regulations requiring registration of laboratories, requirements for gamete donor screening, and requirements for good tissue practices. There are three regulations of particular significance.

The first regulation, Establishment Registration and Listing for Human Cells, Tissues and Cellular and Tissue-Based Products (HCT/Ps) became effective January 21, 2004 [13]. Registration is required within 5 days of beginning IVF operations and annually in December. The second regulation, Eligibility Determination for Donors of Human Cells, Tissue and Tissue-Based Products (HCT/Ps) became effective May 25, 2005 [14]. The third regulation is Current Good Tissue Practice for Human Cell, Tissue and Cellular and Tissue-Based Product Establishments: Inspection and Enforcement which became effective May 25, 2005 [15]. However, reproductive tissues are temporarily exempt from this third GTP regulation and it is not known when they will become subject to the GTP regulations. Although compliance with the Good Tissue Practices is not mandatory, the FDA is urging "voluntary compliance" for reproductive tissue facilities.

To emphasize the mandatory nature and seriousness of these regulations, the FDA performs unannounced on-site inspections of clinics approximately every 2 years. Infractions can result in sanctions including penalties for an individual of up to $100,000 per violation and up to $250,000 if death results from the violation. For organizations, each violation is punishable by a fine of up to $200,000 and if death results from the violation a fine of up to $500,000. Additionally, criminal penalties can involve imprisonment for up to 1 year.

Professional Society Accomplishments Overseeing ART in the USA

The ASRM was founded in 1944 and since that time has been the leading professional organization for reproductive medicine. The SART was formed in 1987 in response to the rapid development of ART technology in the USA and elsewhere. SART began publication of clinic-specific success rates on a voluntary basis in 1989. SART initiated collaboration with the CDC and assisted Congressman Wyden in developing the FCSRCA that was passed in 1992. The American Association of Bioanalysts (AAB) developed proficiency testing for laboratories. SART and ASRM worked with the College of American Pathologists (CAP) to create the Reproductive Laboratory Accreditation Program in 1992. This program set requirements and performed on-site accreditation every 2 years for embryo laboratories. Currently two-thirds of SART programs are accredited through this CAP/SART/ASRM program. The other one-third are accredited through New York State or through the Joint Commission on Accreditation of Healthcare Organizations (JCAHO). SART also has worked with the FDA developing their recently enacted regulations. Furthermore, SART and ASRM have developed dozens of Practice, Laboratory and Ethical guidelines that are widely distributed and implemented and that have dramatically improved the quality of clinical and laboratory ART care [2, 16].

One of the biggest criticisms of regulation in the USA is that it has not controlled the increase in multiple birth rate that has occurred with ART procedures. While some countries have introduced regulations with arbitrary limitations on the number of embryos transferred, the USA has not. This is an extremely complex clinical problem, because limiting the number of embryos transferred does reduce multiple pregnancy rates, but can also reduce overall pregnancy rates and the number of infertile patients who will successfully have a family. Most professionals in the USA do not believe that rigid regulation is the appropriate solution to this problem. Professional societies, however, have actively advocated for limitations on the number of embryos transferred based on evaluation of the evidence regarding number of embryos transferred, multiple pregnancy rates, and individual patient clinical circumstances. Triplet birth rates have been reduced over 80% from 1996 to 2010 as a result of implementation of these guidelines, showing they can be effective. Current efforts are now focused on reducing the twin pregnancy rate. Constant evaluation of data, new technology, new clinical approaches, improved patient understanding, and professional education should assist in continuing to reduce the number of embryos transferred and the multiple pregnancy rate while maintaining the live birth rate. Significant attention is being paid to the possibility of changing the way results are reported in order to encourage replacement of fewer embryos, in particular elective single embryo transfer.

SART has as its mission "setting the standards" for ART. It has established rigorous mandatory requirements for membership, and approximately 85% of the programs performing over 90% of the IVF cycles in the USA have met these requirements and are SART members. These requirements include personnel requirements: the Medical Director must have completed a Board-certified fellowship in reproductive endocrinology and infertility; the Laboratory Director must have a Ph.D. degree, 6 months of training in ART, 2 years' experience in ART, and be certified as a High Complexity Laboratory Director. SART IVF clinics must agree to on-site accreditation of their laboratory by CAP/ASRM, JCAHO, and/or New York State inspectors every 2 years. SART clinics must report their results annually to SART and to the CDC and agree to participate in on-site validation of their results. They also must agree to on-site review of their adherence to SART Practice, Laboratory, Advertising and Ethics Guidelines. There is mandatory participation in SART's Quality Assurance Program for programs with low pregnancy rates, high multiple pregnancy rates, and/or other clinical problems.

In addition to these activities with its members, both SART and ASRM have continued to cooperate with and lead initiatives with other professional, governmental, and patient advocacy organizations and institutions which are stakeholders in ART. ASRM continues to advocate for appropriate insurance coverage also. These activities are intended to improve access, effectiveness and safety of IVF and demonstrate that self-regulation and constructive involvement in the major issues affecting IVF make regulation unnecessary.

The American Bar Association has been actively involved in social issues that would benefit from regulation. The Family Law Section through its Continuing Legal Education program is addressing issues such as posthumous reproduction, international law, donor anonymity, and payment to donors. The Uniform Parentage Act passed by the ABA does not address issues related to cloning. Therefore, a resolution was passed in August, 2004 which opposes reproductive cloning. However, should reproductive cloning occur in the future, it sets forth the rights of the cloned offspring. The ABA passed a resolution in favor of therapeutic cloning (SCNT) in August, 2003.

The International Regulatory Environment

The IFFS Surveillance 2010 is the third and latest document describing the international regulatory environment [3]. It reports a wide range of regulation, guidelines, and hybrid oversight systems affecting many aspects of ART globally.

Some countries have very restrictive regulations. For example, Germany severely restricts the creation and cryopreservation of embryos. Many countries regulate and restrict use of donor gametes. Donor embryos are not permitted in some countries, and approximately one-third of countries require some type of information on gamete donors if requested, with a few of these being non-identifying information. Many countries have laws regarding the right to information about the donor if necessary for the health of the child. In France anonymity is protected, while in Australia lack of anonymity is a major problem for recruitment. The UK, which previously prohibited payment to gamete donors, has now reversed itself because of the lack of donors under the former policy. Canada has a shortage of gamete donors because of prohibition of payment. Fetal reduction is not allowed in some countries. PGD for known genetic conditions is allowed in the majority of regulated countries. PGS to identify "normal" embryos is specifically not allowed in a few countries. The use of gestational carriers is performed infrequently, with limitations in many countries including the need for a panel or court to approve, availability only in altruistic situations and/or with serious medical conditions, and with restrictions on the marital status of the carrier and others involved. Payment to a carrier is illegal in many countries [3].

Although some have hoped that international comparison of regulations and guidelines might lead to standardization of the provision of ART services, it has become clear that this is highly unlikely. Indeed, at most international meetings it has now become recognized that different societies, religions, and cultures need to have their values respected, and that the best approach is to try to understand what works and doesn't work in different settings, and why. In this way, each society can develop approaches most consistent with its own cultural and socioeconomic settings. While the actual situation is not optimal, it does allow for countries to make their own choices, for change to occur over time, and for patients to obtain and physicians to provide reproductive services at least in some situations. When countries are developing regulations or guidelines, it is important to include all the stakeholders in the process. This includes not only policymakers, ethicists, and lawyers, but also physicians, embryologists, their professional organizations and, most importantly, patients [4].

Regulation of ART is extremely variable in different countries around the world, and is changing rapidly, just as it has in the USA. The country that has widely been considered to have the most comprehensive and well thought out regulatory framework has been the UK and their Human Fertilization and Embryology Authority (HFEA) that came into force in 1991 [17]. A comprehensive review of the HFEA by the Department of Health found that licensing of clinics, reporting of results and the use of embryos for research were functional. However, it was quite critical of many aspects, especially regarding those issues not included in the initial Act or that have become controversial: rules on embryo screening, assessing the "welfare of the child," and the "need for a father" which is supposed to be taken into consideration before providing ART services, sex selection, what happens when couple's disagree about an embryo's use, the regulation of web-based gamete donation services and the role of the independent regulator itself, the HFEA. One of the controversial aspects of the HFEA's actions has been the limitation to transfer a maximum of two embryos for women under 40 and three for women over 40. HFEA policy now sets a maximum twin birth rate of 15% for each clinic, but leaves clinics to draw up their own patient selection criteria to meet that target. The HFEA also determined that cryopreservation of embryos that were abandoned could be discontinued after 5 years if serious attempts to locate their creators were unsuccessful. However, after several thousand embryos were destroyed the expressed public concern over this policy caused the time period to be increased to 10 years. It can be learned from the UK that regulation has brought advantages, and also disadvantages, and has not created unanimous agreement among those affected. Their experience also shows that the best regulations require intermittent reassessment since scientific progress and clinical and social changes can render some aspects of regulation irrelevant or detrimental.

Australia, and particularly the state of Victoria, has strongly regulated IVF beginning in 1984 with The Medical Procedures (Infertility) Bill, which was updated in 2008. The bill defined life as starting at the time of fertilization, mandated a 2 year wait for commencement of IVF unless both fallopian tubes were blocked, made a second medical opinion necessary before IVF could be performed, did not allow the physician initially recommending IVF to perform the procedure, and made marriage compulsory before a couple could gain access to reproductive technology [18]. Other Australian states generally have fewer restrictions on the practice of IVF. Many countries have enacted strict laws limiting the number of embryos that can be transferred. In nations with such legislation, the penalties for violation of the laws may be severe; they include withdrawal of the license to practice medicine (in the UK and Sweden), fines or imprisonment (in Germany), and imprisonment with a substantial fine (in Switzerland). Even though double embryo transfer has reduced triplet rates wherever implemented, twin rates still remain at 20–35%. It has been shown that elective single embryo transfer (eSET) can reduce the twin rate to less than 5% (monochorionic twinning still occurs). On the basis of data from Finland, Sweden, and Belgium, the European Society for Human Reproduction and Embryology in 2001 recommended eSET for women less than 34 with a "top-quality embryo" [19] (see Chapter 5). Belgium amended its national embryo-transfer policy to allow the transfer of only one embryo in women less than 36 years of age (on the first attempt). Sweden's national health plan will cover an unlimited number of IVF cycles in which a single embryo is transferred, but only up to four cycles if more than one embryo is transferred. In Finland there is no regulation, but ART clinics, by professional consensus, perform eSET in approximately 70% of patients [20].

Regulating the number of embryos to transfer can be a complex task. In Germany, The Embryo Protection Act of 1990 states that no more than three eggs can be cultured for a patient undergoing IVF, and these must all be transferred [21]. Cryopreservation is allowed only at the pronuclear stage, soon after sperm penetration, before occurrence of syngamy. Overall, this regulation results in lower pregnancy rates because poorer quality embryos are created on average, yet higher multiple pregnancy rates occur because too many good quality embryos must be replaced in some women.

Italy passed regulation in 2003 that is at least as restrictive as that in Germany [22, 23]. The law restricts fertility treatments to heterosexual couples who live together and are of childbearing age, prohibits egg or sperm donation or gestational carrier, forbids freezing embryos for use at a later date and mandates that all, but no more than three, embryos must be implanted at the time of embryo transfer. It also outlaws embryo research, including cloning or genetic therapy. Sanctions include fines up to $726,000 for using donors and 10- to 20-year jail terms and fines up to $1.21 million for doctors who try to clone humans. Parts of this law were eventually overturned and now embryo transfer decisions can be more individualized.

In Spain it is legal to freeze embryos and put them in storage, but it is illegal to destroy them or donate them to research. Since many patients would like to donate them to research, but not to other couples, many embryos remain in storage, some beyond the 5 year storage limit. The central government has also filed a lawsuit contending it has regulatory control over research on embryonic stem cells and that even private research must be supervised by the national government [24].

Canada had no regulation in place until 2004 when a comprehensive act was passed [25]. This Act created the Assisted Human Reproduction Agency of Canada. The objectives of the Agency are to protect and promote the health, safety, and human dignity and rights of Canadians, and to foster the application of ethical principles in relation to assisted human reproduction. The regulations allow some embryo research, prohibits sex selection except to diagnose or treat a sex-linked disease, forbids changing the genome if the change could be transmitted to descendants, prohibits payment to gamete or embryo donors or surrogates, requires written informed consent, sets out confidentiality and disclosure requirements, regulates research, allows for on-site inspections of clinics, and has penalties of up to $500,000 and up to 10 years in prison for violations of the Act. The Act was challenged by the province of Quebec because it was a federal law which Quebec argued interfered with their provincial health care rights. The Supreme Court of Canada agreed with some of their positions and overturned important aspects of the bill leading to the dissolution, early in 2012, of Assisted Reproductive Health Canada which is the government entity which had been established to oversee and enforce the law.

Cross-Border Reproductive Care

The first international meeting on cross-border reproductive care was sponsored by the Government of Canada in Ottawa in January, 2009 [26]. This meeting brought together a broad range of international stakeholders. It was recognized that respect for the very diverse approaches to reproductive care and its regulation was essential for discourse and progress on this important topic. It was also noted that almost no comprehensive data exist on this important area of reproductive health care. No countries have actual cross-border data in their registries. An approximate estimate of the amount of cross-border reproductive care was that about 3–5% of US cycles were performed on European, Canadian, Asian, and other nationals. In Europe approximately 7–10% of care was provided to foreign nationals, mainly from other European countries.

It would appear that most patients seek cross-border care to avoid restrictive regulations in their own country that limited the general availability of services (e.g., payment to gamete donors, sex selection), prevented their own to access services (e.g., age limitations, long waiting times), or intruded on their confidentiality and anonymity (e.g., need to participate in a gamete donor registry). Patients also traveled to access what is perceived as higher quality care (e.g., higher efficacy or safety, more personal, and/or convenient care) and/or to access less expensive treatment [27]. Patients often go to countries in which they have relatives. Geographical proximity of services seemed to be important in at least some cross-border travel situations, for example, Swedish women traveling to Denmark for egg donor services. In other cases cross-border traveling did not seem to deter patients; for example, North Americans and Europeans traveling to India for gestational carrier services. The conclusions from this meeting were that better consent forms for patients and improved information for physicians were needed for patients to enhance the quality and safety of care; much better data were needed on the care provided, and a mechanism was needed to promote further progress in the understanding of cross-border reproductive care. There is concern that high patient motivation levels, poor information, limited informed consent, unfamiliar cultural and healthcare systems, travel and language difficulties increase the possibility of less efficacious and safe reproductive care in foreign countries.

Cross-border care can also create ethical dilemmas for physicians who have patients desiring services they cannot provide for legal or other reasons in their country of origin, or who have unrealistic requests in the country of destination. There is the potential conflict of following national regulations and/or guidelines or social norms versus physicians' professional obligations to their patients. Clearly, laws must be followed. However, the involvement of the physician in providing information, referral services, or supportive medical care before or after foreign treatment can be problematic. It would also be ethically and otherwise difficult for a country to forbid travel of its citizens to another country for care, but it might limit funding for services for those who did on their return, for example, obstetrical care following egg donation. However, it should be noted that Turkey has recently enacted laws that create penalties for citizens traveling abroad to access reproductive services that are illegal in Turkey. Published March 6, 2010 in the Official Gazette, the new law states that any clinic, doctor, or patient using or encouraging the use of overseas sperm or egg banks will be reported to state prosecutors and face possible criminal charges [28]. This has caused some non-

Turkish professionals who provide reproductive services to Turkish citizens to decide not to travel to Turkey because of their concern over the risk of prosecution. Also, the UK and other countries limit access to public funding for foreign patients accessing reproductive services in that country and for their own citizens who travel abroad for reproductive services not available at home. Although cross-border reproductive travel can act as a safety valve for a country with many patients leaving for care in other countries, it can also signal a need for individual countries to evaluate their own health policies to ensure that they reflect the needs of their citizens [4].

Additional issues of major concern with cross-border reproductive care include exploitation of involved parties, informed consent in foreign languages, coordination of services with the home country health care provider, immigration issues with offspring, especially with third party reproduction, and reporting/documentation of services, gametes, embryos, and children that is accurate and truthful but also complies with the laws of multiple countries. Professionals involved in providing such services must be knowledgeable about these issues or seek collaboration with those who are.

Responding to Regulatory and Legal Concerns

Regulations have created many legal concerns for IVF professionals. CMS, FDA, and FTC are regulatory bodies that have authority to make on-site visits, perform assessments and levy sanctions that have financial, licensing, and criminal components. Physicians must make themselves aware of them. The appropriate personnel with necessary qualifications need to be hired to perform specific services. The physical facilities must meet the required standards and be accredited/certified. Internal operating systems, either paper or preferably electronic, need to be created and used. Internal quality assurance systems involving all relevant providers must be set up and followed. All activities need to be documented and reported as required. All of the systems and processes must be regularly reevaluated and updated. Preparation of systems and staff for both announced and unannounced inspections needs to be undertaken and regularly reviewed.

SART and ASRM Practice Guidelines and Ethics Committee Opinions are just that—guidelines and opinions. However, in addition to the risk of sanctions and/or losing membership in SART, it is possible that practitioners could place themselves at medico legal risk if they are not followed—especially if there is a bad outcome. So it is recommended that clinical indications and fully informed consent be documented in the medical record in instances in which patient care deviates from SART or ASRM guidelines.

Informed consent is an area of increasing interest. IVF practitioners function in a complex clinical, scientific, laboratory, surgical, ethical, and emotional area of medicine. It behooves all practitioners to provide comprehensive, understandable, balanced, evidence-linked information to their patients so that together they can share in decision making. Such activities, not just the signing of consent forms, should be well documented.

Bad outcomes dramatically increase medico legal liability and lawsuits. Such actions cost time, money, potential business to the practice and take a large emotional toll on physicians, other professionals and their families. The most preventable bad outcome in IVF is multiple pregnancy, as discussed in Chap. 5. Multiple birth, if not preventable, can be reduced significantly below current rates by reducing the number of embryos transferred. Patients and society will likely be increasingly unsympathetic towards poor outcomes from multiples, including twins, in the future.

Third party reproduction is an area of particular legal risk because of the increased number of individuals involved in a more complicated clinical situation and, often, the vagueness of laws. Comprehensive information and informed consent regarding rights, responsibilities, decisions, and treatment now and in the future need to be provided to all parties. Legal documents from expert attorneys knowledgeable about state and federal laws are mandatory. Psychological counseling to ensure firm understanding of current and future issues in third party reproduction should be mandatory. And, of course, all appropriate laws must be followed. Laws with respect to commitments of anonymity or the nature of the relationship between parties in third party reproduction are often vague or absent, and different jurisdictions often have different laws. If the laws change, future relationships could be affected. Recent developments in Australia in which new regulations require retroactive application of identity disclosure of donors raises new and troubling complexity to third party reproduction.

The legal environment in which IVF is practiced can be vague even in the USA. It is important for practitioners to be aware of federal and state laws and know where there might be issues. Expert attorneys should be utilized in unusual clinical situations to avoid potential liability. This is especially true when agencies or individuals that are not licensed or regulated are involved in third party reproduction.

Many ethical issues are raised even in the routine practice of IVF. These include those associated with third party reproduction, welfare of the child, age of the intended parent(s), unconventional life-style of intended parents, gender selection, intentional exposure to risk (e.g., with respect to multiple births), confidentiality, and many others. Each practice should have in place a documented system for identifying and managing clinical and laboratory situations that raise ethical issues. This system should identify the process, the individuals involved, patient management in ethically challenging situations, and management of discordant views.

Conclusions

ART is a complex and rapidly changing clinical, scientific and ethics-laden field of medicine involving highly visible and emotional issues. It is not surprising that there are many parties interested in the regulation and oversight of ART and that a multitude of country-specific and, in some cases, state or province-specific regulations and/or guidelines currently prevail.

Continuing international communication and cooperation is furthering collaboration, especially in scientific and medical endeavors. Reductions in economic disparities between the developed and developing world should lead to further international standardization of ART services, greater access and some harmonization of regulations. Increased cross-border care can be expected as information about ART becomes more accurate, sophisticated and available through the Internet and other sources. Newer technologies and research opportunities, particularly in stem-cell research, will likely lead to increased cross-border reproductive travel. Differences in quality of care will likely lessen over time, but some differences will undoubtedly remain and cause some cross-border travel along with cost differences. There will likely be increased efforts to regulate cross-border care.

The recognition by the WHO of infertility as a disease and increased utilization of IVF is increasingly causing IVF to be seen as in the mainstream of medicine. This recognition will likely result in better insurance coverage and also closer surveillance and more regulation. Payers will want to ensure not only effectiveness but also safety and practice consistent with societal values. This will result in regulation that mandates access and also payment amounts, limitations on the number of embryos transferred and restricted availability of some services. Genetic services and other areas of technology improvement might also be major areas of regulation.

In the USA, the significant progress in developing regulation and oversight of ART is reflected in the involvement of a great diversity of institutions, organizations, and perspectives on federal, state, professional, and private levels that together, reflect the unique social composition and public and private institutions and values of this country. The current system substantially meets many of the objectives of an ideal regulatory and oversight mechanism. IVF in the USA is highly regulated, except for reproductive choice. It is important for all IVF practitioners to recognize that we will continue to have to represent the interests of our patients and the infertile population against inappropriate and

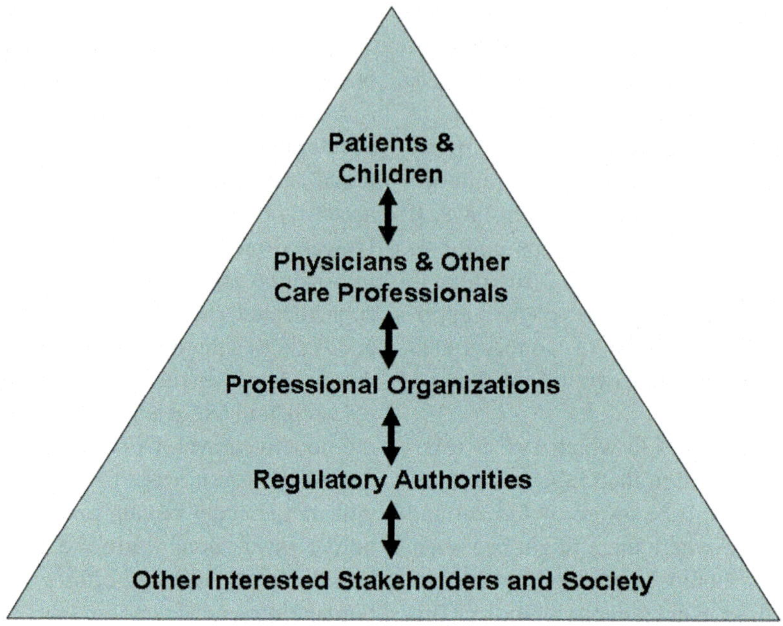
Patients & Children
Physicians & Other Care Professionals
Professional Organizations
Regulatory Authorities
Other Interested Stakeholders and Society

Fig. 16.1 Pyramid showing "hierarchy of interest"

restrictive regulation. Yet we must be sensitive and responsive to legitimate societal concerns regarding safety and proper utilization of the powerful technology that we have developed. In a pluralistic society, it is reasonable to consider a "hierarchy of interest" [29] (Fig. 16.1) in balancing patient reproductive choice, the practice of medicine, research and the values, needs and desires of society. As all aspects of IVF continue to evolve, including regulation, we can also continue to learn from the experiences of the international community.

References

1. Zegers-Hochschild F, Adamson GD, de Mouzon J, Ishihara O, Mansour R, Nygren K, Sullivan E, Vanderpoel S. International Committee for Monitoring Assisted Reproductive Technology (ICMART) and the World Health Organization (WHO) revised glossary of ART terminology, 2009. Fertil Steril. 2009;92:1520–4.
2. American Society for Reproductive Medicine Practice Committee Documents. 2012. www.asrm.org/guidelines/. Accessed 23 Jun 2012.
3. Jones HW, Cooke I, Kempers R, Brinsden P, Saunders D. International Federation of Fertility Societies Surveillance 2010. 2012. http://www.iffs-reproduction.org/documents/IFFS_Surveillance_2010.pdf. Accessed 23 Jun 2012.
4. Adamson GD. Global cultural and socioeconomic factors that influence access to assisted reproductive technologies. Women's Health (Lond Engl). 2009;5(4):351–8.
5. Nygren KG, Sullivan E, Zegers-Hochschild F, Mansour R, Ishihara O, Adamson GD, de Mouzon J. International Committee for Monitoring Assisted Reproductive Technology (ICMART): ICMART world report on assisted reproductive technology 2003. Fertil Steril. 2011;95(7):2209–22. 2222.e1–17.
6. Jones HW, Cohen J, Cooke I, Kempers R. International Federation of Fertility Societies (IFFS) surveillance. Fertil Steril. 2007;87 Suppl 1:S1–67.
7. Baker VL, Gvakharia MO, Rone HM, Manalad JR, Adamson GD. Economic cost for implementation of the U.S. Food and Drug Administration's Code of Federal Regulations Title 21, Part 1271 in an egg donor program. Fertil Steril. 2008;90(3):537–45.
8. Adamson GD. Regulation of assisted reproductive technologies in the United States. American Bar Association Family Law Quarterly. Fall. 2005;39(3):727–44.
9. Public Law 104–191—Health Insurance Portability and Accountability Act of 1996. 2012. http://www.gpo.gov/fdsys/pkg/PLAW-104publ191/content-detail.html. Accessed 23 Jun 2012.
10. Privacy Act System Notice 09-20-0165. 2012. http://www.cdc.gov/SORNnotice/09-20-0165.htm. Accessed 23 Jun 2012.
11. The Fertility Clinic Success Rate and Certification Act of 1992; Public law. Federal Register Notice November 6, 1998;63(215):102–493. Accessed September 20, 2012 at http://wwwn.cdc.gov/dls/art/fcsrca.aspx.

12. Assisted Reproductive Technology (ART). 2012. http://www.cdc.gov/art/. Accessed 23 Jun 2012.
13. Vaccines, blood and biologics. Tissue establishment registration. http://www.fda.gov/cber/tissue/tisreg.htm. Accessed 23 Jun 2012.
14. Eligibility determination for donors of human cells, tissues, and cellular and tissue-based products. 2012. http://www.fda.gov/OHRMS/DOCKETS/98fr/97N-484S-nfr0001.pdf. Accessed 23 Jun 2012.
15. Vaccines, blood and biologics. tissue notices, proposed and final rules. 2012. http://www.fda.gov/cber/rules/gtp.pdf Accessed 23 Jun 2012.
16. American Society for Reproductive Medicine. Ethics committee documents. 2012. www.asrm.org/EthicsReports/. Accessed 23 Jun 2012.
17. Human Fertilization and Embryology Authority. 2012. http://www.hfea.gov.uk/Home. Accessed 23 Jun 2012.
18. Assisted Reproductive Treatment Act 2008 Vic, s.44. 2012. http://www.austlii.edu.au/au/legis/vic/num_act/arta200876o2008406/. Accessed 23 Jun 2012.
19. Prevention of twin pregnancies after IVF/ICSI by single embryo transfer: ESHRE campus course report. Hum Reprod. 2001;16:790–800.
20. Hyden-Granskog C, Tiitinen A. Single embryo transfer in clinical practice. Hum Fertil (Camb). 2004;7: 175–82.
21. Felderbaum R. ART laws put patients at risk and should be changed, warns head of Germany's IVF registry. From European Society for Human Reproduction and Embryology 2003. 2012. http://www.scienceblog.com/community/older/2003/E/20032592.html. Accessed June 23, 2012.
22. European Society for Human Reproduction and Embryology: Italian law on ART brings problems for doctors and patients. 22 Jun 2005. http://www.medicalnewstoday.com/medicalnews.php?newsid=26443. Accessed 23 Jun 2012.
23. Fineschi V, Neri M, Turillazzi E. The new Italian law on assisted reproduction technology (Law 40/2004). J Med Ethics. 2005;31:536–9.
24. Fuchs D. Bank for human stem cells starts ethics debate in Spain. New York Times Feb 15, 2004. http://www.nytimes.com/2004/02/15/international/europe/15SPAI.html?ex=1077823559&ei=1&en=c0095959d6296136. Accessed 23 Jun 2012.
25. House of Commons of Canada. Bill C-6: An Act respecting assisted human reproduction and related research. 2012. http://www.parl.gc.ca/common/Bills_ls.asp?Parl=37&Ses=3&ls=C6. Accessed 23 Jun 2012.
26. Wilson E. Assisted human reproduction Canada. International forum on cross-border reproductive care: quality and safety; 2009 Jan 14–16; Ottawa, Canada. Information note Feb 6 2009.
27. Nygren KG for ICMART. Cross border fertility care. Assisted human reproduction Canada. International forum on cross border reproductive care: quality and safety; 2009 Jan 14–16; Ottawa, Canada.
28. Overseas artificial insemination outlawed in Turkey. 2012. www.bionews.org.uk/page_56782.asp. Accessed 23 Jun 2012.
29. Adamson D. Regulation of the assisted reproductive technologies in the United States. Fertil Steril. 2002;78(5):932–42.

Index

E.S. Ginsburg and C. Racowsky (eds.), *In Vitro Fertilization: A Comprehensive Guide*,
DOI 10.1007/978-1-4419-9848-4, © Springer Science+Business Media New York 2012

CPSIA information can be obtained
at www.ICGtesting.com
Printed in the USA
LVOW02*1732131215
466491LV00003B/85/P